Disease Handbook for Massage Therapists

Disease Handbook for Massage Therapists

Ruth Werner
LMT, NCTMB

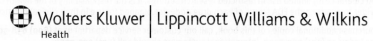

Wolters Kluwer | Lippincott Williams & Wilkins
Health

Philadelphia • Baltimore • New York • London
Buenos Aires • Hong Kong • Sydney • Tokyo

Acquisitions Editor: John Goucher
Product Manager: Linda G. Francis
Design Coordinator: Doug Smock
Compositor: Aptara, Inc.

351 West Camden Street   530 Walnut Street
Baltimore, MD 21201   Philadelphia, PA 19106

Printed in China

9 8 7 6 5 4 3 2 1

Library of Congress Cataloging-in-Publication Data

Werner, Ruth (Ruth A.)
    Disease handbook for massage therapists / Ruth Werner.
      p. ; cm. – (LWW in touch series)
    Includes index.
    ISBN 978-0-7817-5094-3
    1. Massage therapy–Handbooks, manuals, etc. 2. Diseases–Handbooks, manuals, etc. I. Title.
II. Series: LWW in touch series.
    [DNLM: 1. Diagnosis–Handbooks. 2. Massage–Handbooks. 3. Signs and Symptoms–Handbooks.
4. Therapeutics–Handbooks. WB 39 W494d 2010]
    RM721.W47 2010
    615.8'22–dc22

                                                                      2009011069

DISCLAIMER

Care has been taken to confirm the accuracy of the information present and to describe generally accepted practices. However, the authors, editors, and publisher are not responsible for errors or omissions or for any consequences from application of the information in this book and make no warranty, expressed or implied, with respect to the currency, completeness, or accuracy of the contents of the publication. Application of this information in a particular situation remains the professional responsibility of the practitioner; the clinical treatments described and recommended may not be considered absolute and universal recommendations.

The authors, editors, and publisher have exerted every effort to ensure that drug selection and dosage set forth in this text are in accordance with the current recommendations and practice at the time of publication. However, in view of ongoing research, changes in government regulations, and the constant flow of information relating to drug therapy and drug reactions, the reader is urged to check the package insert for each drug for any change in indications and dosage and for added warnings and precautions. This is particularly important when the recommended agent is a new or infrequently employed drug.

Some drugs and medical devices presented in this publication have Food and Drug Administration (FDA) clearance for limited use in restricted research settings. It is the responsibility of the health care provider to ascertain the FDA status of each drug or device planned for use in their clinical practice.

To purchase additional copies of this book, call our customer service department at **(800) 638-3030** or fax orders to **(301) 223-2320**. International customers should call **(301) 223-2300**.

Visit Lippincott Williams & Wilkins on the Internet: http://www.lww.com. Lippincott Williams & Wilkins customer service representatives are available from 8:30 am to 6:00 pm, EST.

This book is dedicated to massage therapists
and bodywork practitioners—people with oily hands
and piles of laundry who take joy in the gift of touch
that they share with others. You make the world a warmer
place, and we are lucky to have you.

Preface

Fast Decisions for Best Benefits

Welcome to the *Disease Handbook for Massage Therapists*, a reference guide designed to provide clear, concise information about hundreds of conditions for massage therapists who need to make decisions quickly and accurately. This resource is the first of its kind to address the fact that many massage therapists work in settings where they need to have information about pathology that is precise, succinct, and accessible. The *Disease Handbook for Massage Therapists* was designed to coordinate with another important reference, the *Drug Handbook for Massage Therapists*. With these resources, practitioners can make fast decisions that promote safe and effective work, even for clients who may live with complex conditions that are treated with an array of medications.

Who Is This Book For?

Picture this: You work in a setting that requires careful timekeeping and efficient turnover of clientele. On a new client's information sheet, she reports that she hopes that a massage will help her with stress because she has just been diagnosed with diverticulosis and her nummular eczema is flaring up again. She takes anti-inflammatory drugs and uses a steroid cream for her rash. Now she's getting on the table, and you have to make some choices about how to give this client the most effective, satisfying, and safest massage possible.

You don't have time to do all the background reading on these conditions; you need information in a streamlined, accessible, massage-oriented format. The *Disease Handbook for Massage Therapists* was created for this situation and others like it. *It is designed specifically for massage therapists and bodywork practitioners who need to make fast decisions for best benefits.*

What Can You Find Here?

It is important to emphasize that the *Disease Handbook for Massage Therapists* does not contain a complete discussion of every condition; it is only a brief synopsis of issues that may inform a short-term decision about massage. Practitioners who want to further pursue topics are strongly encouraged to do so when time permits. The information that is included here falls under five major topics:

- A brief definition and description of the condition. Associated conditions and diseases are indicated with **bold** font to direct readers to the appropriate other entries
- A list of signs and symptoms
- A description of common treatment options, with emphasis on those that might influence choices about massage
- A list of types of medications that are often recommended to treat the condition; this issue can be further pursued in the *Drug Handbook for Massage Therapists*
- A discussion of massage considerations, including possible risks, benefits, and advice for practitioners. Bodywork approaches have been loosely grouped into two types: mechanical, manipulative modalities, such as Swedish massage, and reflexive or energetic techniques. Obviously, this is an oversimplification, but it provides enough information for practitioners to make educated decisions.

Conditions are listed in alphabetical order, and cross-references for subtypes are found throughout the text. For instance, a practitioner wanting some quick information on nummular eczema could look under "N" for nummular or "E" for eczema and be directed to the entry on **dermatitis/eczema**.

Additional Resources

Purchasers of this book can access the searchable full text online by going to the *Disease Handbook for Massage Therapists'* Web site at http://thePoint. lww.com/Werner-handbook. See the inside front cover of this text for more details, including the passcode you will need to gain access to the website.

How Did This Book Come About?

Way back when I was first licensed as a massage therapist, I got a phone call from a woman who had found one of my brand-new business cards, and she wanted to get a massage. I was excited to have a new client for my new business. "By the way," she said, "I have Guillain-Barré syndrome. Can you work on me?"

I didn't even know how to look up this disease (pronounced ge-YAHN bar-RAY) in the dictionary, never mind having an informed opinion about the appropriateness of massage, and I had no resources to help me. Reluctantly, I turned her away.

That conversation happened in the days before any textbooks about massage and pathology existed. Now massage therapists have many references, including my own, *A Massage Therapist's Guide to Pathology*, a textbook for students and practitioners that explores in detail the etiology, demographics, signs, symptoms, diagnostic procedures, and treatment options for more than 200 diseases and conditions. These references are useful for students and practitioners who have the time to do background research to make the best decisions about bodywork, but what about the massage therapist whose client is getting on the table *right now* and who needs to make some decisions in the next few moments? That is the practitioner for whom this book was written.

A Final Note

The practice of massage therapy and bodywork continues to expand into new settings and venues. Our clients continue to ask us to help them with chronic and acute conditions. Consequently, the expectations for massage therapists to be well informed about diseases and pathologies continue to increase. I hope that the *Disease Handbook for Massage Therapists* will be a useful resource in that process and that it will help readers work with accurate and pertinent information. Furthermore, I hope that the *Disease Handbook for Massage Therapists* will inspire readers to gather more information on the conditions their clients live with. In that way, we will work together to serve our clients and our profession with the best possible intentions and commitment to quality. I am proud to be part of that effort.

—Ruth Werner
2009

Acknowledgments

My thanks always to the many people who knowingly or unknowingly have helped me to carve out a small niche in this highly specialized field. This list includes:

- Curtis, Nathan, and Lily: all the time, every minute, no matter what.
- Students at the Myotherapy College of Utah and participants in workshops who generously share their stories: It is a privilege to work with you, and I learn far more from you than you do from me.
- Cherished colleagues and mentors, especially those at Lippincott Williams & Wilkins, the Massage Therapy Foundation, and all the Cool Chicks to whom I regularly vent.

Reviewers

Nicole Benge, DC, BA
Rising Spirit Institute
Dallas, Georgia

Patty Berak, MBA, BHSA, NCBTMB
Baker College of Clinton Township
Center Line, Michigan

Gary Bruce, NCTMB, LMT
Project Special Care
St. Augustine, Florida

Leora Fellus, CMT, BA
Western Institute of Neuromuscular
Massage Therapy
Seal Beach, California

Beth Holmes, CMT
Crozet, Virginia

Robert Peterson-Wakeman, MSc
Professional Institute of Massage
Therapy
Saskatoon, Saskatchewan, Canada

Holly Rasmusson, LMT
Total Look School of Cosmetology &
Massage Therapy
Cresco, Iowa

Chris H. Rivers, MA
Cañon City, Colorado

Bill Ryan, PhD
Slippery Rock University of
Pennsylvania
Slippery Rock, Pennsylvania

Contents

Contents

A

abortion, elective and spontaneous

An elective abortion is the intentional termination of a pregnancy; a spontaneous abortion is an unintentional termination, sometimes called a miscarriage or a stillbirth.

During the first 12 gestational weeks, an elective abortion is usually accomplished by vacuum suction. In the 13th to 15th weeks, a dilatation and curettage (D&C) may be performed. Later terminations are brought about by inducing labor.

Miscarriages, or spontaneous abortions, usually happen in the first 14 weeks of pregnancy, although the risk is reduced after the eighth week. If the fetus dies after the 20th week, the event is called a stillbirth, but the principles are the same.

Conditions that increase the risk for a spontaneous abortion include a history of **pelvic inflammatory disease**, sexually transmitted infections, **diabetes**, clotting disorders, and autoimmune disorders as well as conditions that are treated with medications that may interfere with a healthy pregnancy.

Pregnancy and the end of pregnancy also carry a risk of complications, including **deep vein thrombosis**, infection, and **depression**.

Signs and Symptoms

- Local and referred pain
- Vaginal bleeding

Treatment Options

If the uterine lining is not completely shed, a D&C may be required.

Medications

Antibiotics are prescribed if an infection is present. Analgesics may be recommended for pain control.

🖐 Massage Considerations

Risks

- Avoid deep abdominal work for clients with a recent abortion or miscarriage.
- Watch for signs of hemorrhaging and deep vein thrombosis.

Benefits

- Nurturing, educated, nonjudgmental touch during this time of emotional and physical trauma is appropriate and welcome.
- Massage can improve sleep, reduce pain, and promote the parasympathetic balance.

abscess: see boils

acne rosacea

Acne rosacea is an idiopathic condition in which small blood vessels in the face enlarge, causing bright red areas that may then develop pustules.

This condition is traditionally associated with frequently drinking alcohol or hot liquids or eating spicy foods, but the majority of people with these behaviors have no symptoms of rosacea. Other triggers include exposure to hot or cold wind and emotional stress.

Acne rosacea may progress in stages, leading to permanent changes in the skin of the face. The eyelids are occasionally involved, in a condition called blepharitis. Acne rosacea only rarely affects other areas of the body.

Signs and Symptoms

- Flushed facial skin; redness over nose, forehead, cheeks, chin
- Telangiectasias ("spider veins") on the face
- Papules and pustules
- Rhinophyma: the skin is permanently thick, bumpy, reddened

Treatment Options

Acne rosacea patients are advised to avoid triggers and oil-based moisturizers and makeup. Permanently thickened skin may be treated with cosmetic surgery.

Medications

Patients with acne rosacea may use oral or topical antibiotics for pustules.

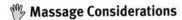 Massage Considerations

Risks
- Acute inflammation locally contraindicates massage.
- Avoid oil-based lubricants on the face.

Benefits
- Massage has no specific benefits for acne rosacea outside of the experience of nonjudgmental, soothing touch.
- Clients who have had acne rosacea can enjoy the same benefits from massage as the rest of the population.

acne vulgaris

Acne vulgaris is a condition in which a person becomes susceptible to small, localized bacterial skin infections that usually appear on the face, neck, and upper back.

This condition is often associated with puberty, but it isn't exclusive to teens. Contributing factors include sudden increases in testosterone production and other hormonal shifts, bacterial activity, stress, suppressed immune system function, and liver congestion.

Signs and Symptoms

- Pimples: red, painful bumps or papules
- Cysts: infections trapped deep in the dermis

- Open comedos ("blackheads"): pimples in which the trapped sebum oxidizes and becomes dark
- Closed comedos ("whiteheads"): superficial infections that are covered with a thin layer of epithelium that traps the sebum and pus

Treatment Options

Acne patients are counseled to avoid touching the face, to wash with astringent but gentle cleaning agents, and to use nonirritating moisturizers.

Medications

People with acne may treat it with topical anti-inflammatory and drying agents, oral antibiotics, or retinoids (which have side effects that include birth defects, joint pain, and hair loss).

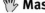 Massage Considerations

Risks

- Avoid touching compromised skin that may be vulnerable to infection.
- Use a water-based lubricant or recommend that the client shower with a gentle astringent soap after the session.
- Don't use alcohol-based drying agents; these may irritate the skin and exacerbate symptoms.

Benefits

- Clients with acne can enjoy nonjudgmental, soothing touch where the skin is healthy.
- Massage may improve liver function, but this shouldn't be claimed as a dependable benefit for clients with acne.

---

acoustic neuroma

Acoustic neuroma, also called vestibular schwannoma, is a benign tumor on a branch of cranial nerve VIII, the vestibulocochlear nerve. The vestibulocochlear nerve transmits information about sound and equilibrium. A tumor may interfere with either of these functions, depending on its location. As it grows, it may also disrupt other cranial nerves or press on the brainstem itself, which can be life threatening.

This condition is usually idiopathic and unilateral. A rare genetic disease, neurofibromatosis type 2, involves bilateral tumors that grow rapidly and carry a high risk of nearby damage.

Most acoustic neuromas are silent. If they grow at all, it happens very slowly over several years. Occasionally, they can grow much faster and interfere with central nervous system function. In this situation, they can mimic several other conditions including **Ménière syndrome**, **vertigo**, **Bell palsy**, and **trigeminal neuralgia**.

Signs and Symptoms

- Often silent and found incidentally
- Hearing loss that develops slowly
- Tinnitus (ringing in the ears)
- Vertigo, disequilibrium
- A feeling of fullness or pressure in the ear
- (If pressing on other tissues): facial numbness, paralysis; severe headache

Treatment Options

Acoustic neuromas are treated with observation, surgery, or radiation. Slow-growing tumors in people who are not good candidates for brain surgery are typically tested regularly with magnetic resonance imaging (MRI) scans to watch for signs of growth. Several surgical approaches have been developed, but they all carry serious risks, including permanent hearing loss and infection. Radiation may shrink tumors and slow their growth, but it rarely eradicates them altogether.

Massage Considerations

Risks

- A client with slowly progressive hearing loss or vertigo needs to seek medical attention.
- A client with vertigo may need assistance in getting on or off the table.

Benefits

- Massage has no specific benefits for acoustic neuroma.
- Clients with acoustic neuroma who can safely get on or off the massage table can enjoy the same benefits from massage as the rest of the population.

---

acromegaly

Acro refers to extremities; *mega* means large. Acromegaly is a disorder involving the production of excessive growth hormone after the epiphyses of the long bones have fused, usually because of a benign tumor on the pituitary gland.

Left untreated, pituitary tumors can lead to several serious complications, including cranial nerve damage, vision problems, **heart failure**, **diabetes**, and **colorectal cancer**.

Signs and Symptoms

- Enlarged hands and feet
- Facial changes (the jaw becomes enlarged with more space between the teeth)
- Headaches
- Hyperhydrosis (excessive sweating)
- Joint pain
- Sleep apnea

Treatment Options

Surgery to remove the pituitary tumor may be performed.

Medications

Acromegaly may be treated with hormones to oppose pituitary secretions.

Massage Considerations

Risks

- Avoid rigorous circulatory massage if the circulatory system is compromised.

Benefits

- Massage has no specific benefits for acromegaly, but it may address some associated symptoms, including joint pain, muscle soreness, and headache.

actinic keratosis: see skin cancer

acute gouty arthritis: see gout

acute idiopathic polyneuritis: see Guillain-Barré syndrome

addiction: see chemical dependency

Addison disease

Addison disease is a deficiency in hormones from the adrenal cortex, leading to low levels of mineralocorticoids and glucocorticoids. It is usually brought about by an autoimmune attack, but it can also be a complication of **tuberculosis, AIDS**, or other disorders.

Addison disease is frequently seen with type 1 **diabetes mellitus, Graves disease**, and **Hashimoto disease**.

Signs and Symptoms

- Weakness
- Fatigue
- Weight loss
- Salt craving
- Hair loss
- Gastrointestinal discomfort
- Decreased cold tolerance
- Increased skin pigmentation
- Depression
- Addisonian crisis: dehydration, hypotension, nausea, vomiting, hypoglycemia

Treatment Options

Underlying conditions that lead to Addison disease must be managed first. After that, a diet that emphasizes adequate water, sodium, and potassium is recommended.

Medications

Clients may take hormones to address the imbalances created by primary Addison disease. Clients with secondary Addison disease may also take medication to manage the underlying condition that is contributing to the adrenal cortex deficiency.

Massage Considerations

Risks

- Clients with Addison disease may have underlying conditions that influence choices about massage.
- Clients with Addison disease may take steroids that decrease bone density and mask the inflammatory response; these side effects require adjustments in the massage session.

Benefits
- Massage has no specific benefits for Addison disease, but it may help promote a healthy sympathetic/parasympathetic balance.

adhesive capsulitis

Adhesive capsulitis, or "frozen shoulder," is an idiopathic problem involving adhesions between the joint capsule at the glenohumeral joint and the head of the humerus. It involves a long, slow, painful onset ("freezing"), followed by a period in which pain is reduced but function is severely restricted ("frozen"), and finally a period during which pain subsides and function is fully or nearly fully restored ("thawing"). The whole process can take anywhere from a few months to well over a year.

This condition is often confused with, or happens concurrently with, other shoulder problems, including **osteoarthritis**, **impingement syndrome**, bone spurs, rotator cuff **tendinopathy**, and **bursitis.**

Signs and Symptoms
- Acute pain in the shoulder
- Limited range of motion, especially medial rotation of the humerus

Treatment Options

Home exercises and physical therapy may be recommended for adhesive capsulitis. Orthopedic manipulation or surgery may be suggested if other methods are unsuccessful.

Medications

People with adhesive capsulitis may treat it with nonsteroidal anti-inflammatory drugs or cortisone injections into the joint capsule.

Massage Considerations

Risks
- Avoid exacerbating inflammation, which may prolong the painful phase of this condition.

Benefits
- Massage may address secondary muscular restrictions seen with adhesive capsulitis.
- Heat with gentle stretching and exercise may help free adhesions.
- Careful massage around the shoulder girdle may be helpful in restoring the best possible range of motion.

alcoholism

Alcoholism is a subtype of **chemical dependency** involving the use of alcohol in such a way that it causes significant mental, physical, or social dysfunction. An alcoholic person shows increasing tolerance to alcohol, withdrawal symptoms when alcohol is withheld, and persistent use despite efforts to stop and the problems that use causes.

Signs and Symptoms
- Repeated unsuccessful attempts to stop substance use
- Difficulty maintaining personal and professional relationships

- Anxiety, depression
- Digestive system signs
    Gastritis, gastric ulcers
    Liver damage, cirrhosis
    Increased risk of esophageal and stomach cancer
    Pancreatitis
- Cardiovascular system signs
    Damage to the myocardium
    Agglutination of the red blood cells, leading to thrombi in the brain and elsewhere
    Poor vitamin K synthesis, leading to decreased clotting factors
- Nervous system signs
    Memory loss
    Slowed reflexes
    Brain damage from toxic metabolic wastes
    Organic brain syndrome: nervous system effects become permanent
- Immune system signs
    Impaired resistance
- Reproductive system signs
    Reduced sex drive
    Erectile dysfunction
    Infertility
    Fetal alcohol syndrome
- Alcoholic families
    Increased risk of substance abuse among children of alcoholics
    Increased risk of depression, anxiety disorders, and phobias among children of alcoholics

Treatment Options

Total abstinence has traditionally been assumed to be the only successful outcome for treating alcoholism. However, it seems that some alcoholism patients can learn to reset their levels of alcohol intake without completely abstaining from it, but the determination of who can handle alcohol successfully and who must completely avoid it is still difficult to make.

Medications

Some medications suppress the craving for alcohol by creating an extreme and painful reaction against it.

✋ Massage Considerations

Risks
- Several complications of alcohol abuse have influence on decisions about massage; these must be addressed first.
- Clients who are intoxicated at the time of an appointment need to reschedule massage.
- Massage can exacerbate nausea.

Benefits
- Clients who are recovering alcoholics who have no underlying contraindications can enjoy the same benefits from massage as the rest of the population.

allergic reactions

An allergy is an immune system response against a trigger (an allergen) that is not inherently dangerous. Allergies often occur on the skin but are also common in the respiratory and digestive tracts.

Allergies occur on a continuum of severity from mildly annoying and easily controlled to debilitating or even life threatening. **Anaphylaxis** and **angioedema** are two extreme allergic reactions. **Hives, eczema,** and **asthma** also involve allergic reactions.

Signs and Symptoms

- Depend on the type of allergy and affected tissues
- Skin reactions: hives, swelling, itching, rashes
- Respiratory reactions: shortness of breath, wheezing, excessive mucus production (itchy eyes and nose may also occur)
- Digestive reactions: nausea, vomiting, diarrhea

Treatment Options

Allergy patients are counseled to avoid triggers whenever possible. Otherwise, allergies are typically treated with medication.

Medications

"Allergy shots" are designed to introduce gradually increasing amounts of identified allergens to the system to desensitize it.

Medications to control allergic reactions include anti-inflammatory drugs, antihistamines, decongestants, and epinephrine. People prone to extreme reactions may carry an EpiPen for a fast dose of epinephrine.

 Massage Considerations

Risks

- Use hypoallergenic lubricants with clients who are prone to allergic reactions.
- Avoid incense and other potential triggers.
- Acutely inflamed areas locally contraindicate massage.

Benefits

- Massage has no specific benefits for clients with allergies.
- If a client with allergies can be comfortable, he or she can enjoy the same benefits from massage as the rest of the population.

altitude sickness

Altitude sickness is a condition in which the body has an insufficient supply of oxygen because of high altitude (usually over 8,000 feet). Rapid breathing that occurs with this change, especially when it is not accompanied by an increase in water intake, can lead to serious problems with pH balance in the blood. Furthermore, high altitude and low air pressure cause fluid to seep out of capillaries. When this happens in the lungs, it is called high-altitude pulmonary edema (HAPE). In the brain, it is called high-altitude cerebral edema (HACE). In extreme cases, either of these conditions can be fatal.

Altitude sickness is seen in its most extreme forms among mountain climbers who ascend over 12,000 feet, but milder forms are common among people who travel from low to high altitudes and then engage in physical activity before acclimatizing to the new conditions.

Signs and Symptoms

- Headache
- Nausea
- Dizziness
- Fatigue
- Decreased coordination

Treatment Options

Mild altitude sickness is treated with adequate hydration and rest. More extreme cases require descending to a safer altitude, diuretics to decrease edema, and oxygen supplementation.

Medications

Severe altitude sickness may be treated with diuretics. Mild cases may be treated with analgesics for headache.

 ## Massage Considerations

Risks

- People with severe cases of altitude sickness require medical intervention, not massage.

Benefits

- People with mild cases of altitude sickness may respond well to gentle circulatory massage with rest and hydration.
- Some aromatherapy techniques may mitigate mild altitude sickness symptoms.

Alzheimer disease

Alzheimer disease is a progressive degenerative disorder of the brain causing memory loss, personality changes, and eventually death.

Two structural changes in the brain, plaques and tangles, are characteristic of Alzheimer disease. Neurofibrillary tangles occur when tau, a protein in supporting glial cells in the brain, breaks down. Without appropriate support, cells cannot transmit messages, and they atrophy and die. Plaques of beta-amyloid then develop on the collapsed neurons and neighboring healthy tissues as well. Plaques and tangles then trigger an inflammatory response that also damages brain cells.

Signs and Symptoms

- Gradual and eventually substantial memory loss
- Deterioration of language skills
- Loss of the ability to accomplish complex and then simple tasks
- Disorientation, confusion, anxiety

Treatment Options

Alzheimer patients may require specialized services and living facilities.

Medications

Cholinesterase inhibitors may improve short-term memory. Antidepressants, antianxiety medications, and tranquilizers may also be used to influence mood and behavior.

Massage Considerations

Risks

- Older clients may have other overlapping conditions that may influence bodywork choices.
- Therapists must be sensitive to nonverbal signals with clients who cannot communicate clearly.

Benefits

- Alzheimer disease patients respond positively to welcomed touch.
- Massage for Alzheimer disease patients has been associated with better orientation, more positive social interactions, and less disruptive behavior.

---

amputation

Amputation is the removal of a limb or portion of a limb as a result of disease, trauma, or birth defect.

In the United States, most amputations are related to complications from disease, especially **diabetes mellitus**. A smaller number are related to trauma or birth defects.

Amputations can lead to several complications. Residual limb pain may be brought about by muscle or **tendinopathy, bursitis**, neuroma, an incomplete surgery, or a poorly fitting prosthesis. Phantom sensation and phantom pain are referred sensory phenomena in which the brain continues to project sensation from nerve endings that have been severed. **Complex regional pain syndrome** may be brought about by the condition that led to the amputation or by the amputation surgery itself. Skin irritation at the wound or at the contact points with the prosthesis is common.

Signs and Symptoms

- Part or all of a limb has been removed.

Treatment Options

A person with an amputation may have difficulties with wound healing or prosthesis function; these should be pursued with the health care team.

Medications

Patients with amputations may use analgesics for pain control.

Massage Considerations

Risks

- If the amputation is related to a disease, other complications may have implications for massage.

Benefits
- Massage, hydrotherapy, and physical therapy are often used to speed or improve healing.
- Massage may improve the symptoms of phantom pain.
- Compensatory distortion (limping, postural adjustments) may be addressed with massage.

amyotrophic lateral sclerosis

Also known as Lou Gehrig's disease or motor neurone disease, amyotrophic lateral sclerosis (ALS) is an idiopathic progressive condition that destroys motor neurons in the spinal cord, leading to the atrophy of voluntary muscles.

After diagnosis, this disease, which has no known cure, usually results in death within 2 to 10 years. Death usually comes about by complications of **paralysis**, particularly systemic infections, such as **pneumonia** or renal infection (**pyelonephritis**). Some ALS patients have, against all odds, survived for decades.

Signs and Symptoms
- Stiffness, weakness, awkwardness in the extremities
- Fasciculations (visible, involuntary muscle twitching)
- Pain as the muscles lose function and the structure begins to collapse
- Usually begins in the extremities and progresses toward the trunk
- Bulbar version begins at the trunk with impaired speech and difficulty swallowing
- Late stage: paralysis of the breathing muscles

Treatment Options

ALS treatment includes moderate exercise and physical therapy to preserve muscle function as much as possible. The use of heat and whirlpools can reduce spasms. The use of braces and wheelchairs can improve mobility.

If the swallow reflex is lost, a gastrostomy (stomach tube) may be used for nutrition.

Medications

ALS patients may use drugs to lower the glutamate levels in the central nervous system. Other drugs to limit muscle spasm, fatigue, and secondary infection may also be used.

 ## Massage Considerations

Risks
- Spastic paralysis limits the applicability of rigorous massage.
- Clients may not be able to communicate verbally, so therapists must be sensitive to their nonverbal signals.

Benefits
- Massage may help with pain and stiffness within limits of client fragility.
- Soothing touch during a difficult and challenging process is always beneficial.

anaphylaxis

Anaphylaxis is an acute, severe, systemic allergic reaction. Some of the most common triggers for anaphylaxis include antibiotics, blood products, the contrast medium used in diagnostic imaging, latex rubber, stings of wasps and honeybees, and some foods (e.g., peanuts and other nuts, soybeans, cow milk, eggs, fish, shellfish, seaweed).

Exposure to a trigger causes a huge reaction mediated by antibodies, complement activation, and mast cell activity, which causes and reinforces inflammation. This happens both at the site of exposure and systemically through the body.

People prone to allergic reactions in general have a higher risk of anaphylaxis. A history of allergic **sinusitis, eczema,** or **asthma** is often associated with this disorder. **Angioedema,** a severe allergic reaction that is localized to the area of exposure, frequently occurs during anaphylaxis.

Signs and Symptoms

- Skin signs: hives, itchiness, flushing
- Respiratory signs: shortness of breath, difficulty swallowing, wheezing, coughing
- Digestive signs: nausea, vomiting, cramps, bloating, diarrhea
- Systemic signs: vasodilation, hypotension, circulatory collapse

Treatment Options

Patients with a history of anaphylaxis are counseled to be especially careful to avoid triggers. Otherwise, this condition is treated with medication.

Medications

Anaphylaxis is a medical emergency that is treated with epinephrine. Other drugs may be used to manage blood pressure.

Massage Considerations

Risks
- Acute anaphylaxis contraindicates massage; this is a medical emergency.

Benefits
- Clients with a history of anaphylaxis can enjoy the same benefits from massage as the rest of the population.
- A hypoallergenic lubricant should be used, and other potential triggers such as heavy scents, incense, and oil additives should be avoided.

anemia

Anemia is the condition of having either an insufficient supply of red blood cells, an insufficient or somehow functionally impaired supply of hemoglobin within those cells, or both. The net result is that the blood has less oxygen-carrying capacity and cells have less access to this vital fuel.

Types of anemia include idiopathic anemia, nutritional anemia (usually caused by a deficiency of iron, folic acid, vitamin B_{12}, copper, or protein), hemorrhagic anemia (caused by chronic blood loss as with bleeding **ulcers, endometriosis,** or other disorders), hemolytic anemia (the premature destruction of erythrocytes), and aplastic anemia (caused by bone marrow suppression). Secondary anemia is frequently a complication of another disorder, such as kidney disease, liver disease, or acute infections.

Signs and Symptoms
- Pallor
- Shortness of breath

- Tachycardia, palpitations
- Fatigue
- Intolerance to cold

Treatment Options

Nutritional anemias are treated with supplements and dietary changes. Other types are treated according to the underlying cause.

Medications

Vitamin or mineral supplements may be recommended. Other medications depend on the subtype of anemia that is identified.

Massage Considerations

Risks

- It is important to determine the causes of a client's anemia before proceeding with massage.
- Pernicious anemia (B$_{12}$ deficiency or poor uptake) can cause neurologic damage, including numbness or weakness.
- Cardiovascular weakness may occur with advanced or severe cases.

Benefits

- Massage may temporarily boost the red blood cell count.
- Massage may help to improve the uptake of nutrients in the digestive system.

---

angina pectoris

This condition describes pain or pressure in the chest brought about by problems in the coronary arteries. It is often discussed as stable angina (symptoms are predictably related to physical exertion) and unstable angina (symptoms are unpredictable).

Some contributing factors to angina include **atherosclerosis** of the coronary arteries, coronary artery spasm, aortic valve stenosis, severe systemic **hypertension**, and pulmonary hypertension.

Signs and Symptoms

- Pain or pressure in chest
- Pain may radiate to the left arm and shoulder and to the left side of the jaw and face
- Dyspnea (shortness of breath), choking sensation

Treatment Options

Treatments for angina are geared toward controlling symptoms while working to solve the problem. Surgery to clear out or replace sections of the coronary arteries is an option when medication is insufficient.

Medications

Angina pectoris patients may take nitrates to manage pain and any combination of anticoagulants, beta-blockers, calcium channel blockers, digitalis, and diuretics to reduce other cardiovascular risks.

Massage Considerations

Risks
- Undiagnosed, untreated chest pain contraindicates rigorous circulatory massage.
- Clients who cannot safely exercise should not receive rigorous circulatory massage.
- Massage strategies may need to be adjusted to accommodate medications used by the client.

Benefits
- Clients with treated and monitored angina pectoris can safely receive massage that doesn't challenge their ability to adapt to rapid changes.
- Noncirculatory techniques that focus on parasympathetic response may offer benefit with minimal risk.

---

angioedema

Angioedema is the rapid onset of localized swelling caused by an **allergic reaction**. The swelling can occur on the skin, genitals, or extremities or in the gastrointestinal tract. If it occurs in the tongue, larynx, or pharynx, angioedema can interrupt airflow, which is potentially life threatening.

Although angioedema is a local condition, it can lead to a systemic reaction called **anaphylaxis**.

Allergens commonly associated with angioedema include peanuts or tree nuts, chocolate, fish, tomatoes, eggs, fresh berries, milk, and food preservatives. Medicines associated with this condition include aspirin, angiotensin-converting enzyme (ACE) inhibitors, and some other hypertension medications.

Signs and Symptoms
- Edematous, hot, sometimes itchy skin
- Often asymmetrical swelling
- Rapid onset; usually resolves within 72 hours

Treatment Options

The highest priority with angioedema is to make sure that the air passageway is open. Patients are counseled to avoid triggers. Localized swellings respond well to cool, moist compresses.

Medications

Angioedema is treated with antihistamines and possibly epinephrine.

 Massage Considerations

Risks
- Acute angioedema contraindicates massage.
- Hypoallergenic lubricants should be used to reduce the risk of allergic reaction.

Benefits
- Clients who have had angioedema can enjoy the same benefits from massage as the rest of the population.

aneurysm

An aneurysm is a permanent bulge in the wall of an artery or the heart. Aneurysms occur most often in the aorta and the arteries at the base of the brain. The damage may be brought about by any combination of injury, genetically weak smooth muscle tissue, **hypertension**, **atherosclerosis**, and compromised connective tissue. If the thinned and delicate wall of the aneurysm ruptures, death will probably occur shortly.

Aneurysms occur in different shapes and sizes. The most common forms are saccular, fusiform, berry, and dissecting.

If a cerebral aneurysm ruptures, the result is a hemorrhagic **stroke**.

Aneurysms in which blood pools, thickens, and then travels again into the circulation may be a source of arterial **emboli**.

Signs and Symptoms

- An aneurysm is often silent until it is a medical emergency.
- A bulge may press on other organs, causing pain.
- Thoracic aneurysms may cause dysphagia (difficulty swallowing), coughing, or hoarseness.
- Abdominal aneurysms may cause a throbbing lump, loss of appetite, weight loss, reduced urine output, and back pain.

Treatment Options

Small, stable aneurysms may be watched for changes. Aneurysms at high risk for rupture are repaired with open or endovascular surgery.

Medications

Clients with a history of aneurysm or aneurysm repair may take prophylactic anticoagulant drugs.

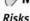 Massage Considerations

Risks

- Identified aneurysms require extreme caution for circulatory massage.
- An unidentified throbbing abdominal bulge may be an early sign; this requires immediate medical attention.
- Abdominal aneurysms, even if they are identified as stable, contraindicate all but the lightest abdominal massage.

Benefits

- A client with a stable aneurysm may receive massage intended to promote relaxation without mechanically impacting circulation.

ankylosing spondylitis

Ankylosing spondylitis (AS) is a progressive inflammatory arthritis caused by an autoimmune reaction, leading to permanently stiff or even fused joints in the spine, usually in flexion. Although AS is usually limited to the spinal joints, the ribs, hips, shoulders, toes, and sternoclavicular joints may also be affected.

Pneumonia related to poor lung capacity is a common complication of this disorder.

Signs and Symptoms

- Runs in cycles of flare and remissions
- During flare: malaise, fever, dry eyes
- Often starts as chronic low back pain
- Referred pain to the buttocks or legs
- Stiffness in the hips, especially after rest

Treatment Options

AS is typically treated with physical therapy to maintain the best function possible. Surgery may address bony misalignment and deformation.

Medications

Clients with AS may take anti-inflammatory drugs, analgesics, and immune-suppressant drugs.

Massage Considerations

Risks

- Avoid massage that may exacerbate inflammation.

Benefits

- Massage along with exercise may help preserve mobility of the spine.
- Carefully given massage can provide pain relief.

anorexia: see eating disorders

---

anterior cruciate ligament injury

These injuries involve damage to the anterior cruciate ligament (ACL), one of the ligaments located inside the knee joint capsule that helps stabilize the knee.

The anterior and posterior cruciate ligaments work with the menisci and the lateral and medial collateral ligaments to keep the femur seated firmly on the tibial plateau. The ACL is damaged most often when the foot is planted but the knee transmits a twisting or pivoting force through the rest of the leg. Soccer, skiing, basketball, and football are activities commonly associated with ACL injuries.

Women are more vulnerable to ACL tears then men for several reasons: they have a wider pelvis, which changes the way weight-bearing force is translated through the knee; they have less muscle mass to support the knee joint from the outside; and estrogen secretion is associated with ligament laxity (a statistical correlation can be found between the ovulatory phase of menstruation and the risk of ACL tears in women athletes).

An ACL injury rarely happens alone; the posterior cruciate ligament, menisci, or collateral ligaments may also be injured at the same time. Similarly, people with a history of ACL tears and poor knee stability have a higher risk of associated injuries, including **meniscus tears** and **osteoarthritis**.

Signs and Symptoms

- Pain and a "popping" noise at the time of trauma
- Rapid swelling, loss of range of motion
- Instability at the knee; it may feel like it will "give way"

Treatment Options

If the ACL is torn but not ruptured, the chance for nonsurgical repair is good. Physical therapy and rehabilitation may take several months, but if the knee can regain stability, the person can again take up demanding activities.

Complete ruptures or injuries that involve other knee structures may require surgery. Typically, a graft of another tendon is installed to take the place of the injured ACL ligament.

Medications

People recovering from an ACL injury are often counseled to use nonsteroidal anti-inflammatory drugs to manage pain and swelling.

Massage Considerations

Risks

- Acute injuries with heat and swelling locally contraindicate circulatory massage.

Benefits

- During the acute phase, lymphatic techniques may help reduce swelling and speed recovery.
- Massage cannot directly access the ACL, but after inflammation subsides, it can address the muscles that cross the joint for pain relief.
- Clients with ACL tears may use crutches, a knee brace, or both; massage can address compensatory limping or other distortions.

anxiety disorders

Anxiety disorders are a group of conditions that have to do with exaggerated, irrational fears and the efforts to control those fears. Some of these conditions come and go; some are chronic, progressive problems; and others reach a peak and then sometimes recede or remain stable.

People with anxiety disorders generally have a higher risk of serious **depression** and **chemical dependency** than the general public. In addition, other stress-related disorders, such as **irritable bowel syndrome, migraine headaches,** and **sleep disorders,** are very common among this population.

Signs and Symptoms

- General anxiety disorder
  - Chronic, exaggerated, consuming worry
  - Constant anticipation of disaster
  - Early onset; slowly progressive
- Panic disorder
  - Panic attacks; sudden onset of extreme sympathetic symptoms
  - A feeling of impending doom that may last for 10 to 60 minutes or more
  - In some cases, agoraphobia: fear of open spaces, or a sense of a shrinking safety zone
- Acute and posttraumatic stress disorder
  - Persistent visceral memories of a specific ordeal relived in nightmares or flashbacks
  - Withdrawal from friends and family; irritability; aggression
  - Hypervigilance; exaggerated startle reflex
  - Dissociation: the detachment of the mind from physical or emotional experience

- Obsessive–compulsive disorder
  Unwelcome thoughts (obsessions) and attempts to control them through ritualized
  activities (compulsions)
  Compulsions can consume many hours each day
  May cycle in flare and remissions; not always progressive
- Social phobia (also called social anxiety disorder)
  Intense, irrational fear of being negatively judged by others
- Specific phobias
  Fear of things that pose little or no real danger (e.g., bridges, elevators, spiders)

Treatment Options

Most anxiety disorders are treated with a combination of medication and psychotherapy.
Strategies depend on which type of anxiety disorder is present.

Medications

People with anxiety disorders may use a variety of antianxiety and antidepressant
medications. People with panic disorder may use beta-blockers to control cardiovascular
symptoms.

Massage Considerations

Risks
- Survivors of touch abuse and other ordeals may be challenged to receive touch in a positive
  way.
- Therapists must be careful to maintain clear and careful boundaries to avoid any perception
  of power differential abuse.

Benefits
- Massage and bodywork may be a useful part of coping skills if massage is perceived as safe
  and welcomed.

appendicitis

Appendicitis is inflammation, usually with infection, of the vermiform appendix.
  Appendicitis resembles several other serious conditions, including **kidney stones, urinary
tract infection, Crohn disease, gastroenteritis, diverticulitis, gallstones, pelvic inflammatory
disease, fibroid tumors**, ectopic **pregnancy**, and **ovarian cysts**.

Signs and Symptoms
- Food aversion
- Nausea, vomiting, diarrhea
- Fever
- Abdominal pain that eventually concentrates in the lower right quadrant
- Rebound pain (pain when the lower right quadrant is pressed and then released)

Treatment Options

After infection in the appendix has been identified, laparoscopic or open surgery is performed
to remove the organ.

Medications

Appendicitis may be treated with antibiotics, but surgery is the more common option.

Massage Considerations

Risks

• Acute appendicitis contraindicates massage.

Benefits

• Clients who have had an appendectomy and are completely healed can enjoy the same benefits from massage as the rest of the population.

Asperger syndrome: see autism spectrum disorders

aspergillosis

Aspergillosis is a fungal infection of the lungs. The fungi that cause aspergillosis are found in dust, decaying plants, and soil. Exposure can simply cause an allergic reaction as the fungus grows in mucous membranes, or the fungus can actively invade the lung tissue.

Aspergillomas, or "fungus balls," may form in cavities caused by **emphysema**, **tuberculosis**, or **lung cancer**. Aspergillosis also carries a risk of becoming invasive when the patient has compromised immunity from a bone marrow transplant, chemotherapy, **HIV** infection, **leukemia**, or other white blood cell shortages.

Signs and Symptoms

• Wheezing
• Productive cough, possibly with bloody sputum
• Possible fever

Treatment Options

Aspergillomas may be surgically removed.

Medications

Allergic aspergillosis is typically treated with bronchodilators and steroidal anti-inflammatory drugs. Invasive disease may be treated with systemic antifungal medications.

Massage Considerations

Risks

• Clients with aspergillosis may not be comfortable lying flat on a table.
• Clients with aspergillosis may have other respiratory problems that influence choices about massage.

Benefits

• Clients with successfully treated aspergillosis can enjoy the same benefits from massage as the rest of the population.

asthma

Asthma is a chronic disorder in which a person is exposed to a stimulus that causes a sympathetic reaction, followed by a parasympathetic overreaction in the lungs, which takes the form of bronchoconstriction. The bronchioles of people with asthma are extremely irritable; they appear to be in a state of constant inflammation, always ready to launch an attack when appropriately stimulated. Asthma is a type of hypersensitivity reaction and is classified by many as an **allergic reaction**.

Signs and Symptoms

- Dyspnea (shortness of breath), wheezing, coughing
- Difficulty expelling air
- Panicky feeling with increased heart rate and anxiety
- Cyanosis (bluish tinge) if oxygen is dangerously low

Treatment Options

Patients are counseled to avoid triggers and to manage their asthma episodes with medication.

Medications

Medical intervention for asthma is available in two forms: anti-inflammatory drugs and bronchodilators that relax the smooth muscles of the bronchiole tubes.

✋ Massage Considerations

Risks

- Clients with asthma are likely to have other allergic reactions as well. Use hypoallergenic lubricant and avoid incense, perfume, or other irritating stimuli.
- An asthma attack may require ending the session.

Benefits

- Massage can be beneficial when a client with asthma is not having an episode; focus on reducing resistance in breathing muscles for more efficient respiration.

arthritis: see gout, psoriatic arthritis, osteoarthritis, reactive arthritis, rheumatoid arthritis, septic arthritis

atherosclerosis

Atherosclerosis is a condition in which deposits of cholesterol and other substances infiltrate and weaken layers of large blood vessels, particularly the aorta and coronary and carotid arteries. The circulatory impairment caused by atherosclerotic plaques is exacerbated by arterial spasm and the blood clots that form at the site of these deposits. Eventually, the arteries become narrowed, inelastic, and vulnerable to having plaques grow until a complete blockage is formed or pieces of debris break off and travel farther into the artery.

Atherosclerosis occurs in conjunction with several other cardiovascular problems. It is both initiated by and a contributor to **hypertension**; it causes **angina pectoris** and increases the risk for **heart attack, aneurysm, heart failure,** and **stroke**.

When atherosclerosis affects distant arteries, **peripheral artery disease** may result.

Signs and Symptoms

- Silent in early stages (up to 80% occlusion)
- Slow onset of poor stamina; fatigue, shortness of breath
- Stable and unstable angina
- High risk of other cardiovascular complications and stroke

Treatment Options

When atherosclerosis is caught early, it may be managed with diet, exercise, and medication. Later interventions include balloon angioplasty, catheter atherectomy, and bypass surgery.

Medications

Medical intervention for atherosclerosis often includes cholesterol-lowering drugs, anticoagulants, and antihypertensive drugs (beta-blockers, calcium channel blockers, diuretics, digitalis). These may require some adjustment by the therapist for best benefit and minimum risk.

🖐 Massage Considerations

Risks

- Clients with a compromised cardiovascular system may be challenged to adapt to changes required by some types of bodywork, especially rigorous circulatory massage.
- Be especially cautious around the sternocleidomastoid to avoid disrupting the carotid arteries.
- Adjustments may be required to accommodate medications; end the session with stimulating strokes and allow extra transition time for the client.

Benefits

- If the client has good homeostatic resilience (i.e., if it is safe for him or her to exercise), massage is probably safe and appropriate.
- Focus on techniques to lower blood pressure and promote parasympathetic response.

athlete's foot: see fungal infections

atopic dermatitis: see dermatitis/eczema

attention deficit hyperactivity disorder

Attention deficit hyperactivity disorder (ADHD) involves inappropriate degrees of inattention, hyperfocus, and impulse control. Attention deficit disorder (ADD) is a similar condition, without the feature of hyperactivity. ADD and ADHD occur among all age ranges, but these disorders are usually diagnosed in children who have trouble managing their schoolwork and their relationships with friends and family.

Signs and Symptoms

- Short attention span
- Poor frustration tolerance
- Impulsivity
- Distractibility
- Hyperactivity
- Symptoms are consistent in varied settings

Treatment Options

ADHD treatment begins with adjusting the patient's surroundings to promote productive behavior and coping skills. It is usually also treated with medication.

Medications

ADHD medications are psychostimulants (dextroamphetamines or methylphenidates) that have a paradoxical calming effect.

 Massage Considerations

Risks

- Massage has no specific risks for clients with ADHD.
- Some clients may not tolerate a full hour of being still.
- ADHD may promote superficial vasodilation.

Benefits

- Massage can offer a valuable and welcomed chance to slow down.

autism spectrum disorders

Autism spectrum disorders are a group of developmental disorders involving problems in speech and language development, the ability to create and maintain relationships, repetitive movements, and complete social withdrawal.

Signs and Symptoms

- Autistic disorder, or severe autism
    Impaired communication
    Poor social interactions
    Repetitive movement patterns
- Asperger syndrome
    Comparatively mild symptoms
    Normal or above normal mental function
    Occasionally, a consuming interest in a single topic
- Pervasive development disorder
    Signs of severe autism but not enough to meet diagnostic criteria

- Rett syndrome
    - Genetic form of autism with severe symptoms among girls
    - Milder forms of Rett syndrome are now recognized among some boys
- Childhood disintegrative disorder
    - Severe form
    - Later onset (age 3 or 4 years)
    - Rapid loss of vocabulary, motor, and communication skills

Treatment Options

Treatment for autism spectrum disorders focuses on developing coping skills for the affected child and his or her family. Most severely autistic children never achieve independence; they will always need an externally structured and sheltered living environment.

Massage Considerations

Risks
- Some people with autism do not tolerate touch well; therapists must accommodate appropriately.
- Some people with autism do not communicate verbally; therapists must be sensitive to nonverbal communication.

Benefits
- If an aversion to touch can be avoided or overcome, massage can provide a positive form of human contact. Use slow, firm, predictable pressure.

avascular osteonecrosis

Avascular osteonecrosis is a condition in which blood supply to an area of bone is interrupted and the bone tissue consequently dies. The resulting weakness leads to a high risk of **fractures, osteoarthritis,** and joint collapse. Avascular osteonecrosis occurs most frequently at the head of the femur.

Avascular osteonecrosis is frequently a complication of some underlying disorder. Decompression sickness ("the bends") can allow nitrogen bubbles in the blood to block flow to bony tissue. Avascular osteonecrosis also frequently accompanies **lupus** and **Raynaud syndrome. Pancreatitis, hemophilia,** and **anemia** can lead to blockages in blood supply. **Alcoholism** and long-term steroid use are also associated with this disorder.

One version of avascular osteonecrosis, called Legg-Calve-Perthes syndrome, is almost exclusively seen in boys between 3 and 12 years old.

Signs and Symptoms
- May be silent in the early stages
- Pain in the affected area (usually the femoral head but can also be elsewhere)
- Arthritis, risk of joint collapse in the affected area

Treatment Options

Treatment for avascular osteonecrosis typically begins with using canes or crutches and electrical stimulation of the affected bony areas. This may be followed by surgery to remove dead tissue and reshape the bone or to rebuild the affected joint.

Medications

Avascular osteonecrosis patients may use analgesics and anti-inflammatory drugs to help manage some symptoms.

 ## Massage Considerations

Risks

- Avascular osteonecrosis locally contraindicates rigorous massage.
- If the bone damage is related to underlying pathologies, they must be addressed in the decision-making process.

Benefits

- Massage may help to address compensatory postural and movement patterns.

avian flu: see influenza

B

Baker cyst

Baker cysts are extensions of the joint capsule of the knee that protrude posteriorly into the popliteal fossa. In children, Baker cysts may accompany trauma; in adults, these cysts are usually associated with other joint inflammations, including **osteoarthritis, rheumatoid arthritis**, and **meniscus tears** at the knee.

Signs and Symptoms

- Often asymptomatic if small
- Feeling of tightness or fullness when the knee is in flexion

Treatment Options

Baker cysts that don't resolve with ice and rest may be aspirated. Cortisone may be injected to resolve joint inflammation. Large cysts may be surgically removed, but they may recur.

Medications

Baker cysts may be managed with anti-inflammatory drugs or cortisone shots.

 ## Massage Considerations

Risks

- Deep work in the popliteal fossa could rupture a Baker cyst; massage in this area is a local contraindication.
- Enlarged Baker cysts may increase the risk of thrombophlebitis or deep vein thrombosis; both of these contraindicate massage.

Benefits

- Massage has no direct benefits for clients with Baker cysts.
- Clients who have had Baker cysts with no other complications can enjoy the same benefits from massage as the rest of the population.

bariatric surgery

Bariatric surgery is not a disorder in itself but is a treatment for **obesity** that is not controllable with diet and exercise. Severe obesity may lead to several serious complications. Bariatric surgery causes weight loss and eliminates or reduces many of the secondary risks associated with obesity.

Several options for this intervention have been developed. Surgery involves stapling off much of the stomach and attaching the jejunum to the functioning portion, which is about the size of a walnut. This allows the stomach to continue producing digestive enzymes but bypasses much of the absorption capacity of the small intestine. Other options include wrapping adjustable bands around the stomach or removing a portion of the stomach and small intestine. Procedures can be conducted as open surgery or laparoscopically.

Bariatric surgery is considered an option only for people whose body mass index (BMI) is over 40 and for those whose BMI is between 35 and 39.9 who also have type 2 **diabetes, hypertension,** or other serious health problems.

Some risks are associated with bariatric surgery. Immediately after surgery, many people experience body aches, fatigue, dry skin, feelings of being cold, thinning or losing hair, and mood swings. Other more serious complications of surgery include vitamin and mineral deficiencies, dehydration, **gallstones,** bleeding **ulcers,** infection at the incision sites or at the internal staples, **deep vein thrombosis, pneumonia,** stricture at the distal end of the stomach, and food intolerance.

Medications

People recovering from bariatric surgery may use analgesics to help manage pain.

Massage Considerations

Risks
- Risks associated with recent surgery include deep vein thrombosis, infection, and other issues; these must be ruled out before massage can be safely performed.

Benefits
- Massage can be a positive experience during the time of rapid change and challenge that accompanies recovery from bariatric surgery.
- Clients who have fully recovered from surgery can enjoy the same benefits from massage as the rest of the population.

Barrett esophagitis: see gastroesophageal reflux disease, esophageal cancer

basal cell carcinoma: see skin cancer

Becker muscular dystrophy: see muscular dystrophy

bedsores: see decubitus ulcers

Behçet disease

Behçet disease is an idiopathic condition involving cycles of inflammation and remission that affect various parts of the body. It is considered to be an autoimmune disease that may be linked to a genetic predisposition along with exposure to some as-yet unidentified triggering pathogen. It is most common in people from the Middle East and Asia and is sometimes called "Silk Road disease."

Behçet disease has many features in common with **herpes simplex**, **Crohn disease**, **AIDS**, **atherosclerosis**, and other diseases, depending on which signs and symptoms are predominant. Part of the diagnostic challenge is ruling out all these other disorders because Behçet disease itself has no definitive test.

Signs and Symptoms

- Painful ulcers in the mouth that may extend into the gastrointestinal tract
- Ulcers on the genitals
- Inflammation of the uvea or retina leading to eye pain or blurred vision
- Rashes or pustules on the skin
- Joint inflammation at the knees, wrists, elbows, and ankles
- Less common: vasculitis with cardiovascular risks; meningitis

Treatment Options

Behçet disease is treated according to the symptoms. It is especially important to resolve inflammation that affects the eyes to avoid permanent damage.

Medications

Behçet disease is treated with nonsteroidal and steroidal anti-inflammatory drugs as well as immunosuppressant drugs.

Massage Considerations

Risks

- Open skin lesions and ulcerations contraindicate massage.
- Acute inflammation contraindicates massage.
- Be aware of potential cardiovascular weakness that may make rigorous circulatory massage inappropriate.

Benefits

- During flare, energetic or reflexive techniques can offer pain relief with minimal circulatory challenge.
- Clients with Behçet disease whose skin is healthy and who have no other complications can enjoy the same benefits from massage as the rest of the population.

Bell palsy

Bell palsy is a type of peripheral neuritis involving damage to cranial nerve VII, the facial nerve. Pressure or other interference with this nerve results in flaccid paralysis on the affected side of the face.

Facial nerve irritation is usually associated with a reactivation of the **herpes simplex** virus, often in conjunction with an **upper respiratory tract infection**. When an infection is active, the inflammatory response can put mechanical pressure on the facial nerve, leading to loss of function. Other contributing factors may include tumors, bone spurs at the cranial foramen, middle ear infections, upper cervical subluxations, **temporomandibular joint dysfunction, diabetes mellitus, Lyme disease**, and **Guillain-Barré syndrome**.

Signs and Symptoms
- Sudden onset of flaccid paralysis of one side of the face
- Difficulty eating, drinking, or closing the eye on the affected side
- Hyperacusis: the ear on the affected side is hypersensitive
- Distorted taste
- Pain associated with inflammation and degenerating muscles

Treatment Options
Bell palsy is usually self-limiting, and most patients have full or nearly full recovery of function. It is important to maintain elasticity of the facial muscles during this time.

Medications
Bell palsy related to herpes simplex may be treated with steroidal anti-inflammatory drugs and antiviral medication to shorten the duration of symptoms.

Massage Considerations

Risks
- If Bell palsy is related to some underlying disorder, massage strategies may have to be adjusted.

Benefits
- After the infection has passed, massage can benefit clients with Bell palsy by keeping the facial muscles as elastic and mobile as possible for the best possible healing.

benign paroxysmal positional vertigo: see vertigo

---

benign prostatic hyperplasia

Benign prostatic hyperplasia (BPH) is a condition in which the prostate gland of mature men becomes enlarged. This growth is not prostate cancer, hence the name "benign."

BPH occurs so frequently that aging men frequently overlook its symptoms. This is problematic because many early diagnoses of **prostate cancer** may be missed this way.

Long-term prostate enlargement can lead to pathologic changes in the bladder, which can become stiff, inelastic, and irritable. The risk of **urinary tract infections, pyelonephritis**, and **bladder stones** is much higher in men who cannot urinate easily; these are common complications of BPH.

Signs and Symptoms
- Problems with urination: weak flow, frequency, leaking, and dribbling

Treatment Options

BPH is treated according to its severity. If it does not seriously impact a man's ability to urinate, it may be left untreated but must be closely monitored for signs of further growth. Surgical options for BPH include a variety of techniques that remove small sections of the prostate gland to relieve pressure on the urethra.

Medications

Medications for BPH include drugs designed to lower hormone levels and alpha-blockers, a group of medications that helps the prostate and bladder relax.

 ### Massage Considerations

Risks

- Any sign of urinary tract or kidney infection (fever, burning pain on urination) requires immediate medical intervention.
- Clients may not be comfortable on a table for a full hour.

Benefits

- Massage has no specific benefits for clients with BPH.
- Clients with BPH who are comfortable on a table can enjoy the same benefits from massage as the rest of the population.

bilharzia: see schistosomiasis

bipolar disease: see depression

bird flu: see influenza

bladder cancer

Bladder cancer is the development of malignant cells in the epithelial lining of the urinary bladder. About half of all bladder cancer cases are believed to be related to cigarette smoking. Other contributing factors include exposure to aromatic amines, which are chemicals used in dry cleaning fluid, hairdressing, and the textile and rubber industries.

People who have undergone pelvic radiation for other problems have an increased risk of developing bladder cancer, as do people who have used a catheter or have had chronic **urinary tract infections** or **bladder stones**.

Signs and Symptoms

- Painless hematuria (blood in the urine)
- Bladder irritability
- Compression of other pelvic organs as tumors grow

Treatment Options

Bladder cancer is treated differently according to the stage at diagnosis. Identified tumors may be surgically excised from the bladder wall, or the whole organ and other nearby tissues may be removed. Bladder cancer has a high rate of recurrence, so radiation, chemotherapy, or both may be used to reduce the risk of metastasis.

Medications

Bladder cancer may be treated with cycles of chemotherapy. Analgesics and other drugs may be used to treat the symptoms of the disease and the side effects of the treatments.

 Massage Considerations

Risks

- Respect the challenges of cancer treatment, including surgery, chemotherapy, and radiation.
- Lymphedema may occur if inguinal nodes are removed.
- Locally avoid any stomas or surgical equipment.

Benefits

- Careful massage can strengthen the immune system, improve sleep, reduce pain, and lower anxiety.

bladder infection: see urinary tract infection

bladder stones

Bladder stones are bits of crystallized minerals from urine. These stones are usually composed primarily of calcium. They develop most often in bladders that don't drain completely, as with a mechanical blockage or a neurogenic bladder (a bladder that must drain passively because of neurologic damage). Bladder stones occur more often in men than in women.

Bladder stones mimic several other disorders, including **urinary tract infection**, **prostatitis**, **benign prostatic hypertrophy**, and **bladder cancer**.

A person with a history of bladder stones will probably have future episodes of this disorder. Bladder stones may also be associated with **gout**.

Signs and Symptoms

- Bladder irritation
- Hematuria (blood in the urine)

Treatment Options

Bladder stones can be broken into small pieces during a cystoscopy or with ultrasound. Very large stones may be removed surgically.

Medications

Bladder stones may be treated with prescription or nonprescription analgesics for pain management.

 Massage Considerations

Risks

- Massage has no specific risks for clients with bladder stones, as long as they are comfortable on the table.

Benefits
- Massage has no specific benefits for clients with bladder stones.
- Clients with bladder stones can enjoy the same benefits from massage as the rest of the population.

blood poisoning: see septicemia

boils

Boils, also called furuncles, are localized staphylococcus infections of the skin. They often occur at hair shafts or in areas that are vulnerable to constant friction. One subtype of boil is caused by a bacterium called **methicillin-resistant *Staphylococcus aureus*** (MRSA).

Signs and Symptoms
- Small, hot, red lesions that enlarge and develop pus
- Often appear at areas of skin friction, such as the axilla (called hidradenitis suppurativa) groin, and around the buttocks (pilonidal cysts)

Treatment Options
Conservative treatment for boils begins with hot compresses, which sometimes help the boils to burst and then drain, relieving the pressure and therefore the pain. If compresses are unsuccessful, a doctor may lance or surgically remove the boil.

Medications
Oral or topical antibiotics may be used to treat boils.

Massage Considerations
Risks
- Acute infections locally contraindicate massage.
- Reschedule the appointment if signs of systemic infection (fever, malaise, inflamed lymph nodes) are present.

Benefits
- If boils are treated and covered, massage may be appropriate elsewhere on the body.
- Clients who have recovered from boils can enjoy the same benefits from massage as the rest of the population.

Practitioner Advice
- If linens have been exposed to boils, separate them from the rest of the laundry and wash them with extra bleach.

bovine spongiform encephalopathy: see Creutzfeldt–Jakob disease

breast cancer

Breast cancer is the development of tumors in the epithelial or connective tissue of the breast. These growths often begin as benign but may become malignant over time. Ductal carcinoma is the most common type of breast cancer followed by lobular breast cancer and then a variety of other rarer possibilities. **Fibrocystic breast disease** can easily be confused with breast cancer; a tissue biopsy is usually called for to distinguish between the two conditions.

As tumors grow (which may take several years), the risk of having some cells invade the circulatory or lymphatic system increases. The proximity of the axillary lymph nodes makes these a common site for the spread of malignant cells.

Signs and Symptoms

- Small lump or thickening in tissue detected during a self-exam or clinical exam
- Asymmetrical breast growth
- Inverted nipple
- Nipple discharge
- "Orange peel" texture of skin on the breast
- Distant symptoms related to tumor growth and spread: bone pain, weight loss, spinal cord compression, lymphedema in the arms

Treatment Options

Four main options for breast cancer treatment are often used in combinations for best results: surgery, radiation, chemotherapy, and hormone therapy.

Medications

Breast cancer patients are often treated with chemotherapy to kill fast-growing cells and hormone therapy to reduce the risk of recurrence.

Massage Considerations

Risks

- The risks for massage in the context of breast cancer relate to both the cancer itself and consequences of cancer treatments.
- Tumors are local contraindications.
- Radiation sites, ports, and medical devices must be avoided.
- Chemotherapy may impair immunity and affect bone density.
- Blood clots and bruising risk increase with cancer and cancer treatments.
- Lymphedema may develop; this contraindicates most types of massage.

Benefits

- Lymphatic techniques can help to manage lymphedema.
- Careful massage can strengthen the immune system, improve sleep, reduce pain, and lower anxiety.

Practitioner Advice

Massage therapists cannot perform breast exams, but they can encourage their female clients to perform monthly self-exams. This is an important way that all massage therapists can support their female clients.

bronchiectasis

Bronchiectasis is a condition involving permanent dilation of the bronchioles and accumulation of mucus in the lungs. Bronchiectasis is usually the result of repeated severe lung infections, often dating from childhood but not showing damage until middle age. Accidentally inhaling a piece of foreign matter (e.g., a small piece of food) into the lung can also lead to bronchiectasis.

People with a history of **cystic fibrosis, tuberculosis, aspergillosis,** or alpha-1 antitrypsin deficiency are at increased risk of developing bronchiectasis. **Gastroesophageal reflux disorder** can also be a factor through the accidental inhalation of corrosive digestive chemicals.

Having this condition increases the risk of developing **pneumonia.** Long-term patients may also face the possibility of right-sided **heart failure.**

Signs and Symptoms

- Chronic, productive cough
- Green or yellow sputum
- Cough is worse when the patient is supine
- Wheezing, cyanosis (bluish tinge), digital clubbing (the ends of the fingers become rounded)
- Rapid heart and respiratory rate
- Anemia, weight loss

Treatment Options

Patients with bronchiectasis must avoid environments that irritate their lungs. In extreme situations, surgery may be conducted to remove the affected area of the lung.

Medications

Clients with bronchiectasis may use bronchodilators. Antibiotics are frequently prescribed to manage lung infections.

Massage Considerations

Risks

- Clients with bronchiectasis are immune compromised; therapists must be careful about spreading infectious agents.
- Clients may not be comfortable lying flat.

Benefits

- Percussion over the thorax may help clear debris from the lungs.
- Massage of the breathing muscles may decrease resistance and improve efficiency of respiration.

bronchitis, acute

Acute bronchitis is an infection of the bronchial tubes. It is often a complication of a primary infection such as a **common cold** or **influenza.** Fungi, air pollutants, and irritating fumes can also cause inflammation and excessive mucus production in the bronchi.

Sinusitis, chronic bronchitis, asthma, and pneumonia can all cause symptoms similar to those of acute bronchitis, so a physician must rule out these conditions for an accurate diagnosis.

Signs and Symptoms

- Persistent, productive cough
- Wheezing, nasal decongestion
- Headache, low fever, fatigue, muscle aches
- Cough that may persist for several weeks after other signs of infection have cleared

Treatment Options

Viral infections of the bronchi are treated with rest; fluids; and warm, humid air.

Medications

Acute bronchitis is treated with antibiotics when the causative agent is identified as bacterial.

🖐 Massage Considerations

Risks

- Acute bronchitis contraindicates massage.

Benefits

- Massage may be appropriate during recuperation if the client is comfortable on the table.
- Percussion over the thorax may help to dislodge debris.
- Clients who have recovered from acute bronchitis can enjoy the same benefits from massage as the rest of the population.

---

bronchitis, chronic

Chronic bronchitis is part of a group of lung problems called chronic obstructive pulmonary disease (COPD). **Emphysema** is the other major condition under this heading, and it occurs frequently with chronic bronchitis. Chronic bronchitis involves long-term irritation of the bronchi and bronchioles, which may occur with or without infection. Inflammation in the bronchial lining destroys elastin fibers and causes the overgrowth of mucus-producing cells, excessive production of mucus, and increased resistance to the movement of air in and out of the system.

Resistance in the pulmonary circuit can stimulate the production of excessive erythrocytes; this is called **polycythemia**. The heart must then push against even more resistance, which may contribute to right-sided **heart failure** and distal edema, especially in the legs and ankles. Chronic lung damage also makes the lungs more vulnerable to infection. **Colds, influenza, acute bronchitis,** and **pneumonia** frequently accompany chronic bronchitis.

Eventually, the damage associated with chronic bronchitis is permanent; this is a progressive disorder that may be halted or slowed but not reversed.

Signs and Symptoms

- Mild cough that persists after other signs of infection have subsided
- Thick, clear sputum
- Frequent throat clearing

- Vulnerability to respiratory infections, especially pneumonia
- Late stage: cyanosis, edema, heart failure

Treatment Options

Patients with chronic bronchitis must avoid respiratory infections if at all possible. Other strategies focus on slowing or preventing the progression of this disease, including quitting smoking, avoiding irritating fumes, and using bronchodilators if necessary. Some patients with chronic bronchitis use supplemental oxygen.

Medications

Patients with chronic bronchitis may use antibiotics to fight bacterial respiratory infections and bronchodilators to reduce resistance in the respiratory tract.

Massage Considerations

Risks

- Clients with chronic bronchitis have a high risk of respiratory infection.
- Chronic bronchitis is associated with a risk of cardiovascular stress and heart failure.
- Clients with chronic bronchitis may not be comfortable lying flat on a table.

Benefits

- If no infection is present and the circulatory system is sufficiently resilient, bodywork may be safe and appropriate.
- Keep modalities within the client's ability to adapt to changes.
- Focus on breathing muscles to reduce resistance in respiration.

bulimia: see eating disorders

bunions

Bunions are also known as hallux valgus, or "laterally deviated big toe." In this condition, the first phalanx of the great toe is distorted toward the lateral aspect of the foot. The joint capsule stretches, a bursa may become inflamed, and a callus grows over the protrusion. A smaller version of the same problem sometimes appears at the base of the little toe; this is called a "tailor's bunion."

Signs and Symptoms

- A large bump on the medial side of the metatarsal–phalangeal joint of the great toe
- Sharp local pain
- May be acutely inflamed

Treatment Options

Bunions are treated first by minimizing irritants that cause pain, in other words, changing footwear. Massage and ultrasound may be used to improve the resiliency of the foot. Cortisone shots may reduce inflammation.

　　If these interventions don't resolve the pain enough to allow normal activity, surgery may be conducted to remove the bunion and realign the joint at the great toe.

Medications

People with bunions may use analgesics to manage their discomfort as they consider whether surgery is a good option.

 ## Massage Considerations

Risks

- Acute inflammation locally contraindicates massage.

Benefits

- Massage within pain tolerance may improve alignment in the foot.
- Massage can help to minimize the effects of limping or postural distortion; this can be done before or after bunion surgery.

burns

When heat, steam, chemicals, electricity, radiation, friction, or other forces kill off exposed skin cells, the resulting damage is called a burn. Skin damaged in this way cannot provide a shield from infection, maintain a stable temperature, or prevent fluid loss. Losing more than 15% of skin function can put a person at risk for serious infection, shock, and circulatory collapse.

Burns are usually classified by how deeply they affect the skin. Superficial burns are first degree; these include mild sunburns or diaper rash. Deep burns can cause scarring and permanent damage to all layers of the skin and accessory organs, including the sweat glands, nerve endings, and hair shafts.

Signs and Symptoms

- First-degree burn: redness, pain, no blistering
- Second-degree burn: redness, blisters, edema, pain
- Third-degree burn: whiteness or charring, leathery skin texture, often less pain than with more superficial burns

Treatment Options

Mild and moderate burns are typically treated with topical cream and analgesics. More severe (third-degree) burns may require wound debridement and skin grafts.

Medications

Clients with recent first- or second-degree burns may use lotion or antibiotic cream over the area. Analgesics may also be used to manage pain.

 ## Massage Considerations

Risks

- Pain and risk of infection contraindicate massage over compromised skin.
- For healed third-degree burns, be cautious around areas of contracted skin with lost sensation.

Benefits

- If fully healed, massage can improve the quality of scar tissue.
- Lymph drainage techniques may minimize local edema.
- Massage can reduce the stress of invasive and painful treatments for third-degree burns.

bursitis

Bursitis is inflammation of the bursae. These tiny synovial sacs generate excess fluid when they are irritated, which causes pain and limits mobility. Most bursae are very small, but the ones that protect the knee and shoulder can be quite large.

Repetitive stress is usually the factor that irritates a bursa, which then manufactures excessive synovial fluid in a tiny amount of space. In response to the pain, the muscles that surround the joint spasm, splinting the injury. This drastically limits the range of motion of the affected joint.

Signs and Symptoms
- Pain on active or passive movement of the affected joint
- Can be acute or chronic

Treatment Options
Bursitis is usually managed with time, rest, and anti-inflammatory drugs. Changing repetitive physical activity to avoid irritating the area is important. If these interventions are insufficient, a surgical bursectomy may be recommended.

Medications
Bursitis is treated with anti-inflammatory drugs and analgesics. Cortisone shots into the inflamed area may also be used.

Massage Considerations

Risks
- Acute inflammation locally contraindicates massage.

Benefits
- Massage may address muscles that cross over the affected joint to relieve some tightness and pressure.
- Massage can help with postural compensation patterns that may also cause pain.

C

candidiasis

Candida albicans is one type of the many yeastlike fungi that normally live in balance with other flora and fauna of the gastrointestinal tract. When *Candida* fungi grow out of control, the condition is called candidiasis. Often the trigger for *Candida* overgrowth is the prescription of antibiotics; these medications are designed to kill harmful bacteria, but they kill beneficial bacteria as well. Other causes of candidiasis include disorders involving genetic immune system dysfunctions, thymus tumors, and hormonal imbalances.

The exact delineation between normal colonization and aggressive infestation is not always clear. Opinions vary about how extensive a candidal colonization has to be before it causes symptoms. Candidiasis may be considered a factor when a person has persistent **headaches,** fatigue, extreme **allergic reactions**, reduced resistance to infection, **vaginitis**, and chronic **urinary tract infections**.

Signs and Symptoms

- Mouth lesions (also called thrush)
- Anal lesions, "diaper rash," "jock itch"
- Vaginitis
- Thickened, discolored fingernails and toenails
- Systemic symptoms (low grade): chemical sensitivities, headaches, chronic yeast infections, recurring urinary tract infections
- Systemic symptoms (severe): fever, leaky gut syndrome

Treatment Options

Re-establishing beneficial internal bacteria to balance yeasts is a high priority. This may be done through dietary changes, but some medications may also be recommended.

Medications

Clients with candidiasis may be treated with topical or oral antifungal medications.

🖐 Massage Considerations

Risks

- The role of massage for a person with candidiasis depends on the client's resilience and whether his or her skin is healthy.
- Some clients may be vulnerable to overtreatment, and rigorous massage may leave them feeling toxic and overwhelmed.

Benefits

- Gentle massage for subtle cases may help to eradicate yeast-related toxins.

carotid artery disease

Carotid artery disease is a type of peripheral vascular disease that involves the development of atherosclerotic plaque in the carotid arteries. This is a subtype of a larger problem, **atherosclerosis**. It frequently occurs with atherosclerosis in other arteries, **hypertension**, and **diabetes mellitus**.

The chief danger with carotid artery disease is the risk of having any debris break loose and travel into the brain, which would cause a transient ischemic attack, ischemic **stroke**, or retinal infarction, depending on the size and location of the obstruction.

Signs and Symptoms

- Often silent
- Carotid bruit (a characteristic sound) may be heard through the stethoscope
- High risk of transient ischemic attack or stroke

Treatment Options

If the carotid stenosis is less than 30%, it is usually treated with medication. Arteries that are 30% to 70% occluded may be treated surgically, and arteries that are more than 70% clogged are almost always treated surgically, either with an endarterectomy or balloon angioplasty with the placement of a stent. The risk of disrupting debris in the days immediately after surgery is fairly high, so this procedure is generally not performed if stenosis can be controlled or reversed with medication alone.

Medications

Carotid artery disease may be treated with antiplatelet or anticoagulant medication, cholesterol-lowering drugs, or a combination of these drugs.

Massage Considerations

Risks

- The carotid arteries are vulnerable to manipulation just medial to the sternocleidomastoid muscle.
- Clients without a diagnosis of carotid artery disease but who have other cardiovascular problems (e.g., hypertension, atherosclerosis, history of stroke) must be considered at risk for this condition.

Benefits

- Energetic or reflexive techniques can maximize parasympathetic effects without challenging the cardiovascular system.

---

carpal tunnel syndrome

Carpal tunnel syndrome (CTS) is a set of signs and symptoms caused by entrapment of the median nerve between the carpal bones of the wrist and the transverse carpal ligament that holds down the flexor tendons. Contributing factors for CTS include edema, subluxation of the carpal bones, and fibrosis (thickened connective tissue at and around the flexor retinaculum).

Many factors can cause pain or reduced sensation in the wrist and hand; these must be considered to get an accurate diagnosis of CTS. The possibilities include (but are not limited to) injured neck ligaments or **disc disease**; nerve **impingement** elsewhere that may lead to **double-crush syndrome**; rotator cuff **tendinopathy**; **thoracic outlet syndrome**; and other wrist injuries, including **osteoarthritis, rheumatoid arthritis, tendinitis,** and ligament **sprains.**

Systemic conditions, such as **hypothyroidism, diabetes, pregnancy,** and **obesity,** can also contribute to nerve pain in the hands.

Signs and Symptoms

- Tingling, paresthesia, burning, or shooting pain in the lateral hand
- Intermittent numbness or weakness in the lateral hand
- Atrophy at the thenar pad
- Symptoms may flare up if the wrist is flexed during sleep

Treatment Options

Management of CTS often begins with a brace that supports the wrist in a neutral position during work and sleep. Acupuncture may be recommended to avoid surgery.

In CTS surgery, the transverse carpal ligament is split, and some of the accumulated connective tissue is scraped away. This can be conducted as open or closed surgery.

Medications

CTS patients may be treated with analgesics and anti-inflammatory drugs.

Massage Considerations

Risks
- Deep work on the wrist may exacerbate the symptoms of CTS.

Benefits
- Edematous CTS may respond to massage that focuses on fluid flow out of the wrist and forearm; mechanical or lymph drainage modalities may be useful.
- Massage of other potential entrapment sites (neck, shoulder, elbow) may also yield good results.

Practitioner Advice
- CTS is an occupational hazard for massage therapists. Taking care not to hyperextend the wrist and to vary how the hands are used can reduce this risk and increase longevity in this career.

---

cataracts

Cataracts are linked to dysfunction of the lens of the eye. The lens is composed of compartments that contain water and highly organized protein molecules. When it functions correctly, light is carried clearly to the retina of the eye and translated into nerve impulses for vision. If the proteins in the lens begin to degenerate, the lens becomes cloudy and discolored. Vision degrades and may become completely obscured because light cannot pass through to the retina.

Most cataracts are related to age. Limited protein degeneration usually begins around age 40 to 50 years, but enough damage accumulates that people with cataracts often develop symptoms in their 60s or 70s.

Other causes of cataracts include a family or personal history of **glaucoma**, **diabetes**, smoking, trauma to the eye, prolonged use of steroidal anti-inflammatory drugs, or exposure to radiation.

Signs and Symptoms
- The need for frequent changes in eyeglass or contact lens prescriptions
- Slowly progressive blurred, cloudy vision
- Perception of faded colors or a brownish tint
- Increased sensitivity to glare; halo around bright lights
- Double vision
- Poor night vision

Treatment Options

If cataracts are mild, they may be treated symptomatically with a changed prescription in glasses or contacts, low-glare sunglasses, brighter light for reading, or using a magnifying glass.

Many cataract patients are eventually treated with surgery, which is usually successful for restoring all or most lost vision.

Medications

Cataracts are not treated with medication.

 ## Massage Considerations

Risks
• Massage has no specific risks for clients with cataracts.

Benefits
• Massage has no specific benefits for clients with cataracts; these clients can enjoy the same benefits from massage as the rest of the population.

causalgia: see complex regional pain syndrome

celiac disease

Celiac disease, also called celiac sprue or nontropical sprue, is a hereditary condition brought about by poor gluten tolerance. Exposure to gluten, a protein found in many grains, creates an inflammatory response that damages and may ultimately destroy the intestinal villi. Fortunately, avoiding food with any gluten allows the villi to grow back; this is the only successful treatment option for celiac disease.

A person with mild celiac disease may not have serious problems, but people with extreme cases have poor access to all nutrients and may eventually develop dangerous malnourishment.

Signs and Symptoms
• In young children: failure to thrive
• Abdominal pain
• Diarrhea, gas, foul-smelling stool
• Muscle and joint pain
• Dermatitis
• Neurologic signs: headache, seizure, dizziness, numbness, tingling
• May be triggered by surgery, infection, or accident

Treatment Options

The only treatment option for celiac disease is to avoid gluten-rich foods. A gluten-free diet gives the villi a chance to heal, and the prognosis is generally that healthy absorption may resume when inflammation in the small intestine subsides.

Medications

Celiac disease is not treated with medication.

 ## Massage Considerations

Risks
• Massage has no specific risks for celiac disease as long as the client is comfortable.

Benefits
- Massage has no specific benefits for celiac disease, although clients may find improved digestion through parasympathetic effect.
- Clients with celiac disease can enjoy the same benefits from massage as the rest of the population.

cellulitis

Cellulitis is an umbrella term for any bacterial infection of the skin. The bacteria usually involved are *Streptococcus pyogenes* or *Staphylococcus aureus*, but some variations may occur. **Erysipelas** is a subtype of cellulitis that affects the superficial layers of the skin. Necrotizing fasciitis ("flesh-eating bacteria") is classified as a type of cellulitis, although the tissues under attack are deep to the dermis; the causative agent in this case is a different type of streptococcus bacterium.

Bacterial infections usually gain access through the skin at the site of some trauma or pre-existing condition. **Athlete's foot**, insect bites, friction blisters, and other lesions provide common portals of entry. Left untreated, cellulitis carries a risk of progressing to **septicemia**.

Signs and Symptoms
- Pain, inflammation of the skin
- Palpable heat
- Possible open wounds, ulcers
- Fever, malaise, inflamed lymph nodes

Treatment Options
Cellulitis is treated with medication.

Medications
The only safe way to treat cellulitis is with appropriate oral or intravenous antibiotics.

Massage Considerations

Risks
- Acute infections are not appropriate for massage; this is a systemic contraindication.

Benefits
- Energetic or reflexive techniques may be appropriate for people recovering from cellulitis.
- Clients who have fully recovered from cellulitis can enjoy the same benefits from massage as the rest of the population.

Practitioner Advice
- Massage therapists are vulnerable to picking up infectious pathogens through tiny lesions on their hands, even from the skin of healthy clients. Cellulitis is one of many reasons massage therapists must be vigilant about taking excellent care of their hands with good hygiene, cuticle maintenance, and always covering open sores.

cerebral palsy

Cerebral palsy (CP) refers to many possible injuries to the brain during gestation, birth, or early infancy. CP is classified into four types: spastic, athetoid, ataxic, and mixed.

Motor consequences of CP include varying levels of **paralysis**. Many CP patients experience partial or total hearing loss. Many have some amount of strabismus (the visual axes of the eyes are not parallel). Although CP doesn't always involve cognitive problems, some patients experience some level of mental disability. About 25% of all CP patients have **seizure disorders**. Finally, the muscles of CP patients can become so chronically tight that they are replaced with tight, restrictive connective tissue; these are called contractures. Contractures can pull on the skeleton so constantly and so powerfully that the patient is at risk for developing **scoliosis**, which can make it painful to sit or stand and difficult to breathe.

Signs and Symptoms
- Vary according to type
- Hypertonicity with contractures
- Hypotonicity
- Poor coordination and voluntary muscle control
- Weak muscles
- Random uncontrollable movements
- Hearing or vision problems
- Seizures

Treatment Options
Physical therapy is recommended for people with CP so that their muscles and joints may be stretched and manipulated to maintain or improve flexibility. Massage therapy may be a valuable adjunct in these cases.

Some surgical interventions have been developed to lengthen contracted muscles, realign vertebrae that have become distorted by scoliosis, and alter nerve pathways in the brain to reduce the severity of tremors.

Medications
Clients with CP may take antiseizure medications, muscle relaxants, or both. Injections of botulinum toxin are used in some CP patients to minimize their motor restrictions.

Massage Considerations
Risks
- Massage must be conducted with caution in clients with spasticity and sensation loss.
- Some clients cannot communicate verbally; it is important to be sensitive to their nonverbal signals.

Benefits
- Positive, non–task-oriented touch has many benefits.
- Proprioceptive facilitation may improve control and range of motion.
- Massage focusing on muscles and connective tissue may improve function.

cerebrovascular accident (CVA): see stroke

cervical acceleration–deceleration: see whiplash

cervical cancer

Cervical cancer is the growth of malignant cells in the lining of the cervix. It is brought about directly by a viral infection, usually with some of the 80 known varieties of human papilloma virus (HPV) family. HPV is a sexually transmitted disease that is transferred by direct skin-to-skin touching.

Exposure to HPV is the central risk factor for developing cervical cancer. However, other factors may also contribute to the likelihood that abnormal cells will become malignant. Smoking increases this risk by close to 100%. Immune system suppression also increases the risk of developing cervical cancer. Finally, socioeconomic standing is a major factor because it often determines whether a woman has adequate access to early detection and care.

Signs and Symptoms
- Early stages: silent, but dysplastic cells are found with the Pap test
- Later stages: vaginal bleeding, spotting between periods, vaginal discharge, pelvic pain

Treatment Options

Early stages of cervical cancer can be treated by removing the abnormal cells and watching carefully for further changes. Surgical interventions to remove cervical dysplasia include cryotherapy, in which cells are frozen off; loop electrosurgical excision procedure (LEEP), in which electricity is passed through a loop of thin wire to slice off the suspicious tissue; laser surgery; and cone biopsy.

Surgical procedures for cancer caught in the later stages may range from full or partial hysterectomies to full pelvic exenteration, in which virtually all the pelvic organs are removed.

Medications

Cervical cancer is usually treated successfully with surgery if it is found early. Radiation and chemotherapy may be used in advanced cases of cervical cancer.

Massage Considerations

Risks
- Use caution in the context of cancer treatment; surgery and chemotherapy are associated with risks for bodywork.

Benefits
- A client who is currently undergoing treatment for cervical cancer may derive supportive benefits from carefully applied bodywork.
- Clients who have been treated for dysplasia or who have a history of cervical cancer can enjoy the same benefits from massage as the rest of the population.

Charcot-Marie-Tooth disease

Charcot-Marie-Tooth (CMT) disease is a collection of inherited genetic mutations that affect the myelin sheath or nerve fibers of peripheral nerves, resulting in a form of **peripheral neuropathy**.

Several types and subtypes of CMT disease have been identified, each linked to a specific genetic anomaly. They all involve dysfunction to peripheral nerves, either to the myelin sheath or to the fibers themselves. The result is varying levels of weakness, muscle atrophy, and sometimes reduced or impaired sensation.

Most cases of CMT disease affect the muscles of the foot and lower leg. CMT disease is frequently associated with foot deformities and **hammertoes**. CMT disease is slowly progressive and may eventually affect the muscles in the hands and arms. Very rarely, it may cause weakness in the muscles of respiration.

Signs and Symptoms

- Onset in adolescence or early adulthood
- Bilateral foot deformities (high arch, flat foot, hammertoes)
- Slowly progressive loss of muscle function in the foot and lower leg
- Weakness, foot drop, frequent tripping, high-stepping gait
- May progress to affect the hand or forearm
- Can involve altered sensation or neuropathic pain

Treatment Options

Because it is a genetic disease, CMT disease cannot be cured or reversed. It is treated with aggressive physical and occupational therapy, assistive orthopedic devices (braces, canes, shoe inserts), and medication to control pain as necessary. Surgery may be conducted to repair significant deformities.

Medications

CMT disease patients who have nerve pain can be treated with analgesics or antiseizure medication.

Massage Considerations

Risks

- Some CMT disease patients may have compromised sensation. In these situations, massage must be adjusted to avoid the risk of overtreatment.

Benefits

- CMT disease is often managed with exercise and physical therapy. Massage therapy can contribute as well to improve muscle and connective tissue function and to manage pain and limit degeneration of muscle cells.

---

chemical dependency

The issue of chemical dependency falls into three categories: use, abuse, and dependence (or addiction). Use means using a substance to change a physical or mental state, abuse means using a substance in a way that damages the user or the people close to the user, and dependency or addiction is identified when the user develops a progressive tolerance so that he or she must use more of the substance to achieve the desired effects.

Addiction is defined in two categories: psychological and physical addiction. Psychological addiction is a dependency on the pleasurable or satisfying sensations that some substance provides—in other words, addicts like the way they feel when they are using. Physical addiction is a dependency arising from the need to avoid withdrawal symptoms, which can range from minor irritability to hallucinations, nausea and vomiting, seizures, and general physical pain. Most addicts have a combination of psychological and physical addiction.

Alcoholism is a specific subtype of chemical dependency.

Long-term substance abuse has several complications, including a high risk of **hepatitis** B or C; **HIV** from shared needles or impaired judgment leading to unprotected sex; and bacterial infections or opportunistic disorders that appear when immunity is compromised, such as **shingles, candidiasis, herpes simplex,** and other infections.

Signs and Symptoms

- Persistent craving for the substance
- Inability to voluntarily control use
- Increasing tolerance
- Alarming or dangerous withdrawal symptoms when use is suspended
- Spending a great deal of time procuring and using the substance
- Neglected responsibilities
- Denial that a problem exists

Treatment Options

Treatment goals for chemical dependency are threefold: abstinence, rehabilitation, and prevention of relapses.

Most programs begin with a detoxification process, during which the drugs are expelled from the body. Detoxification is followed by a process of rehabilitation, during which the patient is educated about the effects of chemical use and often trained in avoidance behaviors to give him or her some alternatives to the tendency to fall back into old habits.

Aftercare has been shown to be the most important part of treatment for chemical dependency; this sets up the patient with a support system that will carry him or her throughout a lifetime choice of drug abstinence.

Medications

Patients undergoing addiction rehabilitation may use tranquilizers or sedatives to address their withdrawal symptoms.

 Massage Considerations

Risks

- Clients who are using drugs at the time of an appointment should not receive massage; bodywork can overload the detoxification processes of the liver.
- Secondary health problems (infection, liver damage) may be present in long-term users; these must be addressed before making decisions about massage.

Benefits

- Massage may help ameliorate withdrawal symptoms during rehabilitation.
- Clients who are in long-term recovery without other health problems can enjoy the same benefits from massage as the rest of the population.

chicken pox: see herpes zoster

chlamydia

Chlamydia is a sexually transmitted disease involving bacteria (*Chlamydia trachomatis*) that inhabit the reproductive tract of men and women. Left untreated, chlamydia infections can persist and be communicable for several years.

Chlamydia is spread through direct sexual contact. The inflammation it causes can lead to significant problems in the reproductive tract. It is a leading cause of **pelvic inflammatory disease**, it increases the risk of infertility and ectopic **pregnancy,** and it increases susceptibility to the transmission of **HIV** in both men and women.

Signs and Symptoms

- In women:
    - Often silent
    - Burning, painful urination
    - Vaginal inflammation and discharge
    - Pelvic pain
    - Vaginal bleeding after intercourse
- In men:
    - Often silent
    - Burning, painful urination
    - Penile discharge

Medications

Chlamydia is sensitive to antibiotics. The partner(s) of the diagnosed person must be treated as well, even if no symptoms are present.

Massage Considerations

Risks

- If chlamydia has been diagnosed, deep abdominal massage should be avoided until treatment is complete.

Benefits

- Massage has no specific benefits for clients with chlamydia.
- Indirect benefits of massage include immune system support during and after treatment.

cholecystitis: see gallstones

chronic fatigue syndrome

Chronic fatigue syndrome (CFS), also called chronic fatigue immune dysfunction syndrome (CFIDS) or myalgic encephalomyelitis (ME), is a collection of signs and symptoms involving extreme fatigue that is not restored by rest, among other symptoms that affect multiple systems in the body. It varies in severity from mildly limiting to completely debilitating.

Although once thought to be a sign of immune system activity that outlasts exposure to a triggering pathogen, CFS is now considered to be the result of a combination of triggers, including viral exposure, stress, central nervous system problems, and any combination of other factors.

CFS frequently occurs along with **fibromyalgia** and **irritable bowel syndrome.**

Signs and Symptoms

- Unrelenting fatigue not relieved by sleep
- General muscle or joint pain, morning stiffness
- Low-grade fever, swollen lymph nodes, sore throat

- Short-term memory loss, problems with concentration
- Abdominal bloating, nausea, diarrhea, cramping
- Chest pain, irregular heart beat
- Dry eyes and mouth
- Night sweats
- Depression

Treatment Options

CFS is managed by making choices that support the body as fully as possible. This means avoiding stress as much as possible; moderating dietary choices to minimize the use of stimulants (caffeine, sugar) and depressants (alcohol); and exercising very gently within tolerance to avoid exacerbating symptoms.

Medications

Some CFS patients are treated with immunosuppressant drugs and low-dose antidepressants.

 ## Massage Considerations

Risks
- Clients with CFS may be vulnerable to overtreatment; work conservatively at first.

Benefits
- Clients with CFS may enjoy an improved quality of sleep with massage.

chronic obstructive pulmonary disease: see chronic bronchitis, emphysema

chronic pelvic pain syndrome: see prostatitis

Churg-Strauss syndrome: see vasculitis

circadian rhythm disruption: see sleep disorders

cirrhosis

Cirrhosis involves the crowding out and replacement of healthy liver cells with nonfunctioning scar tissue. It is the result of long-term underlying liver disease.

The leading cause of cirrhosis in the United States is **hepatitis** C infection, although other types of hepatitis, **alcoholism, chemical dependency, pancreatic cancer,** and **gallstones** can also increase the risk. Some inherited liver diseases can also cause it. Long-term exposure to environmental toxins can contribute to cirrhosis, as can **heart failure**.

Signs and Symptoms
- Nausea, vomiting, weight loss
- Red patches on the skin

- Splenomegaly
- Ascites
- Excessive bleeding and bruising
- Muscle atrophy
- Jaundice
- Hormone disruption
- Renal failure
- Central nervous system toxicity

Treatment Options

The main treatment objective for cirrhosis is to stop the damage to the liver. This can involve medications as well as immediate lifestyle changes if appropriate.

Transplants are recommended only when patients have not developed extensive damage to other organs and when they are in long-term recovery (6 months or more) from any drug or alcohol abuse.

Medications

Medications for cirrhosis address the serious symptoms and complications of this disorder. Levulose may be given to bind with ammonia for excretion. Diuretics, antacids, steroids, and vitamins may also be used. Interferon is used for cirrhosis caused by viral infection.

Massage Considerations

Risks

- Advanced cirrhosis contraindicates circulatory massage because the ability to adapt to challenges in fluid flow is impaired.

Benefits

- Energetic or reflexive techniques may be helpful and supportive for clients with cirrhosis.

claudication: see peripheral artery disease

Clostridium difficile infection

Clostridium difficile is a spore-bearing bacillus that attacks the gastrointestinal (GI) tract. The bacteria release two potent toxins that kill healthy cells and result in the development of inflammatory membranelike plaques on the intestinal wall. A synonym for this infection is pseudomembranous colitis.

C. difficile bacteria are everywhere, and subclinical (asymptomatic) exposure is common. Under normal circumstances, the beneficial bacteria in the GI tract keep *C. difficile* under control. But when a person—especially someone who is older and otherwise immune compromised—uses antibiotics, antiviral medication, or antifungal medication or undergoes chemotherapy, beneficial bacteria may be destroyed, allowing *C. difficile* bacteria to become active.

C. difficile is spread through oral–fecal contamination and is most prevalent in hospitals and nursing homes. It is becoming an increasing public health threat because it now appears commonly outside of hospital settings, and the causative bacteria are becoming increasingly toxic and resistant to antibiotic treatment. Complications of this infection are serious and include severe dehydration, **renal failure**, perforation of the colon with subsequent **peritonitis**, toxic megacolon with a risk of rupture, **septicemia**, and death.

Signs and Symptoms
- Mild to severe diarrhea with watery stools
- Inflammation of the colon
- Fever
- Blood or pus in the stool
- Nausea
- Dehydration
- Symptoms can appear weeks or months after antimicrobial medication use

Treatment Options
This infection is usually treated with medication. If structural damage to the intestines or colon is significant, surgery to remove the affected sections may be conducted.

Medications
C. difficile is sensitive to some specialized antibiotics, but it is becoming increasingly resistant, so antibiotic use in this situation is often strictly controlled.

✋ Massage Considerations

Risks
- An acute *C. difficile* infection with nausea, fever, and diarrhea contraindicates massage.
- Clients who are being treated for this infection may receive massage, but any abdominal work must be conducted conservatively.

Benefits
- Massage has no specific benefits for clients with a *C. difficile* infection.
- Clients who are being treated for or who have recovered from *C. difficile* infections and who have no discomfort or symptoms can enjoy the same benefits from massage as the rest of the population.

Practitioner Advice
- Hygiene is always important in a massage setting, but for clients at risk for *C. difficile*, the stakes are even higher. This is a spore-bearing bacteria, which means it can live on surfaces for weeks or months, waiting for a chance to find a new host.

cluster headache: see headache

colorectal cancer
Colorectal cancer is the development of tumors anywhere in the large intestine from the ascending right side to the rectum. The majority of colorectal cancers begin with the development of adenomas, which are small polyps in the bowel. If the polyps are present for a long period, these benign growths may become malignant and invade deeper tissues or the lymph system.

People with a history of **Crohn disease** or **ulcerative colitis** have a higher risk of developing colorectal cancer than the general population.

Signs and Symptoms

- Small polyps visible with colonoscopy
- Anemia
- Constipation, narrowed stools
- Blood in the stool
- Lower abdominal pain
- Unintended weight loss

Treatment Options

Surgery to remove the affected section of the bowel is the usual recommendation for stage I or II colorectal cancer. The remaining bowel may be reattached if possible or the healthy section may be connected to a colostomy bag for exterior storage and disposal of wastes.

Stage III colorectal cancer requires surgery to remove the affected length of bowel and chemotherapy to reduce the chance of metastasis through the lymph system.

Stage IV colorectal cancer is also treated with surgery, but more aggressive chemotherapy is used, with radiation to limit growths at distant sites.

Medications

Colorectal cancer may be treated with chemotherapy.

Massage Considerations

Risks

- Massage must respect the challenges that cancer treatment involves; chemotherapy, radiation, and surgery all have cautions for bodywork.
- If a client has a colostomy bag, avoid the stoma and enlist the client's participation to minimize discomfort.

Benefits

- Carefully given massage can help improve the quality of life for clients who are being treated for cancer.
- Colorectal cancer survivors can enjoy the same benefits from massage as the rest of the population; make adjustments for a colostomy bag as necessary.

common cold

The common cold, also called an upper respiratory tract infection (URTI), is a viral infection of the mucous membranes. No single infectious agent causes the "common cold," and the viruses themselves keep mutating and changing.

Common colds leave the body vulnerable to a bacterial onslaught that can include **ear infections, laryngitis, acute bronchitis, sinusitis,** and **pneumonia.** Although the symptoms often resemble **influenza,** colds tend to be less severe and shorter in duration.

Signs and Symptoms

- Runny nose
- Coughing, sneezing
- Mild fever, headache
- Sore throat

Treatment Options

Getting extra rest; drinking lots of fluids; and isolating oneself away from family, classmates, and coworkers who could get infected are all high priorities to treat and limit the spread of common cold. Using a humidifier may relieve some of the irritation to the mucous membranes, although some types of humidifiers can be breeding grounds for bacteria, so it is important to keep them scrupulously clean.

Alternative health care strategies for dealing with colds include taking vitamin C, echinacea, lysine (an amino acid with antiviral properties), zinc lozenges (which also has antiviral properties), and licorice root as an expectorant. Some of these interventions have been shown to reduce recovery time, but their efficacy as cold preventatives has yet to be proven.

Medications

Many people treat their colds with over-the-counter analgesics and fever reducers. These drugs can minimize symptoms but may increase the communicability of the cold virus.

Massage Considerations

Risks
- Avoid bodywork before cold symptoms peak.

Benefits
- Clients who have recovered from a cold can enjoy the same benefits from massage as the rest of the population.

Practitioner Advice
- If a client who is still recovering from a cold receives massage, he or she may find that the symptoms are temporarily exacerbated and then clear up faster than they might have otherwise. This can be a benefit, but only if the client knows what to expect.

compartment syndrome: see shin splints

complex regional pain syndrome

Complex regional pain syndrome (CRPS) is a collection of signs and symptoms that involve changes to the skin, muscles, joints, nerves, and blood vessels of the affected areas. Over the years, this condition has had several names, including causalgia and reflex sympathetic dystrophy syndrome. It usually (but not always) begins after some trauma or injury to an extremity that initiates a sympathetic reflex response. For reasons that are unclear, the injury triggers a self-reinforcing loop of pain and circulatory changes that lead to problems in tissue nutrition and growth.

CRPS is often (but not always) a complication of some initiating trauma, such as a car accident or a gunshot wound. It can also occur after a **stroke**, as part of **disc disease**, or as a postsurgical complication.

Signs and Symptoms
- Stage 1: severe pain at the site; muscle spasms; excessive hair and nail growth; hot, red, sweaty skin
- Stage 2: intense pain, proximal spread of swelling, lack of hair growth, cracked nails, blue tinge to the skin

- Stage 3: thin, brittle bones; fused joints; spreading pain
- Stage 4: self-sustaining pain, central nervous system dysfunction

Treatment Options

Early CRPS may be treated with simple analgesics. Patients benefit from heat, especially moist heat applications such as paraffin baths or hot packs. Later-stage patients may use morphine pumps, transcutaneous electrical nerve stimulation (TENS) units, calcium channel blockers, or a sympathectomy (the surgical severing of parts of the sympathetic nervous system to stop the endless cycle of repeating pain signals).

Medications

Analgesics for CRPS range from over-the-counter painkillers to morphine.

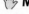 Massage Considerations

Risks
- CRPS contraindicates any stimulus that exacerbates symptoms.

Benefits
- If massage is perceived as pleasant anywhere else on the body, it could certainly add to the quality of life of a person who has some extremely challenging problems.

congenital torticollis: see torticollis

conjunctivitis

Conjunctivitis is a condition in which the conjunctiva (the clear membrane that covers the eyes) is inflamed. Inflammation could be from allergies or chemical irritants, but it is usually attributed to viral or bacterial infection. Bacterial conjunctivitis is often called pinkeye.

Conjunctivitis may also be a complication of another disorder, such as **herpes simplex** or a staphylococcus or streptococcus infection. When it occurs in newborns, it may be from exposure to a maternal vaginal infection with **chlamydia** or **gonorrhea**.

A viral or bacterial infection of the conjunctiva can lead to corneal ulcers or scarring, so it is important to treat these conditions as quickly as possible.

Signs and Symptoms
- Dilatation of the capillaries on the sclera
- Swelling and itching of the conjunctiva
- Excessive tears
- Unilateral if infectious; bilateral if allergic
- Clear or cloudy discharge
- Crusty deposits on the eyelid

Treatment Options

Nonmedical interventions for conjunctivitis include measures to prevent communicability. Face cloths, towels, makeup, and other personal items of a patient with conjunctivitis must be isolated. Contact lenses should be avoided while the infection is present. The best way to prevent the spread of the infection to other people is with frequent hand washing.

Medications

Bacterial conjunctivitis is treated with topical antibiotics. Viral infections must be treated with eye drops and compresses for comfort. Allergic conjunctivitis is typically treated with antihistamines.

Massage Considerations

Risks
- Infectious conjunctivitis is highly contagious; encourage clients to reschedule when the infection has resolved.
- If a client with conjunctivitis keeps an appointment, locally avoid the area, isolate the client's linens for extra bleach in the laundry, and take extra care to swab surfaces.

Benefits
- Massage has no specific benefits for clients with conjunctivitis.
- Clients who have recovered from conjunctivitis can enjoy the same benefits from massage as the rest of the population.

contact dermatitis: see dermatitis/eczema

coronary artery disease: see atherosclerosis

corpus luteum cysts: see ovarian cysts

costochondritis

Costochondritis is inflammation at the costal cartilages (anywhere between the ribs and the sternum). It happens most often at ribs 2 through 5, and most patients have tenderness at multiple levels.

Costochondritis often appears to arise spontaneously without any precipitating event. Occasionally, it may be traced back to a recent respiratory infection or a specific trauma or overuse pattern.

Several other problems can cause chest pain, including trauma to the ribs or acromioclavicular joint, **pleurisy**, or cardiovascular problems. It is important to rule out these conditions so that important symptoms are not ignored.

Signs and Symptoms
- Pain on palpation of the costal cartilage
- Pain with deep breathing
- May persist for weeks or months

Treatment Options

People with costochondritis are advised to treat it with rest, gentle stretching, and local applications of heat.

Medications

Costochondritis is typically treated with nonsteroidal anti-inflammatory drugs.

🖐 Massage Considerations

Risks

- Rule out other causes of chest pain that may contraindicate massage.
- Avoid irritating hypersensitive areas.

Benefits

- Massage within pain tolerance may help restore function.
- Lymphatic techniques may help resolve inflammation.

crabs: see lice

cramps: see dysmenorrhea, spasms/cramps

CREST syndrome: see scleroderma

Crohn disease

Crohn disease is a progressive inflammatory disorder that can affect any part of the gastrointestinal (GI) tract, from the mouth to the anus. It appears in disconnected, unpredictable patches. Eventually, these ulcers can cause accumulations of scar tissue that partially block the intestine, or they can stimulate the development of perforations or fistulas (abnormal connecting tubes from the colon to other organs).

Crohn disease can lead to **peritonitis**, can cause abscesses to form in the GI tract or around the anus, and can cause intestinal hemorrhage if the ulcers erode into blood vessels. If fistulae form into the bladder, leaking fecal material can cause **urinary tract infections**. Chronic irritation to the epithelial cells in the GI tract also increases the risk of developing **colorectal cancer**.

Along with **ulcerative colitis**, Crohn disease is classified as an inflammatory bowel disease. Although the two disorders share many common patterns, they are etiologically different.

Crohn disease has been linked to problems outside the GI tract as well. It can cause inflammation at the bile duct, leading to **cirrhosis** and **jaundice**. It has been linked to acute inflammation affecting the liver, eyes, and joints. It can cause an outbreak of ulcers called aphthae in the mouth and characteristic lesions on the skin as well; these open sores most often appear around the ankles and lower legs.

Signs and Symptoms

- Cycles of flare and remission
- Abdominal pain, cramping, diarrhea, bloating
- Anal fissures
- Weight loss, signs of malnutrition
- Joint pain
- Ulcers in the mouth and throat
- Ulcerations on the legs

Treatment Options

Many Crohn disease patients eventually have surgery to remove affected sections of intestine, but this surgery is not curative; new patches of inflamed tissue may arise in other places, which then requires further surgery.

Crohn disease patients have to be extraordinarily careful about their diet, especially during flare-ups. In extreme cases, the patient may take in all nutrients by an intravenous line to give the whole system a break from the stress of digesting food.

Medications

Crohn disease treatment includes steroidal anti-inflammatory drugs and immunosuppressant drugs.

Massage Considerations

Risks
- Avoid rigorous massage during flare.
- A client's surgical history may influence choices about massage.

Benefits
- Energetic or reflexive techniques may be welcome during Crohn disease flare, as long as the skin is healthy.
- During remission, clients with Crohn disease can receive any massage that is comfortable.

Creutzfeldt-Jakob disease

Creutzfeldt-Jakob disease (CJD) is a brain disease involving proteins called prions. CJD may be contracted in several ways. It can be spread through contaminated surgical equipment. Some cases are hereditary, whereas other cases seem to be spontaneous mutations within the brain. Other cases are the result of eating beef infected with bovine spongiform encephalopathy ("mad cow disease").

Prions destroy material in the brain, leading to a characteristic spongy appearance and many variable neurologic symptoms. It takes 15 to 20 months for the infection to incubate and symptoms to develop, but after they begin, degeneration happens very quickly.

The dementia of CJD has some similarities to **Alzheimer disease,** but its onset is usually in young to middle adulthood, and the muscle twitches that are common to CJD are not usually part of the Alzheimer disease picture.

Signs and Symptoms
- Silent in the early stages
- Myoclonus: uncontrolled spasmodic contractions of the arm and leg muscles
- Loss of cognition
- Personality changes
- Rapidly progressive dementia

Treatment Options

CJD has no cure. Symptoms are treated with medication.

Medications

CJD is treated palliatively with analgesics and anticonvulsives to limit myoclonus.

Massage Considerations

Risks
- Clients with advanced CJD may not be able to communicate verbally; be sensitive to nonverbal signals.

Benefits
- Massage has no specific benefits for clients with CJD, although it may improve their general quality of life.

Cushing syndrome

Cushing syndrome is a condition in which too much cortisol is produced in the adrenal cortex.

Cushing syndrome is associated with several other disorders. It is a complication of long-term steroid use, so it is often seen with organ transplant recipients, people with autoimmune diseases, and others who may have to take steroidal anti-inflammatory drugs for a prolonged time.

Benign and malignant tumors of the pituitary or adrenal gland and **lung cancer** may increase cortisol secretion, either by affecting the adrenal glands directly or by secreting high levels of adrenocorticotropic hormone. When Cushing syndrome is related to a pituitary tumor, **hypothyroidism** may also be involved.

Signs and Symptoms
- Glucose intolerance, risk of type 2 diabetes mellitus
- Fluid retention, hypertension
- Fat deposits around the face and shoulders
- Skin becomes thin and delicate; poor wound healing
- Stretch marks
- Weakness in the muscles of the shoulders and hips
- Osteoporosis
- Depressed immunity

Treatment Options
Cushing syndrome is treated according to the underlying cause. If it can be traced to an operable tumor, surgery is performed to remove it. Medications to suppress adrenal cortex secretions are not often successful.

Medications
Medications for Cushing syndrome depend on the underlying cause.

 Massage Considerations

Risks
- Complications, including hypertension, osteoporosis, delicate skin, and easy bruising, may make rigorous Swedish massage impractical.
- Underlying causes of Cushing syndrome must be understood to make fully informed decisions about bodywork.

Benefits
- Very gentle energetic or reflexive techniques can offer relaxation benefits for Cushing syndrome patients without challenging their homeostatic processes.

cystic fibrosis

Cystic fibrosis (CF) arises from a genetic anomaly that makes exocrine secretions dangerously viscous and sticky. This is particularly true for mucus, pancreatic enzymes, bile, and other digestive and reproductive secretions.

When these secretions don't function correctly, a number of problems ensue including dangerous gastrointestinal (GI) obstructions, poor absorption of nutrients, and liver congestion. CF that affects the GI tract may lead to adhesions and intestinal obstructions along with poor absorption of nutrients. Thickening of the bile may lead to **cirrhosis** or **gallstones**.

In the lungs, CF can lead to chronic pulmonary infections (**pneumonia**) from stagnant, sticky mucus that clings to bronchioles instead of moving up the respiratory tract for normal expulsion. Other complications may include **bronchitis, bronchiectasis**, and right-sided **heart failure** as the heart tries to push blood through a pulmonary circuit that is resistant.

Males with CF are usually sterile; their epididymal secretions are too viscous to allow the passage of sperm.

Signs and Symptoms
- Abdominal pain, failure to thrive
- Greasy, foul-smelling stool
- Chronic respiratory tract infections
- Sinus polyps
- Clubbing (rounding and broadening) of the fingertips

Treatment Options

CF has no cure, so treatment focuses on improving lung health and function. Physical therapy is often used to mechanically loosen deposits of mucus in the lungs.

Medications

CF is treated with bronchodilators, anti-inflammatory drugs, and medication to soften the mucus. Bacterial respiratory infections are aggressively treated with antibiotics.

✋ Massage Considerations

Risks
- Clients with CF are extremely vulnerable to respiratory infections.
- Avoid deep abdominal work if the client has GI problems.

Benefits
- Massage with physical therapy may help loosen mucus deposits.
- Massage won't change the course of CF but may help with resilience and quality of life.

cystitis: see urinary tract infection

cytomegalovirus infection

Cytomegalovirus (CMV) is one of the herpes family of viruses. Many adults test positive for exposure to this pathogen, but most people never have significant symptoms related to CMV infection. Similar to other herpes viruses, CMV stays in the body forever, although the risk of its return as an active infection is low for most people with healthy immune systems.

Acute CMV infections are always associated with underlying disorders that compromise immune system function. Transplant recipients and people with **leukemia, lymphoma,** and **AIDS** are all at risk for this situation.

Signs and Symptoms

- Often silent
- In immunocompromised people: inflammation of the colon, retina, salivary glands, lungs, kidneys, and liver
- High risk of damage to the fetus if a pregnant woman has active CMV

Treatment Options

Mild CMV infections in healthy people are simply treated with rest and reduced activity.

Medications

Acute infections in high-risk populations are treated with antiviral medications.

✋ Massage Considerations

Risks

- Acute symptoms appear in immunocompromised people; rigorous circulatory work is inappropriate in these situations.

Benefits

- Energetic or reflexive techniques may help support a compromised immune system for people undergoing active CMV infections.
- Clients who have recovered from CMV infections can enjoy the same benefits from massage as the rest of the population.

Practitioner Advice

- Most adults have a history of exposure to CMV; communicability is not an important issue for this population.
- If a therapist is pregnant and has never been exposed to CMV, she may wish to avoid contact with clients who have active CMV infections.

D

decubitus ulcers

This condition, which is also known as bedsores, pressure sores, and trophic ulcers, is a problem stemming from inadequate blood flow to the skin that stretches over bony or otherwise prominent areas. It almost always occurs in an area that has constant contact with a surface such as a backboard, a bed, a wheelchair, a cast, or a splint.

Left unchecked, a decubitus ulcer can destroy the epidermis, the dermis, and the superficial fascia, eroding tissues down to the bone. The heels, buttocks, sacrum, and elbows are the most common places for bedsores to appear.

Decubitus ulcers come about because of an injury or disorder that leads to immobilization. Secondary infection of the open wound can lead to **gangrene**, **septicemia**, and death.

Signs and Symptoms
- Early: change in skin temperature, reddish or purplish color, pain, itching
- Later: purple color, necrosis, possibility of infection

Treatment Options

Treatment for pressure sores depends on their stage and location. Topical antibiotics and dressings can be effective for some lesions; bigger, more advanced sores may require debridement and plastic surgery.

Decubitus ulcers are much more expensive to treat than to prevent, so many efforts are made with massage, movement, and changing the position of immobilized patients to prevent the ulcers before they start.

Medications

Decubitus ulcers may be treated with topical or oral antibiotics

Massage Considerations

Risks
- Decubitus ulcers carry a high risk of infection, even around the edges of the lesion.

Benefits
- Massage can help prevent decubitus ulcers.
- Clients who have healed decubitus ulcers can enjoy the same benefits from massage as the rest of the population.

deep vein thrombosis: see thrombophlebitis/ deep vein thrombosis

degenerative joint disease: see osteoarthritis, spondylosis

dementia: see Alzheimer disease, Creutzfeldt-Jakob disease, Lewy body disease, Pick disease

depression

Depression is a central nervous system disorder involving a genetic predisposition and neurochemical changes, often with a triggering event, that results in a person's losing the ability to enjoy life. Depression can be a long-lasting, self-propagating, and ultimately debilitating disease.

The most obvious and most serious complication of depression is suicide. In addition to suicide risk, a history of depression has a statistical correlation to several other conditions, notably **heart attack, stroke,** and other forms of cardiovascular disease.

Many distinct types of depression have been identified and described. Six of them are relatively common:

- Major depressive disorder involves severe symptoms with a specific onset for periods longer than 2 weeks. Left untreated, episodes of major depression may last from 6 to 18 months. People with a history of major depressive disorder are at increased risk for repeat episodes.
- Adjustment disorder is depression related to a specific event that triggers an emotional response with symptoms outlasting what might be considered a normal recovery or grieving period.
- Dysthymia involves less severe symptoms but has a duration of months or years.
- Bipolar disease is also called manic depression. It is marked by mood swings from major depression to mania (a state defined by heightened energy, elation, irritability, racing thoughts, increased sex drive, decreased inhibitions, and unrealistic or grandiose notions).
- Seasonal affective disorder (SAD) is related to inadequate exposure to sunlight. Incidence in the general population increases according to the distance from the equator.
- Postpartum depression occurs in women after giving birth. Women with postpartum depression have all the symptoms of major depression along with the deep-rooted fear of having harm come or of actually doing harm to the baby.

Signs and Symptoms

- Persistent sad or empty feelings
- Lack of enjoyment in activities
- Sense of guilt or disappointment with oneself
- Sense of hopelessness
- Irritability
- Change in sleeping habits
- Poor concentration
- Change in eating habits
- Physical pain: muscle aches, headaches, indigestion
- Suicidal thoughts or actions

Treatment Options

Most types of depression are treatable. A combination of medical intervention and various types of psychotherapy seems to be the most effective way to treat most types of depression.

Other therapies for depression may include light therapy, electroconvulsive therapy, St. John's Wort, and others.

Medications

Antidepressants include several classes of drugs, including selective serotonin reuptake inhibitors (SSRIs), serotonin norepinephrine reuptake inhibitors (SNRIs), and tricyclic antidepressants (TCAs). Patients may take any combination of these drugs to manage their disease.

Massage Considerations

Risks
- Massage has no specific risks for depression.

Benefits
- Massage improves stress response, which is often inefficient with depression.
- Massage promotes relaxation and a feeling of well-being; this is especially valuable for people with depression.

Practitioner Advice
- A depressive client may wish to change his or her medication and may enlist the therapist in that decision, but it is important that this decision be made with the primary care provider.

De Quervain tenosynovitis: see tenosynovitis

dermatitis/eczema

Dermatitis is an umbrella term for skin inflammation of the skin that is not caused by infection. Two main types of dermatitis are contact dermatitis and atopic dermatitis.

Contact dermatitis is skin inflammation caused by an external irritation or allergen. Atopic dermatitis, or eczema, is a systemic **allergic reaction** that is expressed in the skin.

People with dermatitis are particularly susceptible to secondary infection because their skin may be scratched or blistered. **Impetigo**, **herpes simplex**, and **fungal infections** are all common complications for dermatitis and eczema patients.

Signs and Symptoms

Symptoms of dermatitis or eczema depend on what subtype of disorder is present.
- Contact dermatitis: red, itching, irritated skin at site of contact with allergen (e.g., nickel, latex) or irritant (e.g., harsh cleansers)
- Atopic dermatitis (eczema): red, itching skin, often at the joints
- Dyshidrosis: intensely itchy, weepy blisters on the palms and soles
- Nummular eczema: small, circular, itchy lesions on the legs and buttocks
- Seborrheic eczema: yellowish, oily, peeling skin around the scalp and face

Treatment Options

Self-help measures for people with contact dermatitis and eczema begin with identifying and avoiding irritating substances. Good skin care with a nonirritating emollient is important.

Medications

People with dermatitis or eczema may use corticosteroid cream, which suppresses itching but may cause skin damage. Other options include antihistamines, topical immunomodulators, and oral steroids.

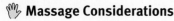 **Massage Considerations**

Risks
- Acutely inflamed areas contraindicate massage.
- Skin that is compromised by bleeding, blisters, or other openings contraindicates massage.
- Avoid using lubricants with allergenic ingredients.

Benefits
- Areas that are dry and flaky but not acutely inflamed may benefit from the application of a hypoallergenic lubricant.
- Clients with dermatitis or eczema but no current symptoms can enjoy the same benefits from massage as the rest of the population.

---

diabetes insipidus

Diabetes insipidus is a disorder involving damage to the pituitary gland or kidneys, leading to excessive urination and thirst. Damage to the pituitary leads to insufficient secretion of antidiuretic hormone (ADH). This can occur as a complication of radiation or as part of a head wound, a tumor, or an infection. A genetic form also exists. The result of insufficient ADH production is that a person with diabetes insipidus may urinate up to 20 L every 24 hours.

Diabetes insipidus is not a type of diabetes mellitus; the only thing these conditions have in common is frequent urination. Diabetes insipidus is sometimes a complication of a pituitary tumor, a **traumatic brain injury**, or a central nervous system infection, such as **encephalitis** or **meningitis**.

Signs and Symptoms
- Frequent urination
- Unquenchable thirst
- Headaches
- Dry skin
- Constipation

Treatment Options
If this condition is severe enough to cause dehydration, synthetic ADH may be prescribed until (if ever) the pituitary begins to produce this hormone again. Patients are counseled to follow a low-salt diet. If the disorder has been caused by a pituitary tumor, surgery is necessary to remove it.

Medications
Clients with diabetes insipidus may be treated with synthetic ADH.

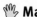 **Massage Considerations**

Risks
- Avoid rigorous circulatory massage for clients who have difficulty managing body fluids.
- Clients with diabetes insipidus may not be comfortable lying on a table for a full hour; they may need shorter sessions to accommodate for their needs.

Benefits
- Clients with successfully treated diabetes insipidus can enjoy the same benefits from massage as the rest of the population.

diabetes mellitus

Diabetes mellitus involves poor insulin production, insulin resistance, or both. The result is hyperglycemia and muscle cells that cannot use sugar as a primary fuel source.

Type 1 diabetes is an autoimmune disorder. In this situation, the immune system attacks insulin-producing cells in the pancreas. The destruction of these cells leads to a lifelong deficiency in insulin.

Type 2 diabetes is much more common. It involves insufficient secretion of insulin, insulin resistance, or both.

Gestational diabetes is transient and occurs during **pregnancy**. This condition can cause birth defects in the fetus and a high risk of cesarean section surgeries. Women who have gestational diabetes and their children also have an increased risk of developing type 2 diabetes later in life.

Secondary diabetes may develop with damage or trauma to the pancreas or as a symptom of some other endocrine disorder such as **acromegaly** or **Cushing syndrome**.

The complications of diabetes mellitus include vision loss with **cataracts**, cardiovascular disease, skin ulcers, **renal failure**, and **peripheral neuropathy**. The onset of some of these complications may lead a person to be diagnosed with the condition. People with diabetes also have a high incidence of **candidiasis**, gingivitis, and **urinary tract infections**. A consequence of supplementing insulin but not eating enough sugar may be a rapid decrease in blood glucose, which is called **hypoglycemia**.

Signs and Symptoms
- Early: excessive thirst, excessive hunger, and frequent urination
- Late: heart disease, kidney disease, vision loss, and skin damage
- Ketoacidosis: related to hyperglycemia and metabolism of proteins and fats
- Hyperosmolality: similar to ketoacidosis; seen in patients with type 2 diabetes
- Insulin shock: hypoglycemia related to the use of insulin with insufficient food intake

Treatment Options

Type 1 diabetes is treated with insulin supplementation, diet, and exercise.

Type 2 diabetes is first addressed with changes in diet and exercise, along with hypoglycemic agents. Some patients with type 2 diabetes are treated with insulin supplementation as well. The high risk of cardiovascular disease for diabetes patients requires that this disease be managed carefully and conscientiously.

If the kidneys experience extensive damage, dialysis may be recommended. Dialysis of any kind is usually a stop-gap measure while a person is waiting for a kidney to become available for transplant.

Medications

Type 1 diabetes is treated with insulin supplementation.

Type 2 diabetes may be treated with medications that improve insulin uptake, inhibit the liver's release of glycogen, or both. Some type 2 diabetes patients are treated with insulin supplementation as well.

Massage Considerations

Risks
- Many complications of diabetes contraindicate massage; consult with the health care team for best results.

- Avoid insulin injection and pump attachment sites.
- Massage may rapidly decrease blood glucose; time sessions to occur when insulin is not at the peak of activity and have a sugar-based snack available for diabetic clients who might feel hypoglycemic after a massage.

Benefits

- Diabetic clients who have healthy, responsive tissue with good blood supply can enjoy the same benefits from massage as the rest of the population.

disc disease

Disc disease is identified when the intervertebral discs extend beyond their normal borders. This can occur if the soft nucleus pulposus bulges or if the brittle annulus fibrosis cracks. If this puts pressure on the spinal cord or spinal nerve roots, pain will be present. Pain is also generated by the inflammatory reaction that accompanies disc damage.

Discs that cause pain usually bulge posterolaterally. Occasionally, a disc bulges directly posteriorly, which puts pressure on the spinal cord rather than nerve roots. This is a very serious situation that can lead to permanent damage. In the lumbar spine, this is called cauda equina syndrome.

Discs may be injured as part of a **whiplash** incident or low back injury, but similar symptoms can be created if nearby ligaments are injured. This is an important distinction because disc lesions are out the reach of bodyworkers but spinal ligaments are not. The primary distinctions are that ligament injuries don't cause complete numbness or specific muscle weakness.

Signs and Symptoms

- Nerve pain that is exacerbated with movement or compression forces
- Local and radicular pain
- Weakness in the muscles supplied by a damaged nerve root
- Paresthesia, reduced sensation, numbness

Treatment Options

Chiropractors and osteopaths work to correct bony alignment to create a maximum of space for the bulging disc to retreat. Other interventions include chemonucleolysis (the injection of protein-dissolving enzymes into the area of the protrusion), transcutaneous diskectomy (the removal of disc material through a tiny incision), or open surgery to remove the posterior arch of the vertebra.

Physical therapy and training in correct posture and body mechanics are often recommended for people recovering from disc problems.

Medications

Drugs for herniated discs include muscle relaxants and painkillers. Cortisone is sometimes injected into the area.

Massage Considerations

Risks

- Avoid techniques and positions that exacerbate symptoms.
- Clients with damaged discs may need extensive bolstering or other adjustments to be comfortable on the table.

Benefits
- Disc disease symptoms may be relieved with techniques that focus on elongating the affected part of the spine.
- Massage can address secondary muscle spasms that are common with disc disease.

discoid lupus: see lupus

dislocations

When the bones in a joint are separated so that they no longer articulate, the joint is said to be dislocated. This situation can be brought about by trauma, congenital weakness of the ligaments, or other diseases that weaken joint structures. The glenohumeral joint and fingers are the most common sites of dislocations.

A person with a permanently unstable joint is likely to develop trigger points connected to **myofascial pain syndrome** in the muscles that surround that joint. Unstable joints also carry a risk for developing **osteoarthritis** and further injury.

Signs and Symptoms
- Swelling or discoloration of the affected joint
- Severe pain at the site of injury
- Loss of function of the affected joint
- Later: laxity or instability of the affected joint

Treatment Options

Acute dislocations must be reduced within a few minutes of the trauma to avoid muscle spasms. Then the joint is splinted until it is capable of weight-bearing stress. Physical therapy to strengthen and rebuild muscles around the joint follows.

Surgery to tighten damaged structures is sometimes recommended when ligaments are too lax to support a joint.

Proliferant injections are designed to stimulate the growth of new collagen fibers that, with appropriate stretching and exercise, will lie down in alignment with the original fibers. This procedure can tighten stretched-out ligaments, thus reducing the chance of future injury.

Medications

Acute dislocations may be treated with anti-inflammatory drugs, analgesics, and muscle relaxants.

Massage Considerations

Risks
- Acute dislocations contraindicate massage.
- A joint with a history of dislocation (especially the shoulder) may dislocate again without trauma; take care to position the client and move the affected joint with caution to prevent this from happening.

Benefits
- Subacute injuries may benefit from massage to address muscular splinting and scar tissue.
- Clients with a history of dislocation and no current symptoms can enjoy the same benefits from massage as the rest of the population.

diverticular disease

Diverticular disease is a condition of the colon in which the inner layers of the colon bulge through the outer muscular layer to form a small sack or diverticulum. These bulges may become infected, leading to diverticulitis.

Most diverticulae form in the sigmoid flexure or descending colon, but they have also been seen throughout the alimentary canal all the way up to the esophagus. They can range from about the size of a kernel of corn to the size of a walnut or even larger.

Complications of diverticulitis are rare but they can be serious. They can include bleeding, abscesses, perforation of the colon, blockage of the colon, and the formation of fistulae (passageways that allow fecal matter to leave the colon and enter another hollow organ, such as the small intestine, urinary bladder, or uterus).

Signs and Symptoms

- May be silent
- If infection is present: nausea, fever, cramping, pain

Treatment Options

Although diverticulae are not reversible, further protrusions can be prevented with changes toward a higher fiber diet and exercise.

Treatment for diverticulitis starts with antibiotics and a strictly controlled diet. If substantial tissue damage has occurred, including a bowel obstruction, uncontrolled bleeding, perforation, large abscesses, or fistulae, surgery may be performed to resolve the situation.

Medications

Clients with diverticular disease may use fiber supplements or laxatives to help the colon work more efficiently. Acute diverticulitis may be treated with antibiotics and antispasmodics.

✋ Massage Considerations

Risks

- If a client has been diagnosed with diverticular disease, conduct deep abdominal work with caution.
- Acute infection (diverticulitis) contraindicates massage.

Benefits

- Bodywork may enhance parasympathetic effects and improve the efficiency of the digestive system.

dizziness: see vertigo

double-crush syndrome

Double-crush syndrome is a disorder in which a peripheral nerve is irritated at multiple sites. Research indicates that a lesion at the proximal end of a nerve can increase the chance for other entrapments to occur. The reasons for this are not clear, but experts suggest that a combination of a disturbance in axonal flow and changes in the architecture of involved neurofilaments can be contributing factors.

Double-crush syndrome may be an issue with several nerve impingement diagnoses, including **carpal tunnel syndrome,** foot drop, tarsal tunnel syndrome, and **thoracic outlet syndrome.**

Signs and Symptoms

- Sharp, shooting, electrical pain in a radicular pattern
- Paresthesia, reduced sensation, numbness
- Weakness and atrophy in the muscles supplied by the affected nerve

Treatment Options

Double-crush syndrome is most successfully treated by identifying all the places that a nerve might be trapped or irritated and then working to reduce that irritation. In brachial plexus nerves, this can involve adjustments in neck alignment as well as treating entrapment at the thoracic outlet, cubital fossa, and carpal tunnel. In the lumbosacral plexus, a similar pattern examines the spine and other possible entrapment sites all the way to the ankle.

It is important to be precise about where nerves are compressed because this information influences treatment options. Carpal tunnel surgery, for instance, tends to have a poorer outcome when double-crush syndrome is identified as a factor in median nerve entrapment.

Medications

Double-crush syndrome is not treated with medication other than to control pain and inflammation.

 ## Massage Considerations

Risks

- It is possible that rigorous deep massage at the site of a nerve entrapment could exacerbate symptoms of double-crush syndrome.

Benefits

- Carefully and sensitively applied massage can help reduce nerve irritation where soft tissues are involved.

Down syndrome

Down syndrome, or trisomy 21, is a birth defect in which a person has three copies of chromosome 21 instead of two. It is a common cause of mental disability and other problems.

Down syndrome is frequently accompanied by other problems, notably congenital weakness of cardiac valves, **hypo-** or **hyperthyroidism,** bowel obstructions, a higher than average risk of **leukemia,** and early onset of **Alzheimer** disease. Alzheimer plaques are found in 100% of the brains of people with Down syndrome older than 20 years of age.

Signs and Symptoms

- Upward-sloping eyes with epicanthic folds
- Small, low-set ears
- Enlarged tongue
- Short, broad hands with a single palmar crease
- Cognitive disability

Treatment Options

Down syndrome can be identified early in pregnancy but not prevented. Children with Down syndrome need to be monitored for heart, thyroid, and gastrointestinal health, but as long as these issues are controlled, they may be as active as any other person.

Down syndrome patients may learn to be somewhat independent, but most require some level of assisted living.

Medications

Medications for people with Down syndrome depend on which complications are present.

 Massage Considerations

Risks
- Clients with Down syndrome have a high risk for cardiovascular weakness, which may contraindicate rigorous massage.

Benefits
- Massage may be beneficial if bodywork is within the challenges of the client's activities of daily living.

drug abuse: see chemical dependency

drug-induced lupus: see lupus

Duchenne muscular dystrophy: see muscular dystrophy

Dupuytren contracture

This condition, also called palmar fasciitis, is an idiopathic thickening and shrinking of the palmar fascia that limits the movement of the fingers.

Signs and Symptoms
- May be mildly painful
- Fibrous bumps on the palmar surface of hands
- In extreme cases, severely bent, unusable fingers
- Usually affects the ring and little fingers most severely
- Bilateral in about 50% of cases

Treatment Options

If this condition is left untreated, the connective tissue may strangle the muscles and nerves until the affected fingers eventually lose all function.

Surgery for Dupuytren contracture is generally not recommended until the fingers become too stiff to move. The surgery involves making several zig-zag cuts in the palm to release the fascia, followed by skin grafts, physical therapy, and massage to limit the growth of scar tissue. Even when surgery is successful, Dupuytren contracture recurs in about one third of all cases.

Medications

Dupuytren contracture may be treated with cortisone or collagenase injections.

 ## Massage Considerations

Risks

- Avoid deep work in any numb areas.

Benefits

- Massage may help mobilize the fascia and slow the progress of Dupuytren contracture.
- Massage may be useful after surgery to limit scar tissue and promote mobility.

dysmenorrhea

Dysmenorrhea is a technical term for painful menstrual periods. Primary dysmenorrhea is usually attributable to some combination of three contributing factors: prostaglandin secretion that exacerbates inflammation, the pain-spasm cycle, and ligament irritation as the uterus tugs on the uterine ligament and the broad ligament.

Secondary dysmenorrhea is a complication of some other pelvic disorder. Some of the most common situations that cause menstrual pain include **pelvic inflammatory disease, fibroid tumors, endometriosis, ovarian cysts,** and the use of an intrauterine birth control device. Pelvic adhesions, deposits of scar tissue from previous surgeries, or trauma may also contribute to menstrual pain.

Signs and Symptoms

- A dull ache in the abdomen, low back, and groin during menstruation
- Sharp pain and cramping in the abdomen
- Headache, nausea, vomiting
- Constipation, diarrhea

Treatment Options

The first step in treating dysmenorrhea is to rule out underlying pathologies such as endometriosis and fibroid tumors.

A thorough nutritional analysis may reveal strategies for dealing with menstrual pain; this is a useful course for many women, but no specific nutritional supplements have been found to alleviate all cases of dysmenorrhea. Exercises and stretches can also relieve the pain caused by the irritated uterine ligament.

Medications

For most cases of dysmenorrhea, painkillers such as ibuprofen and naproxen work by inhibiting the secretion of prostaglandins.

For more serious situations low-dose birth control pills prohibit ovulation, which in turn prohibits the secretion of prostaglandins in the uterus.

 ## Massage Considerations

Risks

- Avoid deep abdominal massage for women experiencing menstrual pain.

Benefits
- Women with menstrual pain can benefit from the relaxation and pain relief that massage offers.
- Massage that focuses on the low back and sacrum can often result in reflexive relaxation of the uterus.

dyshidrosis: see dermatitis/eczema

dysphonia: see dystonia

dysthymia: see depression

dystonia

Dystonia is a group of movement disorders that result in involuntary and sometimes painful contractions of the skeletal muscles. The action of various neurotransmitters on the movement control centers in the basal ganglia is dysfunctional in these patients. Dystonia ranges in scope from affecting only one isolated muscle or area to affecting the whole body.

Dystonia is frequently discussed as individual syndromes, depending on which part of the body is affected.
- Torsion dystonia is the most severe form of the condition. This genetic disorder is systemic and can be debilitating.
- Cranial dystonia affects the muscles of the head, face, and neck.
- Blepharospasm dystonia affects the orbicularis oculi muscles, causing uncontrolled blinking. This condition may become severe enough to cause functional blindness, although no damage to the eyes themselves occurs.
- Cervical dystonia is a synonym for spasmodic torticollis.
- Laryngeal dystonia, also called dysphonia, affects the muscles of speech and sound.
- Writer's cramp is a type of focal dystonia that affects the hand and forearm muscles. It is also called musician's cramp or typist's cramp.
- Dopa-responsive dystonia is a type that affects children. It is easily misdiagnosed as cerebral palsy (CP), but it responds to drug treatment in ways that CP does not.

Signs and Symptoms

The primary symptom of dystonia is an involuntary and sometimes painful contraction of the skeletal muscles. Contractions may be transitory or persistent. The longer a person has had dystonia, the more severe and tenacious the spasms become, but this condition does not tend to spread to other muscles or areas of the body.

Treatment Options

Treatment for dystonia depends on the type and severity of the dysfunction. If medications are unsuccessful, surgery is performed to cut the dysfunctional motor nerves, but this is considered a "last-ditch" option.

Medications

Medications that mimic or restore dysfunctional neurotransmitters are successful for some patients. Sedatives to limit involuntary contractions are used, as well as injections of botulinum toxin to temporarily paralyze the affected muscles.

Massage Considerations

Risks
- Touch or passive stretching may exacerbate dystonia symptoms, so it should be avoided when possible.
- Massage has no other specific risks for clients with dystonia.

Benefits
- Massage can improve recovery from fatigue.
- Massage may improve the mobility of fascial restrictions.
- Massage may improve proprioceptive function to reduce hypertonicity.

earache: see otitis

eating disorders

Eating disorders include a variety of destructive eating habits. They often begin as an emotional coping mechanism but become a serious impairment to health. Women with eating disorders outnumber men by a wide margin.

- Anorexia nervosa is the use of any combination of fasting, severely restricted eating, and compensatory activities to drastically reduce the number of calories that enter the digestive system. In restrictive anorexia, a person doesn't take in enough calories to sustain him or her. In purge-type anorexia, the person's calorie intake may be adequate for sustenance, but it is negated by compensatory activities, including vomiting; the use of laxatives, diuretics, or enemas; and excessive exercise.
- Bulimia nervosa involves normal or higher-than-normal calorie consumption followed by compensatory activities to prevent the absorption of calories.
- Binge eating involves the consumption of large amounts of food for reasons other than hunger. Eating is not followed by compensatory activity, leading to weight gain.

    Many eating disorder patients struggle with **depression, sleep disorders**, and **anxiety disorders**, especially obsessive–compulsive disorder. In addition, heart problems, **osteoporosis**, infertility, tooth damage, esophageal erosions, and electrolyte imbalances are seen with anorexia and bulimia. Binge eaters are at risk for type 2 **diabetes** and **osteoarthritis**.

Signs and Symptoms
- Anorexia: thinness (often hidden by baggy clothes); lanugo (the growth of fine, downy body hair)
- Bulimia: no obvious signs, but the complications are potentially dangerous
- Binge eating: inability to control eating; obvious weight gain

Treatment Options
Treatment for eating disorders is most successful when the emphasis is not on gaining or losing weight but on resolving the issues that contribute to the behaviors in the first place.

Research revealing neurotransmitter imbalances in the brains of many eating disorder patients has opened the door to medications that may help.

Medications

Eating disorders may be treated with any combination of antidepressants and antianxiety medications.

Massage Considerations

Risks

- Complications of eating disorders include osteoporosis, irregular heart beat, and electrolyte imbalances; massage must be adjusted accordingly.

Benefits

- Massage is nonjudgmental, affirmative touch for a person who may not have positive feelings about his or her body.
- Clients who have recovered from eating disorders with no long-term consequences can enjoy the same benefits from massage as the rest of the population.

Practitioner Advice

- Our culture puts a high value on physical attractiveness, including being thin. People who feel isolated in this context sometimes compensate by overeating, or "hugging their inner skin." Massage, which stimulates the outer skin so positively, can be a wonderful substitute for overeating behaviors.

eclampsia: see pregnancy-induced hypertension

ectopic pregnancy: see pregnancy

eczema: see dermatitis/eczema

---

edema

Edema is the accumulation of excessive fluid between cells, usually in association with inflammation or poor circulation. It isn't generally noticeable until the interstitial fluid volume is about 30% above normal.

Edema can have several causes; most of them are a combination of chemical and mechanical factors. Mechanical factors may involve a weakened heart or a physical obstruction to lymph or venous flow. Chemical causes of edema are usually related to the accumulation of proteins in the interstitial fluid, which causes the area to retain water. **Lymphedema** is an associated condition.

Signs and Symptoms

- Congested, boggy tissue
- May be local or systemic, depending on the cause
- Affected area is usually soft; may become indurated with time

Treatment Options

Edema is treated according to its underlying cause.

Medications

Depending on the cause, edema may be treated with anti-inflammatory drugs, diuretics, or other drugs to control water retention.

 Massage Considerations

Risks

- Systemic edema, especially with pitting, shows that the circulatory or lymph systems are impaired; this contraindicates rigorous circulatory massage.
- Be cautious about the risk of edema caused by thrombophlebitis.

Benefits

- Edema related to acute musculoskeletal injury may benefit from lymphatic work that reduces local fluid retention.
- Edema related to subacute or postacute musculoskeletal injury may benefit from a variety of massage modalities to reduce inflammation and speed healing.

Ehlers-Danlos syndrome

Ehlers-Danlos syndrome (EDS) is a group of genetic disorders that affect the formation of connective tissue proteins, including collagen, elastin, and other components of the extracellular matrix.

EDS occurs on a continuum of severity, depending on the specific genetic anomaly. Mild cases involve skin that is stretchy, delicate, and prone to bruising. More extreme cases involve easily dislocated joints, ligament laxity, a high risk of mitral valve prolapse, and extreme **postural deviations**.

Signs and Symptoms

- Vary, depending on subtype
- Stretchy, delicate skin
- Poor wound healing
- Ligament laxity
- Risk of aneurysm
- Postural deviations

Treatment Options

EDS is treated according to the symptoms. Patients are educated to preserve their joint function and are discouraged from overstretching their joints. Skin wounds are usually treated with bandages and wound glue rather than sutures. Other accommodations for connective tissue weakness are made as needed, but individual requirements may vary.

Medications

If a patient is at risk for mitral valve problems, prophylactic antibiotics may be prescribed to prevent infection of the endocardium. Some EDS patients may be treated with high doses of vitamin C to boost their connective tissue strength and health.

 Massage Considerations

Risks

- Any massage or bodywork for a client with EDS must be adapted to meet skin and connective tissue fragility issues.

- Passive stretching or range of motion exercises must be conservative for EDS patients.
- Clients with EDS have a higher than average risk for blood vessel fragility; this may make rigorous circulatory massage inappropriate.

Benefits
- Massage that stays within the limitations of a client's activity levels can be supportive and may contribute to an improved quality of life.

ehrlichiosis

Ehrlichiosis is an infection with a tick-borne leukocytic rickettsia called *Ehrlichia sennetsu*. It can resemble other tick-borne infections, which sometimes makes accurate identification and treatment difficult. It is sometimes misdiagnosed as babesiosis, **Lyme disease**, or **Rocky Mountain spotted fever**.

Signs and Symptoms
- Tick bite
- Fever, chills
- Diarrhea
- Headache

Treatment Options

Ehrlichiosis is treated with medication.

Medications

Antibiotics are effective for ehrlichiosis infections.

Massage Considerations

Risks
- Acute infection contraindicates massage.

Benefits
- Clients who have had ehrlichiosis and have fully recovered can enjoy the same benefits from massage as the rest of the population.

embolism, thrombus

An embolism is a traveling clot or collection of debris, and a thrombus is a lodged clot that accumulates onsite. Where an embolism lands depends on whether it formed on the venous or arterial side of the systemic circuit.

When clots form on the venous side of the systemic circuit, they may fragment and travel to the lungs; this is a pulmonary embolism. When clots or other debris collect on the arterial side of the systemic circuit, they may grow to completely occlude the artery (thrombosis), or they may break up and travel further into the arterial system (arterial embolism). The brain, heart, kidneys, and legs are statistically the most common sites for arterial emboli to lodge.

Pulmonary embolism is usually related to **thrombophlebitis** or **deep vein thrombosis** that develops as a complication of surgery or trauma.

Clots that grow in the carotid artery contribute to **carotid artery disease**. Arterial emboli may lead to progressive **renal failure** if they collect in the kidneys, a transient ischemic attack or a **stroke** if they collect in the brain, or a **heart attack** if they obstruct the coronary artery.

Signs and Symptoms

- For pulmonary embolism: shortness of breath, chest pressure, coughing with bloody sputum
- For arterial thrombosis or embolism: depends on the site of obstruction

Treatment Options

Pulmonary emboli may be removed with a vacuum, and a vena cava filter may be inserted to prevent future lung damage. Arterial emboli are treated according to what tissue they affect.

Medications

People with a tendency toward thrombi or emboli may use anticoagulant or thrombolytic drugs to reduce the risk of heart attack, stroke, and other complications.

Massage Considerations

Risks

- Known blood clots or other obstructions contraindicate massage.
- Anticoagulant medication increases the risk of bruising.

Benefits

Reflexive or energetic techniques can offer many benefits of relaxation and pain relief without challenging the circulatory system.

Emery-Dreifuss syndrome: see muscular dystrophy

---

emphysema

Emphysema is part of a group of disorders called chronic obstructive pulmonary disease (COPD). In this condition, the alveoli become inelastic and fill up with mucus. This interferes with the alveoli's ability to exchange oxygen and carbon dioxide. The alveolar walls eventually merge with each other, forming larger sacks, called bullae.

Other conditions in the COPD group include **chronic bronchitis, bronchiectasis**, and some types of **asthma**.

Emphysema patients are extremely vulnerable to **influenza** and **pneumonia** because they have lost much of their ability to resist secondary infection. If the bullae rupture, air enters the pleural space, leading to **pneumothorax**, or lung collapse. The stress to the circulatory system if the lungs sustain this kind of damage is enormous. The right ventricle, trying to pump blood through the partially collapsed pulmonary circuit, enlarges and may develop **heart failure**. The risk of blood clots forming somewhere in the circuit is also high, which results in **pulmonary embolism**.

Signs and Symptoms

- Shortness of breath
- Dry cough, wheezing

- Fatigue, poor stamina
- Unintended weight loss
- "Barrel chest": the intercostal muscles lock into a position that holds the rib cage out as wide as possible

Treatment Options

Emphysema can be slowed or stopped, but it is irreversible. Treatment options include quitting smoking and working to dilate the bronchi and reduce the risk of secondary infection. Oxygen supplementation may be recommended during sleep or after exercise. In rare cases, a heart and lung transplant may be necessary.

Medications

People with emphysema may use bronchodilators, mucolytic drugs, and diuretics to manage fluid accumulation in the lungs. Lung infections are treated aggressively with antibiotics when appropriate.

Massage Considerations

Risks
- Emphysema increases the risk of heart failure; this systemically contraindicates massage.
- Clients with emphysema are especially vulnerable to respiratory infections; practitioners must be careful not to work when they are fighting a cold or flu.
- Some emphysema patients find that lying flat exacerbates their cough; a reclining chair or massage chair may be more comfortable.

Benefits
- Back, neck, and chest massage may be especially helpful to help reduce muscular resistance to the movement of air in and out of the body.
- Massage may help address the fatigue that many emphysema patients experience.

---

encephalitis

Encephalitis is an infection of the brain or spinal cord that is usually caused by a virus. It is a vector-borne illness, which means that although it can be spread by infected mosquitoes or other insects, it is not transmissible directly from person to person.

Encephalitis is an inflammation of the brain; **meningitis** is an infection of the meninges. Viral meningitis can be discussed alongside with encephalitis, but it is not always synonymous. West Nile disease is a subtype of encephalitis.

Signs and Symptoms

- Range from mild to severe
- Sudden onset of headache, drowsiness, fever
- Double vision
- Confusion
- Changes in personality, memory, intellect
- Convulsions
- Paralysis
- Can progress to stupor, coma

Treatment Options

Encephalitis is treated with medication, rest, and supportive therapies.

Medications

Antiviral medications are prescribed for encephalitis patients to slow viral activity along with steroids to limit inflammation and sedatives to moderate convulsions.

Massage Considerations

Risks

- Sudden onset of headache and fever contraindicates massage.
- Clients who have had encephalitis may have long-term consequences that affect sensation and motor control; these have implications for decisions about massage.

Benefits

- Clients who have recovered from encephalitis with no long-term consequences can enjoy the same benefits from massage as the rest of the population.

---

endometriosis

Endometriosis is a condition in which cells from the endometrium, the inner lining of the uterus, become implanted elsewhere in the body.

Endometrial growths usually become established on the outside of the uterus, uterine tubes, broad ligaments, ovaries, bladder, or colon. Growths continue to respond to hormonal command by growing and then contracting, but they are never shed. Instead, the body attempts to build connective tissue walls around them to isolate them.

Endometriosis is frequently identified when a woman is being treated for **dysmenorrhea**. Scar tissue deposits can create adhesions in or on the uterine tubes and ovaries, which causes infertility or ectopic **pregnancy**. The development of endometrial capillaries in these extra unintentional deposits routes blood away from where it can be useful, resulting in **anemia**. Uterine hyperplasia occasionally accompanies endometriosis; in this condition, the normal endometrial lining becomes pathologically thickened, leading to excessive bleeding and further difficulties with fertility.

Signs and Symptoms

- Painful menstrual cramps
- Infertility
- Premenstrual spotting

Treatment Options

Four main goals are the focus of medical intervention for endometriosis. These are to relieve pain, stop the progression of established growths, prevent the establishment of any new growths, and maintain or restore fertility if that is the patient's wish.

Surgical interventions may include the use of lasers or electrocauterization to ablate or cut out visible growths and to reduce adhesions between the pelvic organs.

Medications

Nonsteroidal anti-inflammatory drugs or other analgesics may be adequate for pain relief. Hormone therapy that disrupts the secretion of estrogen may be provided to limit growths.

Massage Considerations

Risks
- Deep abdominal work is contraindicated for clients with endometriosis, especially during menstruation.

Benefits
- Massage may help with the stress, frustration, and anxiety involved with this condition.
- Massage and relaxation techniques can relieve menstrual pain.

epilepsy: see seizure disorders

epistaxis: see nosebleed

---

erectile dysfunction

Erectile dysfunction (ED) is the inability to achieve or maintain an erection sufficient for sexual intercourse. It is a common disorder that affects young men as well as mature ones, but it has increasing prevalence with age.

The mechanism of achieving an erection is complicated, requiring strong psychological, neurologic, and circulatory function. Until recently, it was assumed that ED was usually a psychological disorder. Now, especially when it occurs in men older than 40 years of age, a physical cause (circulatory or nerve impairment) is usually found. Risk factors for ED include **diabetes**; cardiovascular disease with **atherosclerosis** and **high blood pressure**; long-term **alcoholism**; a history of spinal surgery (especially in the low back); and a history of radiation for **prostate, colorectal,** or **bladder cancer.** Some medications, including those used to treat high blood pressure and **depression,** can contribute to ED. A fairly rare risk factor for ED is low testosterone levels; this usually accompanies unusually small or atrophied testicles.

ED can start as a mechanical problem and develop into a psychological disorder. The stress of not having an erection at the appropriate time can make it more difficult to achieve one. This "performance anxiety" can make ED a self-fulfilling prophecy.

Signs and Symptoms
- The inability to achieve an erection sufficient for intercourse

Treatment Options
ED is a highly treatable condition, and most men find a method that is ultimately satisfactory. In addition to medication, treatment options include use of a vacuum pump or a surgically implanted prosthesis.

Medications
The most popular medications for ED belong to a class of drugs called phosphodiesterase-5 inhibitors. These medications work by boosting signals that prolong and amplify erections. However, they are associated with a risk of interaction with nitrates, which can dangerously lower the blood pressure, so men who take nitroglycerin for heart disease must not use these drugs.

Massage Considerations

Risks

- Confusion about sex, touch, and intimacy may lead clients to think that a massage therapist can help them sexually.

Benefits

- Massage has no specific benefits for ED, but clients with this disorder can enjoy the same general benefits as the rest of the population.

---

erysipelas

Originally called St. Anthony's fire, erysipelas is a streptococcal infection of the cells in the skin. The redness that characterizes this condition is caused by the enzymes produced by streptococcus bacteria, which break down and kill skin cells.

Erysipelas is a superficial form of **cellulitis**. It can lead to a potentially dangerous infection of the lymph system (**lymphangitis**) or the circulatory system (**septicemia**).

Signs and Symptoms

- Tender red area, usually on the face or lower leg
- A sharp margin around the edges of redness
- Red streaks running from the wound toward the nearest lymph nodes
- Chills, fever, malaise

Treatment Options

Erysipelas is treated with medication.

Medications

Antibiotics are used to treat erysipelas; these should be administered as quickly as possible to avoid dangerous complications.

 Massage Considerations

Risks

- Acute infection systemically contraindicates massage.

Benefits

- Clients who have had erysipelas and have no further signs of infection can enjoy the same benefits from massage as the rest of the population.

Escherichia coli *infection: see gastroenteritis*

F

facioscapulohumeral muscular dystrophy: see muscular dystrophy

fatigue

Fatigue is a state in which the body doesn't function at its best levels because of lack of recovery time. Fatigue can be discussed as two types: mental (or emotional) fatigue and physical fatigue (brought about by overexertion). These two phenomena are inextricably linked; one could hardly occur without the other.

Fatigue is often (but not always) related to **sleep disorders**. Fatigue can cause a person to move inefficiently or clumsily, thus increasing the chance of musculoskeletal injury. Fatigue that is not relieved with a reasonable amount of rest and recovery time may be a warning sign of another condition, such as **fibromyalgia**, **chronic fatigue syndrome**, **anemia**, **candidiasis**, **depression**, or **hypothyroidism**.

Signs and Symptoms

- Unusual tiredness or physical exhaustion

Treatment Options

Treatment options vary according to the cause of the symptoms.

Medications

Fatigue may be treated with nutritional supplements, sleep aids, or other interventions depending on the underlying causes.

🖐 Massage Considerations

Risks

- Massage may temporarily mask the symptoms of a serious disorder. If fatigue persists, it is important that the client seek help from his or her primary health care provider.

Benefits

- Massage can promote an improved balance between the sympathetic and parasympathetic states.
- Massage improves the quality of sleep.
- Massage may assist in the metabolic exchange of wastes and nutrients for faster recovery from physical exhaustion.

fever

Fever is an abnormally high body temperature, usually brought about by bacterial or viral infection but sometimes stimulated by other types of tissue damage and inflammation. It is an effective mechanism for creating a hostile internal environment for bacterial or viral invasion.

Fever may occasionally progress to a dangerous situation, particularly when the temperature increases above 104°F. The most common complications are dehydration, acidosis, and brain damage. Death from fever occurs somewhere around 112°F to 114°F for adults.

If a fever develops too quickly, it can lead to circulatory shock, which can be dangerous, especially in older patients.

Signs and Symptoms
- Elevated temperature

Treatment Options
When fever is treated, a variety of antipyretic medications may be used.

Medications
Aspirin, ibuprofen, and acetaminophen all work to inhibit fever.

Massage Considerations
Risks
- Acute fever systemically contraindicates massage; the client may not be ready for the circulatory challenge, and the therapist is better off avoiding the risk of contagious infection.

Benefits
- Reflexive or energetic techniques may help a client get through an illness as long as the therapist takes precautions against the risk of infection.

fibrocystic breast disease
The vast majority of growths in breast tissue are cysts or benign tumors. These are so common (present in more than half of mature women) that they are sometimes called fibrocystic breast changes rather than disease. Some factors that can cause breast changes include infection, trauma, surgery, and radiation that can lead to fat necrosis. Breast infections and fat necrosis can be serious situations that require medical intervention for the best outcomes.

A small number of breast cysts have a risk of becoming **breast cancer**; all changes in the quality of breast tissue should be investigated.

Signs and Symptoms
- Gross cysts: large enough to be palpable; may come and go with the menstrual cycle
- Fibroadenomas: small cysts that grow in clusters and come and go with the menstrual cycle
- Atypical hyperplasia: also called proliferative breast disease; increases the risk of breast cancer
- Fibrosis: firm, painless areas of thickened connective tissue
- Phyllodes tumors: relatively rare; involve the epithelial and connective tissue; associated with some risk of breast cancer
- Papillomas: tiny warts that grow in ductal tissue

Treatment Options

After they have been identified as nonmalignant, cysts may be surgically removed or aspirated, but they are often left alone because they pose no imminent threat.

 Massage Considerations

Risks
- Massage has no specific risks regarding breast cysts.

Benefits
- Women who have this condition may benefit from lymph drainage techniques to reduce congestion around the breast area.

---

fibroid tumors

Fibroid tumors, or leiomyomas, are benign tumors that grow in or around the muscular wall of the uterus. Fibroids vary in size from microscopic to weighing several pounds and completely filling the uterus.

Fibroids can cause heavy periods, sometimes leading to **anemia** and **dysmenorrhea**. They can cause infertility by obstructing the fallopian tubes or interfering with the implantation of a fertilized ovum. They can also interfere in pregnancies brought to term; if a fibroid is large enough, it can crowd the growing fetus or may block the exit through the cervix.

Pedunculate fibroids can twist on their stalks, which causes extreme pain and requires surgery. It is also possible for very large fibroids to outgrow their blood supply, leading to tissue death. The necrotic mass is usually slowly reabsorbed by the body, but it can be painful in the process; more often, surgery is required to remove the growth.

Signs and Symptoms
- Often silent
- May cause secondary pressure on other pelvic organs, leading to urinary frequency or constipation
- Infertility
- Heavy menstrual bleeding
- Occasional bleeding between cycles

Treatment Options

Fibroids seldom require treatment unless they cause pain and excessive bleeding or if they interfere with pregnancy. Surgical options include procedures to shrink the growths with liquid nitrogen, block off the supplying arteries; laser surgery; and a partial or full hysterectomy.

Medications

Hormone therapy can shrink fibroids, but the fibroids will grow back when the medication is stopped.

 Massage Considerations

Risks
- Large fibroids may displace the pelvic organs and make them vulnerable to injury; identified large fibroids contraindicate deep abdominal massage.

Benefits
- Massage has no specific benefits for clients with fibroid tumors. Clients with fibroids can enjoy the same benefits from massage as the rest of the population.

fibromyalgia

Fibromyalgia syndrome (FMS) is a group of signs and symptoms that involve chronic pain in the muscles, tendons, ligaments, and other soft tissues. Several factors, including sleep disorders, neurotransmitter imbalance (predominance of pain-sensitizing chemicals), fatigue, pain, and tender points (hypotonic areas of local tenderness distributed all over the body) seem central to the development of fibromyalgia.

Many patients diagnosed with fibromyalgia meet the criteria for a diagnosis of **chronic fatigue syndrome** and vice versa. Other conditions that frequently overlap with fibromyalgia include **restless leg syndrome, migraine headaches, irritable bowel syndrome, hypothyroidism, sleep disorders, myofascial pain syndrome,** and **temporomandibular joint dysfunction.**

The tender points of FMS can be confused with the trigger points seen with myofascial pain syndrome. The phenomena are etiologically very different, however, and must be treated differently.

Signs and Symptoms
- Tender points in all four quadrants of the body
- Widespread, shifting pain
- Stiffness after rest
- Poor stamina
- Sensitivity amplification: all senses are magnified, especially regarding pain

Treatment Options

The first priority in fibromyalgia treatment is to educate the patient as completely as possible about his or her condition, emphasizing that although he or she may feel incapacitated, fibromyalgia is not a progressive or life-threatening disease. Nutrition, sleep, exercise, stretching, and reducing emotional stress are all important as well.

Medications

Fibromyalgia patients may take tricyclic antidepressants to help improve their mood, sleep, and pain sensation. Other drugs are now being applied in this context as well, including Parkinson disease drugs to help manage restless leg syndrome, which is common among fibromyalgia patients, and anticonvulsive drugs that may interrupt nerve pain. Other pain-killing drugs are generally avoided because they interfere with sleep and can be habit forming.

Massage Considerations

Risks
- Clients with fibromyalgia are easily overtreated; be cautious with rigorous massage.
- Trigger points seen with myofascial pain syndrome can be resolved with specific pressure; tender points seen with fibromyalgia can be irritated with the same techniques.

- Fibromyalgia patients don't usually tolerate cold well; avoid using ice and cold types of hydrotherapy.

Benefits
- Massage improves sleep, which is an important issue for fibromyalgia patients.
- Massage can reduce anxiety, depression, and perceived pain.
- The experience of being even temporarily painfree can improve the quality of life for fibromyalgia patients.

flesh-eating bacteria: see cellulitis

flu: see influenza

focal dystonia: see dystonia, torticollis

follicular cysts: see ovarian cysts

folliculitis

Folliculitis is the inflammation of the hair shafts. It is usually related to an infection but can also be the result of chemical or physical irritation of the skin.

The pathogens that cause folliculitis include several varieties of bacteria, fungi, herpes simplex, and the virus associated with **molluscum contagiosum**. Infections are usually superficial but can go deep into the hair shaft, which may cause permanent scarring and hair loss.

Folliculitis has several names, depending on where it develops.
- Sycosis barbae, also called barber's itch, is a bacterial infection of hair shafts in areas that are shaved; tinea barbae is a fungal infection of the same area.
- Pseudofolliculitis barbae is a condition in which coarse, curly beard hair grows back toward the skin, irritating it without actually causing an infection.
- Hot tub folliculitis is self-explanatory; it typically appears where bathing suits hold contaminated water close to the skin.
- Folliculitis of the eyelid is called a sty.
- Folliculitis is a particular risk for people who have **HIV/AIDS** or **diabetes**. It is unusual but possible for untreated folliculitis to progress to a more serious problem, such as **boils** or **cellulitis**.

Signs and Symptoms
- Usually appears in areas with coarse hair: face, groin, axilla
- Red bumps or pustules with central hair
- Often in clusters or a gridlike pattern
- May be itchy or painful

Treatment Options
Some types of folliculitis are self-limiting (i.e., they clear up with no intervention).

People with folliculitis are counseled to wash with antibacterial soap, stop shaving or use an electric razor (soaking the head for at least 1 hour in alcohol every day), and isolate their towels and bedding from other people. Linens should be washed separately and frequently in hot, soapy water.

Medications

Bacterial folliculitis is usually treated with topical or oral antibiotics. Fungal infections are treated with topical antifungal medications.

 Massage Considerations

Risks
- Acute infections at least locally contraindicate massage.
- Oil-based lubricants may exacerbate folliculitis.

Benefits
- Massage has no specific benefits for folliculitis, but if lesions are avoided or are no longer present, clients with this condition can enjoy the same benefits as the rest of the population.

---

food poisoning: see gastroenteritis

---

fractures

Fractures are any variety of broken bone, from a hairline crack to a complete break with protrusion through the skin.

Ankle **sprains** and **shin splints** are two conditions that frequently hide small bone fractures. Having **osteoporosis** increases the risk of fractures that occur with only minor trauma or no trauma at all; this is called "spontaneous fracture."

Signs and Symptoms
- Depends on the severity of the injury
- Can be masked by a soft tissue injury
- Can make the bone and nearby joints unusable

Treatment Options

Most fractures heal well if they are casted to immobilize the bones. Some fractures need more support than a standard cast can offer, especially if the break involves a joint, as in the wrist or ankle. Pins or plates may be introduced to further stabilize the joint, but they carry the risk of introducing infection to the site.

Several grafting procedures using a variety of materials for permanent or temporary scaffolding have been developed to speed healing of broken bones.

Medications

Acute fractures may be treated with analgesics.

 Massage Considerations

Risks
- Acute, undiagnosed, or unset fractures contraindicate massage.

Benefits
- Lymphatic work around the area may help resolve excessive edema and speed healing.
- Massage can address compensation patterns and pain associated with limping or the use of crutches.

frostbite

Frostbite is the destruction of cells caused by hypothermia. When a body part (usually the fingers, toes, nose, or cheeks) is exposed to cold temperatures for a prolonged period, two things may happen: ice crystals may form in cells in the extremities, which causes the cells to rupture and die, or ice crystals and sticky red blood cells and platelets may prevent the flow of blood into the affected area, causing the cells to die. If the damage reaches deeper tissues, it may affect the blood vessels, muscles, and nerve tissue.

The people most at risk for frostbite are those with poor circulation, smokers, people with **Raynaud disease**, and people who are intoxicated and unable to tell when they are in danger from the cold. Frostbite has a high risk of progressing to wet or dry **gangrene** with a subsequent need for **amputation**.

Signs and Symptoms

- Hard, cold, white area
- During rewarming: blotchy, swelling, pain
- Blisters filled with clear fluid accompany superficial injury
- Blisters filled with blood accompany deep injury

Treatment Options

Treatment for frostbite depends on the extent and depth of the damage. Emergency measures include slow rewarming of the area and other care for systemic hypothermia. If gangrene is present, steps to limit the spread of infection must be taken.

It often takes several days or weeks to fully evaluate the permanent tissue damage caused by frostbite. Amputations and other corrective surgeries are usually delayed until the damaged skin has stopped shedding.

Medications

Frostbite is treated with analgesics and antibiotics during the healing process.

Massage Considerations

Risks

- Acute frostbite contraindicates massage; friction further damages cells.
- Areas that have had frostbite may have permanent numbness; this contraindicates any massage that might damage tissues because of a lack of sensation.

Benefits

- Clients who have recovered from frostbite can enjoy the same benefits of massage as the rest of the population.

frozen shoulder: see adhesive capsulitis

fungal infections

Fungal infections of human skin involve several different types of fungi called dermatophytes. The lesions the infections create are called tinea. The term *ringworm* is frequently used to refer to several types of tinea.

Fungal infections are transmitted through touching contaminated surfaces or infected people or animals. It takes anywhere from 4 to 14 days for lesions to appear, and during that time, the carrier is infectious, which makes this condition very difficult to control.

Fungal infections often resemble other skin conditions, including some that are not contagious (atopic **dermatitis**, nummular **eczema, psoriasis**). Therefore, it is especially important that massage therapists avoid all undiagnosed skin lesions.

Signs and Symptoms

- Tinea corporis (body ringworm)
    - Small, round, scaly, itchy patch
    - Pale in the middle; flaky around the edges
    - Gradually increase in size
- Tinea capitis (head ringworm)
    - Itchiness and flaking of the scalp
    - Temporary or permanent hair loss
- Tinea pedis (athlete's foot)
    - Usually starts between the third and fourth toes
    - Burning, itching, weeping blisters
    - Cracking, peeling skin; possibility of infection
    - "Moccasin distribution": dry, scaly, itchy lesions on the heel and sole of the foot
- Tinea cruris (jock itch)
    - Lesions on the groin, upper thigh, and buttocks.
    - May be caused by yeast infections in the gastrointestinal tract
- Other varieties
    - Tinea manus: on the hands
    - Tinea barbae: in the beard area
    - Tinea versicolor: changes in the pigmentation of the skin
    - Tinea unguium: under the fingernails or toenails

Treatment Options

Fungal infections are usually treated with medication.

Medications

External applications of fungicide are the typical treatment unless the infection is under the nail. In this case, oral doses of fungicides may be prescribed.

🖐 Massage Considerations

Risks

- Fungal infections contraindicate massage, but small, treated lesions may be covered and considered a local contraindication only.

Benefits

- Massage has no specific benefits for fungal infections.
- Clients with a history of fungal infections can enjoy the same benefits from massage as the rest of the population.

G

gallstones

Gallstones are crystallized formations of cholesterol or bile pigments in the gallbladder. When either cholesterol or bilirubin occurs in higher than normal concentrations in the bile, it can precipitate out of the liquid to become either tiny granules called "bile sludge" or larger stones. Gallstones can be as small as grains of sand or as large as a golf ball.

A lodged gallstone that obstructs the cystic or hepatic duct may cause **jaundice**. If the blockage is distal to the pancreatic ducts, acute **pancreatitis** may occur. The pooling of stagnant bile can also lead to infection of the gallbladder. It is possible for an infected gallbladder to rupture, releasing its contents and causing **peritonitis**.

Signs and Symptoms
- Mostly silent unless a stone is lodged in a duct
- Excruciating right-sided abdominal pain
- Pain may subside if the stone moves out of the duct
- Possible pain referral to the right shoulder or between the scapulae

Treatment Options
Most identified gallstones are removed with laparoscopic surgery. Loss of gallbladder function may require supplements to assist in the absorption of fat-soluble vitamins.

Medications
Gallstones are not treated with medication.

Massage Considerations

Risks
- Gallbladder attacks contraindicate massage; this is a medical emergency.
- If gallstones are known to be present but are not causing symptoms, the right costal angle is a local caution for deep massage.

Benefits
- Clients with a history of gallstones or gallbladder surgery but no current symptoms can enjoy the same benefits from massage as the rest of the population.

Practitioner Advice
- The gallbladder can refer pain between the shoulder blades and over the right shoulder. This may prompt clients to seek massage, but the problem needs to be addressed by a medical professional.

ganglion cyst

Ganglion cysts are small connective tissue pouches filled with synovial fluid. They grow on joint capsules or tendinous sheaths, usually on the wrist, hand, or top of the foot.

Ganglion cysts are not inherently dangerous, but when they appear on the distal phalanges of the fingers, they can interfere with normal fingernail growth. They may also interfere with joint capsule function at the distal interphalangeal joint.

Signs and Symptoms

- Small, round, nonpainful bumps on the tendinous sheaths or joint capsules
- Range from pea sized to golf ball sized
- May limit normal range of motion at the affected joint

Treatment Options

Ganglion cysts may be aspirated or surgically excised, but they frequently grow back.

Medication

Ganglion cysts are not treated with medication.

Massage Considerations

Risks

- Ganglion cysts locally contraindicate deep specific massage, which may irritate them.

Benefits

- Clients with ganglion cysts can enjoy the same benefits from massage elsewhere on the body as the rest of the population.

---

gangrene

Gangrene is a general term for infection of necrotic tissues. Typically, this tissue death is related to a gradual or sudden loss of blood supply. Gangrene can also occur when a wound is infected with a particular type of bacterium (usually *Clostridium perfringens*).

Much of the tissue damage associated with gangrene is not brought about by bacterial growth but by the toxins the bacteria produce. These enzymes may dissolve cell membranes and weaken fascial sheaths, allowing the bacteria to spread rapidly and possibly fatally through the body.

Gangrene is rare outside of some very specific circumstances. It is usually the result of an interruption in blood supply, as may occur with **frostbite, thrombophlebitis,** or **atherosclerosis.** Most people who develop gangrene are immune compromised with other disorders such as **diabetes, liver failure, leukemia, lymphoma, myeloma,** or **colorectal cancer.**

Some types of gangrene are aggressive and fast moving. Left untreated, they can overwhelm a person, leading to shock and **septicemia** within hours.

Signs and Symptoms

- Wet gangrene: skin appears bruised, swollen, and blistered
- Dry gangrene: skin appears dark; tissues are shriveled
- Gas gangrene: the area is swollen; the skin is bronze colored with large, painful blisters

Treatment Options

The first priority is to remedy the situation that led to the infection. Surgery may be performed to remove necrotic tissue and prevent the spread of bacteria to the rest of the body.

Medications

Broad-spectrum antibiotics are prescribed for gangrene to limit the infection.

 ## Massage Considerations

Risks
- Acute gangrene contraindicates massage; bodywork may allow the infection to penetrate deeper into the system, and the bacteria may be contagious.

Benefits
- Clients with a history of gangrene but no risk of current infection can enjoy the same benefits from massage as the rest of the population.

gastric bypass surgery: see bariatric surgery

gastroenteritis

Gastroenteritis is inflammation of the gastrointestinal (GI) tract, specifically the stomach or small intestine. It is usually caused by viral or bacterial infection, although parasites, fungi, and food sensitivities may also cause symptoms. When the GI tract is damaged or inflamed, absorption of nutrients and water is severely limited, leading to a loss of water and valuable electrolytes through diarrhea and vomiting.

The most serious complication of gastroenteritis is dehydration from the massive fluid and mineral loss. Some gastroenteritis factors can cause other complications as well. *Campylobacter* bacteria have been linked with **Guillain-Barré syndrome**, and *Salmonella* can progress to **meningitis** or **septicemia**. Some forms of *Escherichia coli* are highly toxic and can lead to **renal failure**.

If symptoms of gastroenteritis persist longer than 2 or 3 weeks, it is no longer considered an acute infection but a chronic condition. This should lead the medical professional to look for an underlying problem such as food **allergies, irritable bowel syndrome, diverticulitis, ulcers, Crohn disease, ulcerative colitis,** or **HIV/AIDS**.

Signs and Symptoms
- Nausea, vomiting, diarrhea
- Extreme dehydration
- Bloating, abdominal cramps, gas
- Mucus or blood in the stools

Treatment Options

Gastroenteritis is usually treated with rest and fluid replacement. If supplementing fluids by mouth aggravates vomiting, it may be necessary to use intravenous fluid replacement in a hospital setting.

Medications

Antiemetic medications may be used to limit vomiting. Antidiarrheals are often avoided because by interfering with digestion, they may prolong infection. Antibiotics are ineffective for viral and parasitic infections and can exacerbate the symptoms of bacterial infections.

Massage Considerations

Risks
- Acute infectious gastroenteritis contraindicates massage because of client comfort and communicability issues.

Benefits
- Gastric distress that is not related to infection or disease may respond positively to the parasympathetic effects of massage.
- Clients who have recovered from gastroenteritis can enjoy the same benefits from massage as the rest of the population.

---

gastroesophageal reflux disease

Gastroesophageal reflux disease (GERD) is a condition involving damage to the squamous epithelial lining of the esophagus when it is chronically exposed to digestive juices released from the stomach. It is sometimes called reflux esophagitis. GERD is usually associated with weak muscular action at the lower esophageal sphincter and the possibility of a hiatal **hernia**.

Chronic irritation of the esophageal lining can cause several problems. Respiratory injury may occur if gastric secretions reach the larynx. **Ulcers** may form in the esophagus. A stricture may form, making it difficult to swallow normally. Barrett's esophagitis, a precancerous condition leading to **esophageal cancer**, may develop.

Signs and Symptoms
- Chronic, repeated heartburn
- Indigestion, bloating, abdominal pain
- Dysphagia (difficulty swallowing)
- Chronic cough, possibly with bloody sputum
- Chest pain that may resemble angina or a heart attack
- Symptoms are aggravated by lying down

Treatment Options

Managing GERD includes strategies such as losing weight if the patient is overweight; eating smaller portions so the stomach doesn't get stretched; not lying down within 2 hours after a meal; avoiding caffeine, alcohol, and nicotine; raising the bed about 6 inches at the head; and putting a heating pad on the stomach when it is painful.

Surgery for GERD usually focuses on strengthening the esophageal sphincter and taking pressure off the stomach. This can include repairing a damaged sphincter and reducing a hiatal hernia.

Medications

Medication for GERD can work in a variety of ways. Antacids neutralize stomach acid, but over-the-counter brands may also cause the stomach to expand with gas, putting more pressure on the esophageal valve. Proton pump inhibitors block receptors in the stomach that stimulate acid production.

Massage Considerations

Risks
- Long sessions with the client lying flat may exacerbate symptoms.

Benefits
- Clients who have GERD but who are comfortable receiving massage can enjoy the same benefits from massage as the rest of the population.

Practitioner Advice
- Some clients with GERD may find that massage exacerbates their symptoms by promoting gastric activity. To minimize potential problems, schedule sessions to occur more than 2 hours after the client's last meal and consider shorter sessions or working in a massage chair to minimize the risk of heartburn symptoms.

general anxiety disorder: see anxiety disorders

genital warts

Genital warts are viral infections of the genitals, rectum, and perineum in both genders. They are caused by several varieties of human papilloma virus (HPV), although these are different from the strains that cause common **warts**.

Genital warts are highly contagious; one sexual encounter with an actively infected person carries a significant risk of spreading the virus. The viruses penetrate the skin through tiny abrasions around the genitals, and the first outbreak usually occurs within 3 months of exposure. Men may develop growths inside the urethra, around the rectum, or on the scrotum; women may have warts in the labia or vaginal canal or around the rectum.

The most important complication of genital warts is a significantly increased risk of **cervical cancer** in women. The most common types of warts carry a low risk, but the less common HPV warts cause up to 80% of all diagnosed cases of cervical cancer. Unfortunately, it is impossible to tell which kind of virus is present without testing, so all suspect tissue must be examined for signs of dysplasia, or abnormal growth.

A vaccine is now available that prevents the spread of the most common forms of HPV that are associated with both genital warts and cervical cancer. The vaccine doesn't protect against all forms, however, so women who use this vaccine must still adhere to a schedule of regular pelvic exams.

Signs and Symptoms
- Often silent
- May be tiny, gray growths
- May occur in clusters
- May itch or bleed
- May obstruct the male urethra

Treatment Options
The most common initial treatment options for genital warts include surgical excision, cryotherapy (killing the wart with liquid nitrogen), or both. If these are unsuccessful, other options (which are more expensive and have more possible complications) include laser excision, electrodissection, and antiviral drugs.

Medications
A person with genital warts may be treated with antiviral drugs.

Massage Considerations

Risks
- Massage has no specific risks relating to genital warts.

Benefits
- Clients with genital warts can enjoy the same benefits from massage as the rest of the population.

gestational diabetes: see pregnancy

giant cell arteritis: see polymyalgia rheumatica, vasculitis

Giardia *infection: see gastroenteritis*

glaucoma

Glaucoma is an umbrella term used to describe circumstances in which the aqueous humor of the eye holds too much fluid, leading to optic nerve damage. It is usually classified as angle-closure glaucoma or open-angle glaucoma. Typically, glaucoma develops because channels that drain the aqueous humor are blocked or because the channels may be open but fluid accumulates more rapidly than it is removed.

Signs and Symptoms
- Progressive vision loss
    Blind spots in the peripheral vision
    Blurred vision
    The appearance of halos around light sources
- Increased intraocular pressure (IOP)
- Headaches and nausea

Treatment Options

The damage from glaucoma can be stopped but not reversed. Strategies include the use of medications and a variety of surgeries that relieve pressure or drain the aqueous humor.

Medications

A wide variety of medications may be used to reduce IOP. Some of these medications are taken orally; others are applied as eye drops. Possibilities include beta-blockers, alpha-agonists, prostaglandin analogs, and others.

Massage Considerations

Risks
- Massage has no specific risks related to glaucoma as long as the client is comfortable. Avoid putting pressure on the eyes with a face cradle.

Benefits
- Clients with glaucoma can enjoy the same benefits from massage as the rest of the population.

glomerulonephritis

Glomerulonephritis is a disorder involving inflammation and scarring of the glomeruli (microscopic knots of circulatory capillaries surrounded by the Bowman capsules in the kidneys).

Glomerulonephritis is a common complication of **lupus** and other autoimmune diseases. It may also be part of a delayed reaction against certain kinds of streptococcal infections, especially in young children. Many people who have glomerulonephritis have also been exposed to environmental toxins (notably hydrocarbons, silicon, mercury, and lithium).

Although acute glomerulonephritis may resolve with no long-term effects, chronic glomerulonephritis may lead to **hypertension** and **renal failure**.

Signs and Symptoms
- Hematuria (blood in the urine)
- Abnormally high levels of protein in the urine
- Hypertension
- Signs of renal failure, including malaise, skin discoloration, rashes, itching, low urine output, systemic edema, lethargy, confusion, coma

Treatment Options
Glomerulonephritis is treated according to the predisposing factors.

Medications
If the glomerulonephritis is related to an autoimmune or other inflammatory problem, steroidal anti-inflammatory drugs may be used to limit damage to the nephrons. Cytotoxic drugs are also used to inhibit the damaging effects of an immune system attack against the kidneys. Antihypertensive drugs may be used to control kidney stress; antibiotics are reserved for identified renal infections.

Massage Considerations

Risks
- Glomerulonephritis systemically contraindicates rigorous circulatory massage because it is a sign of a severely compromised ability to adapt to changes in fluid levels.

Benefits
- Reflexive or energetic modalities can offer the benefits of relaxation and pain relief without circulatory challenge.
- Clients who have fully recovered from glomerulonephritis can enjoy the same benefits from massage as the rest of the population.

gonorrhea

Gonorrhea is infection with a bacterium called *Neisseria gonorrhoeae*. Gonorrhea is spread through intimate contact. It can infect the throat, vagina, and rectum. It is rarely transmitted in any contact other than sex; for instance, it is unusual for a pregnant woman with gonorrhea to pass it to her child.

After it is inside the body, gonorrhea often affects the joints in a type of **septic arthritis** called gonococcal arthritis. Gonorrhea, which often coexists with **chlamydia**, can also lead to **pelvic inflammatory disease**. Infection with gonorrhea increases the risk of transmission for **HIV**.

Signs and Symptoms

- For women:
    Often silent
    Vaginal discharge
    Urinary discomfort
    Painful intercourse
    Oral infection: sores in the mouth, sore throat
- For men:
    Burning on urination
    Penile discharge
    Orchitis (swelling of the testicles)

Treatment Options

Gonorrhea is treated with antibiotics, although it has become resistant to penicillin.

Medications

A number of powerful, single-dose antibiotic therapies have been developed that can successfully and quickly eradicate a gonorrhea infection. This condition frequent appears with chlamydia, which requires a different antibiotic.

✋ Massage Considerations

Risks

- Clients with diagnosed gonorrhea should begin antibiotic therapy before receiving massage.
- Clients with septic arthritis need special care; consult with the health care team for best results.

Benefits

- Clients in recovery from septic arthritis may benefit from massage and stretching that complement their other forms of therapy; work with the health care team for best results.
- Clients with treated gonorrhea or a history of this infection can enjoy the same benefits from massage therapy as the rest of the population.

gout

Gout is a type of inflammatory arthritis brought about by the presence of uric acid crystals that irritate and inflame the joint capsules from the outside. When uric acid consolidates, it forms sharp, needlelike crystals that usually accumulate in the foot, grinding on and irritating synovial capsules, bursae, tendons, and other tissues. The foot may be the primary target because of gravity, but it may also have to do with the lower temperature found in extremities that aids in the crystallization process.

The complications of gout are usually indications that the kidneys are not functioning at adequate levels. Gout may occur in conjunction with **kidney stones**. If the kidneys are sufficiently blocked by kidney stones, the result may be **renal failure**. Impaired kidneys can't process adequate fluid, causing **hypertension**, which can result in **atherosclerosis** or **stroke**.

Signs and Symptoms
- Sudden onset of symptoms, usually in the feet
- The affected joint is red, hot, shiny, and excruciatingly painful
- Moderate fever and chills may be present

Treatment Options
Gout is treated in the short term with medication. In the longer term, preventive measures include other drugs, increasing fluid intake, and limiting gout-promoting substances (alcohol, legumes, sardines, mushrooms, asparagus, cauliflower, spinach).

Medications
Pain relief is a high priority for gout, with analgesics other than aspirin. Anti-inflammatory drugs may be used, and drugs that modify uric acid excretion are recommended for long-term use.

Massage Considerations
Risks
- Gout at least locally contraindicates any firm massage; manipulating uric acid crystals can exacerbate symptoms.
- A client with repeated episodes of gout may have other kidney problems; these can influence massage decisions.

Benefits
- Clients with acute gout may benefit from lymphatic techniques that may reduce inflammation.
- If clients with active gout can be comfortable and the affected area is avoided, they can enjoy the same benefits from massage as the rest of the population.

Graves disease: see hyperthyroidism

Guillain-Barré syndrome

Guillain-Barré syndrome (GBS) is a condition involving acute inflammation and destruction of the myelin layer of peripheral nerves, specifically in the extremities. Its synonym is acute idiopathic polyneuritis. It is a severe, extreme inflammation of multiple peripheral nerves that develops for reasons that are not fully understood; it is believed to be related to immune system hyperactivity.

Regardless of what initiates the disease process, the end result is that the myelin sheaths on peripheral nerves are attacked and destroyed. The damage progresses proximally and may also affect the cranial nerves. This can be a life-threatening situation if the nerves that control breathing are damaged; many GBS patients spend time on a ventilator. Most people who develop GBS have a full or nearly full recovery, although the process may take 18 months or more.

Signs and Symptoms

- Fast, severe onset
- Symmetrical presentation
- Weakness, tingling in the affected limbs
- Diminished reflexes
- Progresses proximally
- If in cranial nerves of face: pain, difficulty with speech
- May affect the nerves that control breathing
- Symptoms peak at 2 or 3 weeks after onset and then subside

Treatment Options

Two treatment options for GBS have been used successfully to shorten recovery time; these include plasmapheresis and injections of high concentrations of immunoglobulin or gamma globulin (donated antibodies).

Other interventions for GBS patients are dictated by individual needs. Many patients require the use of a ventilator for a period of time until the respiratory nerves regain full function.

Medications

GBS patients may use a variety of drugs in their recovery to alter their immune system activity, reduce the risk of infection and blood clots, and ameliorate the challenges of plasmapheresis.

 Massage Considerations

Risks

- Acute GBS contraindicates rigorous massage simply because the body is already taxed and does not need further challenge.
- During recovery, it is important to establish that sensation is present and accurate to avoid the risk of overtreatment.

Benefits

- Clients in recovery from GBS may use physical and occupational therapy to help regain function; massage may have a valuable role here as well.
- Clients with a history of GBS but no current symptoms can enjoy the same benefits from massage as the rest of the population.

gynecomastia

Gynecomastia is the enlargement of breast tissue in males. True gynecomastia involves hypertrophy of glandular breast tissue, and pseudogynecomastia involves excess fat in the breast area.

Most cases of gynecomastia are idiopathic or are related to temporary hormonal imbalances that occur in infancy and again in adolescence. Some drugs may also cause abnormal growth of breast tissue. When gynecomastia is pathologic, it usually indicates the loss of balance between testosterone and various types of estrogens. This can be brought about by endocrine disease, some types of cancer, or liver dysfunction.

When gynecomastia occurs in mature men, the possibility of ductal carcinoma (**breast cancer**) must be considered. Outside of other fairly rare endocrine disorders, gynecomastia is usually a benign, if sometimes embarrassing condition.

Signs and Symptoms
- Excessive growth of male breast tissue
- May be unilateral or bilateral

Treatment Options
Men with idiopathic gynecomastia may pursue plastic surgery to reduce the size of the affected breast or breasts.

Massage Considerations

Risks
- Massage has no specific risks for gynecomastia that is unrelated to underlying disorders.

Benefits
- Massage has no specific benefits to offer men with gynecomastia; they can enjoy the same benefits from massage as the rest of the population.

hammertoes

Hammertoes are a condition in which an imbalance in the muscles of the toes leads to permanent flexion at the interphalangeal joints. It usually happens to toes other than the great toe and is especially prevalent in toes that are longer than the great toe.

Hammertoes are usually related to genetics, including **Charcot-Marie-Tooth disease, osteoarthritis,** or injuries to the toes (often caused by tight or ill-fitting shoes).

Signs and Symptoms
- Permanent involuntary flexion of the affected toe or toes
- May be painful
- Eventually becomes rigid with bony adaptation

Treatment Options
Early treatment interventions for hammertoes include stretching, exercises, and physical therapy. If the distortion is fixed, surgery to correct and realign the joints may be recommended.

Medications
If hammertoes are painful, they may be treated with nonsteroidal anti-inflammatory drugs.

Massage Considerations

Risks

- Deep specific work on the affected joints may be irritating. Otherwise, massage has no specific risks for clients with hammertoes.

Benefits

- Massage may help reverse hammertoes if it is used very early in the process.
- Massage within pain tolerance may improve the function of the affected foot.
- Massage can help with pain related to postural distortions or limping in connection with hammertoes.

Hansen disease

Hansen disease, also known as leprosy, is an infection of a variety of bacteria that grow best in skin and nerves that are cooler than core body temperature. For this reason, the condition usually affects the hands, feet, mucous membranes, nose, ears, or testes. The bacteria invade the skin and nerve cells, leading to the atrophy of skin and small muscles and loss of sensation. Secondary infection and trauma may lead to serious tissue loss.

The bacteria associated with Hansen disease often grow very slowly. They may incubate anywhere from several months to 4 decades before producing symptoms, but most cases show lesions within 2 to 3 years of exposure. The method of transmission is unclear, although it is suspected that the bacteria may be spread through mucous secretions. Most people have inborn immunity to Hansen disease; it infects only a small percentage of those exposed.

Several different subtypes of this disease have been identified, each with a particular presentation, prevalence among certain races, and risk of permanent damage.

Signs and Symptoms

- Vary according to subtype
- Patches of hyper- or hypopigmentation of the skin
- Progressive numbness of the infected areas
- May go into remission with later flares
- Eventually, neuritis, muscle atrophy, contractures of the hands and feet, damage from secondary trauma and infection

Treatment Options

Hansen disease is a treatable infection. In addition to drug interventions, surgery may be conducted to repair contractures or reconstruct damaged extremities. Protective gear to guard against injury to the hands and feet is highly recommended.

Medications

Hansen disease is sensitive to several antibiotics. Chemotherapeutic drugs may also be prescribed to limit secondary inflammation and tissue damage.

 Massage Considerations

Risks

- It is unlikely for a massage therapist in the United States to have a client with Hansen disease. If this occurs, consultation with the medical team is necessary to avoid causing further damage.

Benefits
- Massage has no specific benefits for Hansen disease.
- Clients who have recovered from this infection can enjoy the same benefits from massage as the rest of the population.

Hashimoto thyroiditis: see hypothyroidism

hay fever: see sinusitis

headache, cluster

Cluster headaches are a fairly rare, not well-understood variety of vascular or congestive headache. Reliable triggers for cluster headaches have not been identified. They may occur seasonally, once or twice a year, or just once in a lifetime. Cluster headaches affect men more often than women.

Cluster headaches are similar to **migraines** in etiology because they both involve excessive fluid in the cranium. But although migraines tend to make people want to retreat into a warm, dark, small space, cluster headaches seem to be exacerbated by stillness, with patients often preferring constant movement to quell their symptoms.

Signs and Symptoms
- Repetitive episodic headaches lasting days or weeks at a time
- Often begin at night
- The eye and nostril of the affected side may water
- May cause facial swelling or unilateral sweating

Treatment Options

The most proactive and least invasive way to treat cluster headaches is to avoid known triggers.

Medications

Some medications that are used with migraine headaches have success with cluster headaches as well. These include nonsteroidal anti-inflammatory drugs (often in combination with caffeine), serotonin agonists, and smooth muscle constrictors.

Massage Considerations

Risks
- Clients in the midst of a cluster headache episode will probably not tolerate massage well.

Benefits
- Clients who get cluster headaches can enjoy the same benefits from massage as the rest of the population, as long as no symptoms are present.

headache, migraine

The word *migraine* comes from the French, *hemi-craine*, or "half-head." This is because migraine headache has a characteristic unilateral presentation. Migraine headaches begin with extreme vasoconstriction followed by vasodilation in the affected hemisphere of the brain. This creates pressure against the blood vessel walls and meninges, which causes excruciating pain.

Some migraine triggers have been identified. They include the consumption of red wine, cheese, chocolate, coffee, tea, and any kind of alcohol. Abnormal levels of stress can bring them on, as can hormonal shifts such as menstruation, pregnancy, and perimenopause.

Migraine headaches share a vasoconstriction–vasodilation pattern with **cluster headaches**, but migraines affect women more often than men, and the coping mechanisms people tend to use (going to bed in a quiet, dark room) are different from those often used with cluster headaches (staying in constant movement as a distraction from the pain).

Signs and Symptoms

- Throbbing pain on one side; the eye and nose may water
- Hypersensitivity to light
- Nausea, vomiting
- Pain may be preceded by blurred vision, the perception of flashing lights, or auditory hallucinations
- May last several hours to several days

Treatment Options

Migraines are often treated medically, but other interventions include relaxation therapy, biofeedback, acupuncture, and hydrotherapy (specifically, cold packs on the forehead or neck).

Medications

Medications for migraine headaches include prophylactics to reduce the frequency of headaches and other drugs to shorten the duration of headaches. Options include nonsteroidal anti-inflammatory drugs (often in combination with caffeine), serotonin agonists, and smooth muscle constrictors.

Massage Considerations

Risks

- Any stimulus can exacerbate symptoms; migraine headaches contraindicate massage until the episode has passed.

Benefits

- Massage as a stress management tool may help decrease the frequency of migraine headaches.

Practitioner Advice

- Migraines are easily confused with severe tension headaches. It is useful to know the difference because although massage is typically not useful for someone in the midst of a migraine, it can be a valuable intervention for tension headaches.

headache, tension

Tension headaches are headaches triggered by mechanical stresses that initiate central nervous system changes in serotonin levels and blood vessel dilatation.

Triggers for tension headaches are numerous because the cranium is so delicately balanced on the atlas, and it is held there by structures pulling in many opposing directions simultaneously. Some of the major factors for tension headaches include muscular, tendinous, or ligamentous injury to the head or neck; inefficient muscle tension at the suboccipital triangle or at the jaw; **temporomandibular joint disorders**; subluxation of cervical vertebrae; misalignment of the cranial bones; trigger points of the neck and head muscles (**myofascial pain syndrome**); poor ergonomics; and eyestrain.

Very severe tension headaches can mimic **migraines**. It is useful to know the distinction, however, because they respond to massage and other interventions differently.

Signs and Symptoms
- Usually triggered by biomechanical stresses
- Vary in location and severity
- Can be diffuse or localized to a specific area
- No throbbing or excessive watering of the eyes or nose

Treatment Options
Tension headaches can be treated with drugs, but they often also respond well to rest, relaxation techniques, postural adjustments, and massage.

Medications
Nonsteroidal anti-inflammatory drugs are usually sufficient to treat tension headaches.

Massage Considerations
Risks
- Massage has no particular risks for tension headaches unless a technique or position exacerbates symptoms.

Benefits
- Massage can be a useful preventive strategy to reduce the frequency of tension headaches.
- Massage can help unravel some of the biomechanical forces that contribute to tension headaches, even in the midst of an episode.

Practitioner Advice
- Severe headaches with a sudden onset; a new pattern; or accompanied by fever, disorientation, or speech problems constitute a medical emergency.

---

heart attack

A heart attack is damage to some portion of the cardiac muscle as a result of ischemia, which starves and kills some of the muscle cells. The ischemia is usually caused by atherosclerosis in the coronary arteries, which supply the cardiac muscle with oxygen and nutrition. When these arteries are completely occluded by plaque, thrombi, or any combination of the two, some piece of the muscle dies. The muscle tissue is replaced by inelastic, noncontractile scar tissue. The damaged area is referred to as an infarct. Another term for heart attack is myocardial infarction.

Heart attacks are part of a large, interrelated group of disorders that include **hypertension**, **atherosclerosis**, and damage to the arteries. Other disorders in this group include **aneurysm**, stroke, **renal failure,** atrial or ventricular fibrillations, and **heart failure.** Unstable **angina** is one of the few early warning signs for the risk of heart attack.

Signs and Symptoms

- Crushing pain and pressure in the chest
- Pain spreading to the left arm and shoulder
- Possible pain in the neck or jaw
- Lightheadedness, nausea, sweating

Treatment Options

The first priority with heart attack patients is to identify where the blockage is and to eradicate it as quickly as possible. This is done with clot-dissolving drugs or with immediate balloon angioplasty. Coronary bypass surgery may be recommended to remove occluded sections of the coronary arteries after the patient is stable.

Treatment in heart attack recovery embraces lifestyle changes that support a healthier future; eating sensibly, exercising regularly, controlling high blood pressure, and quitting smoking are the most important factors.

Medications

In the short term, heart attacks are treated with oxygen, thrombolytics, and pain management drugs that may include nitroglycerin and morphine.

Heart attack survivors are likely to use a variety of cardiovascular drugs, including cholesterol management drugs, antiplatelet drugs, antihypertensives, and diuretics.

🖐 Massage Considerations

Risks

- Heart attack survivors may or may not be able to keep up with the challenges offered by various types of bodywork; choose modalities that stay within the parameters of activities of daily living.
- Cardiovascular disease has many connected problems; obtain the client's full health history to avoid the risks of associated conditions.

Benefits

- Heart attack survivors who have good resilience and activity levels can enjoy the same benefits of massage as the rest of the population.
- Heart attack survivors who have a permanently compromised circulatory system can enjoy the benefits of reflexive or energetic techniques to promote relaxation without circulatory challenge.

---

heart failure

Heart failure is a term for the progressive loss of cardiac function that accompanies age, congenital problems, or a history of cardiovascular disease.

Heart failure is classified according to which side of the heart is affected. In left-sided heart failure, the left ventricle cannot push out enough blood through the aorta into the systemic circuit, leading to a backup of fluid in the lungs and pulmonary edema. Left-sided heart failure is closely connected to **atherosclerosis** and **hypertension.**

In right-sided heart failure, a history of lung disorders (especially **emphysema** and **chronic bronchitis**) creates resistance for the right ventricle. The result is a backup of fluid throughout the systemic circuit, which is seen as pronounced **edema** in the legs and feet. A person may have left- and right-sided heart failure simultaneously.

Heart failure is one of several closely interlinked cardiovascular disorders, including **aneurysm**, **stroke**, **renal failure**, and **heart attack**. Most heart failure patients have a history that includes at least some of these other issues.

Signs and Symptoms

- Shortness of breath (exacerbated by lying down), pulmonary edema
- Distal edema
- Low stamina
- Chest pain
- Indigestion
- Arrhythmia
- Distended veins in the neck
- Cold, sweaty skin
- Restlessness

Treatment Options

Early interventions for heart failure include rest, changes in diet, drugs, and modifications in physical activity so the heart can be exercised without becoming overly stressed.

If a patient doesn't respond well to these noninvasive treatment options, surgery may be considered. Surgery can range from repair to damaged valves to a complete heart or heart and lung transplant.

Medications

Drugs for heart failure include beta-blockers, digitalis, diuretics, and vasodilators.

Massage Considerations

Risks

- Heart failure contraindicates rigorous circulatory massage, which adds challenge to a system that cannot keep up with the patient's needs.

Benefits

- Energetic or reflexive modalities of bodywork may help reduce blood pressure and perceived stress, which may be useful for heart failure patients.

heat exhaustion, heat stroke

Heat exhaustion and heat stroke are disorders involving dehydration, loss of electrolytes, and failure of thermoregulation. They occur on a continuum of severity from very mild situations to life-threatening loss of function.

Radiation and evaporation are by far the most efficient mechanisms for heat loss from human bodies. When ambient temperatures exceed 95°F and humidity approaches 100%, neither radiation nor evaporation works well. Internal processes to shunt blood away from internal organs and out to the periphery to lower core temperature fail, so blood rushes back to the core and brain. This leads to cerebral edema, intracranial pressure, and a risk of brain damage. When core temperatures approach and exceed 106°F, cellular metabolism speeds to the extent that even more heat is produced. At these temperatures, the proteins that make up cells may begin to degenerate, ultimately leading to organ failure, especially of the kidneys and liver.

Heat exhaustion can lead to painful and alarming muscle **spasms**. This is an issue at many summertime sporting events.

Malignant hyperthermia is a related condition that involves an **allergic reaction** to certain types of anesthetics. This is a rare but dangerous condition that is often not discovered until a person has a surgery or dental work that involves using a triggering substance. It is an inherited condition, so if one family has it, other members are likely to have it as well.

Signs and Symptoms

- Heat exhaustion
  - Fatigue, weakness
  - Headache
  - Nausea, vomiting
  - Muscle cramps
  - Dizziness
  - Irritability
  - Tachycardia (rapid heart rate)
  - Internal temperature below 106°F
- Heat stroke
  - All signs of heat exhaustion
  - Internal temperature above 106°F
  - Central nervous system symptoms, including hallucinations, seizures, coma
  - Possible organ failure with hemorrhage

Treatment Options

The highest priority with hyperthermic injuries is to lower the person's core temperature, maintain the airways, and replace fluids. Tepid showers or baths along with ice packs on the neck, groin, and axillae and use of a fan to move air are typical strategies.

Aspirin and acetaminophen must be avoided during heat exhaustion and heat stroke because both of these substances can exacerbate the complications of heat-related illness.

Massage Considerations

Risks

- Heat exhaustion and heat stroke contraindicate massage. Athletes showing signs of these conditions at sporting events must be referred to the medical team.

Benefits

- People recuperating from a hyperthermic event may experience a shortened recovery period with gentle massage.
- Clients with a history of heat exhaustion or heat stroke but no current symptoms can enjoy the same benefits from massage as the rest of the population.

heat rash: see miliaria rubra

HELLP syndrome: see pregnancy-induced hypertension

hematoma

Hematoma refers to extensive bleeding and pooling of blood between muscle sheaths. The simple leakage of blood from damaged capillaries that causes the familiar discoloration of the skin known as a bruise is called ecchymosis. Bruises and hematomas are considered together here.

An occasional complication of hematoma is **myositis ossificans**. A subdural hematoma is a type of **stroke**. A tendency to bruise easily is an early indicator of **hemophilia** or **leukemia**. Easy bruising is also a side effect of many medications.

Signs and Symptoms

- Bruise: reddish or purplish discoloration; fades to greenish yellow
- Hematoma: inflammation with discoloration and pain, usually in large fleshy areas

Treatment Options

Small bruises do not require medical intervention, but they respond well to alternating hot and cold applications. Larger bleeds can be aspirated or drained. If they go without treatment, they may congeal from the concentration of clotting factors in the blood. At that point, only time, hydrotherapy, and gentle movement will help break up the pooled blood into a form that the body can reabsorb.

Medications

Painful bruises or hematomas may be treated with analgesics.

Massage Considerations

Risks

- Acute hematomas and bruises locally contraindicate massage, which can make the situation worse by bringing more blood to an already painful and congested area.

Benefits

- Subacute or postacute hematomas and bruises are appropriate for massage within pain tolerance; this may help promote faster healing and recovery.

hemophilia

Hemophilia is a collection of genetic disorders involving the absence of some plasma proteins that are crucial in the clot-forming process.

As an X-linked genetic anomaly, hemophilia is primarily seen in boys and men. It is possible that a girl could have hemophilia if she received a positive X chromosome from both her father and mother, but this is a rare circumstance. One type of mild hemophilia, von Willebrand disease, occurs in women as well as men.

When a hemophiliac bleeds into a joint, debilitating **osteoarthritis** may develop. Blood products contaminated with **HIV** or **hepatitis** are another risk. Although screening processes have made the blood supply much safer than it used to be, hemophilia patients are recommended to be vaccinated against hepatitis A and B.

Signs and Symptoms

- Signs are clear in early childhood
- Can range from mild to severe

- Extensive bruising and prolonged bleeding with only minor trauma
- High risk for nosebleeds, hematuria (blood in the urine), bleeding into the joints
- Bleeding may be spontaneous or related to minor trauma

Treatment Options

Hemophilia is treated with clotting factors that match the missing substances in the patient. These may be derived from plasma donations or through recombinant DNA. If these are insufficient, blood transfusions may be required.

Medications

Pain relievers must be chosen carefully because several common analgesics interfere with blood clotting. Acetaminophen is usually the preferred option for hemophilia patients.

Massage Considerations

Risks

- Hemophilia contraindicates rigorous circulatory massage and any other modality that may cause bruising.

Benefits

- Energetic or reflexive techniques can help with pain relief and quality of life for clients with hemophilia.

---

hemorrhoids

Hemorrhoids are the result of varicosities of a group of veins around the anus called the hemorrhoidal plexus. They occur most frequently in mature people, especially those who sit for long periods and who also have chronic constipation or diarrhea or who must strain vigorously to pass a bowel movement.

Varicosities of the hemorrhoidal veins can occur outside or inside the anus. They can range from being very mild to severe. They tend to recur, so even when a person has had hemorrhoidal surgery, he or she may continue to have a risk of future problems.

Pregnancy and **obesity** both increase the risk of hemorrhoids. **Colorectal cancer**, chronic constipation, and advanced age with loss of muscle tone are other contributing factors.

Signs and Symptoms

- Local pain
- Itching after defecation
- Bleeding with bowel movements
- Feeling of incomplete evacuation
- Possible ulcers around the anus

Treatment Options

Dietary changes or fiber supplements can soften the stool for better evacuation. More advanced hemorrhoids with pain and bleeding may be surgically removed; a number of different surgical procedures have been developed to work with different types and locations of hemorrhoids.

Medications

Topical creams can reduce pain and itching. If these along with dietary changes are insufficient, surgery may be considered.

 Massage Considerations

Risks
- Massage has no specific risks for clients with hemorrhoids.

Benefits
- Massage has no specific benefits for clients with hemorrhoids, but careful abdominal work may promote overall better colon function.

hepatitis

Hepatitis is usually a viral infection of the liver. Although seven types of viral hepatitis have been identified, about 90% of all cases in the United States are caused by hepatitis viruses A, B, and C.

Hepatitis B and C both significantly increase the risk for developing **cirrhosis** or **liver cancer**. The risk is higher when hepatitis infection is present along with **HIV/AIDS** or **alcoholism**.

Chronic hepatitis infections can also lead to ascites and varicosities in the stomach and esophagus, which may rupture and bleed.

hepatitis A

Hepatitis A is communicable primarily through oral–fecal contamination, although intimate contact can also spread the infection. Up to 30% of Americans have antibodies for hepatitis A, showing that they've been exposed to this virus.

hepatitis B

Hepatitis B is communicable through shared fluids, specifically through unprotected sex and shared intravenous needles or contaminated tattoo or piercing equipment. It occurs in high viral loads, so even a limited exposure may lead to a new infection. Most people who are exposed to hepatitis B recover fully with immunity and no serious problems, but about 5% develop chronic infections and may be long-term carriers of the virus. Within that group of patients, the risk of developing liver cancer or cirrhosis later in life is higher than that of the general population.

hepatitis C

Similar to hepatitis B, hepatitis C is spread through shared fluids and causes long-term chronic infections. Only 15% to 25% of people infected with hepatitis C recover spontaneously; the other 75% to 85% experience chronic infection. Although it may take many years for symptoms to develop, many people infected with hepatitis C develop cirrhosis within 10 to 20 years, and the risk of liver cancer is much higher than that for the general population.

Signs and Symptoms
- Varying severity and duration, depending on which type of virus is present
- Weakness, fatigue, malaise
- Fever

- Food aversion
- Dark urine, pale stools
- Jaundice

Treatment Options

Treatment for hepatitis A is a combination of rest, fluids, and good sense. Hepatitis B and C are treated with various antiviral medications. Almost half of all the liver transplants conducted in the United States every year are related to hepatitis C infections.

Medications

Gamma globulin shots may be recommended for people infected with hepatitis A. Antivirals, including types of interferon and lamivudine, are recommended for those with hepatitis B and C.

Massage Considerations

Risks

- Acute hepatitis with severe symptoms contraindicates rigorous circulatory massage because the liver may not be able to keep up with the changes that massage brings about.

Benefits

- Clients with a chronic form of hepatitis that is well controlled may benefit from massage that stays within their capacity for resilience and adaptation.
- Massage promotes immune system efficiency and parasympathetic balance.

Practitioner Advice

- Hygienic practices have been developed to help minimize the risk of spreading infections in health care settings. Hepatitis B is a virus that is particularly stable outside of a host. This pathogen, more than most, is a target for hygienic practices that include careful laundering and cleaning of surfaces that clients directly or indirectly contact.

hernia

Hernias are holes in tissue through which something protrudes. Abdominal hernias can be caused by a number of different factors, including congenital weakness of the muscular wall; childbirth; and abnormal straining, which increase internal abdominal pressure. Hiatal hernias involve an enlargement of the diaphragmatic hiatus that allows the stomach to protrude into the thoracic cavity.

Most hernias are reducible, which means that the protrusion can easily be put back where it belongs manually, but the hole tends to get bigger, with a risk of future bulges. Therefore, after a hernia has been identified, surgery to tighten up or close the hole is usually recommended sooner rather than later.

The most common type of hernia is an inguinal hernia. In this situation, the opening for the spermatic cord to enter the abdomen is a structural weak spot. A sudden change in internal abdominal pressure caused by coughing, sneezing, or heavy lifting may force a section of small intestine into the opening at this point.

Untreated hernias can lead to strangulation of intestinal tissue. Nausea, vomiting, and dangerous infections of the obstructed material may result. Hiatal hernias are frequently linked to **gastroesophageal reflux disorder**.

Signs and Symptoms

- Hiatal hernia: gastric reflux
- Epigastric hernia: split in the linea alba; protrusion superior to the navel
- Femoral hernia: mostly occur in women; protrusion of abdominal contents into the inguinal ring
- Inguinal hernia: most common type; protrusion through the abdominal wall at the site of the spermatic cord

Treatment Options

Surgery is frequently recommended even for mild hernias because they tend to get worse as time goes on. The standard surgical technique involves inserting a small piece of mesh at the site of the tear. This helps to distribute the force of abdominal pressure more evenly than do stitches or staples alone, reducing the risk of subsequent hernias at the site of the surgery.

Medications

Hernias are not treated with medications except analgesics to help manage pain.

Massage Considerations

Risks

- Unrepaired hernias locally contraindicate any massage that may stretch the weakened abdominal wall.

Benefits

- Clients with a history of hernia can enjoy the same benefits from massage as the rest of the population.

herniated disc: see disc disease

herpes simplex

Herpes simplex is a virus that causes painful blisters on a red base. Oral herpes occurs anywhere around or inside the mouth, and genital herpes can occur anywhere around the groin, sacrum, or buttocks. Other herpes simplex infections can affect other parts of the body.

A person's first outbreak, which usually 2 to 20 days after exposure, is called primary herpes. All subsequent outbreaks are called recurrent herpes. A primary herpes outbreak may be almost unnoticeable. Most cases of oral herpes are contracted during childhood, and the new carrier may never be aware of his or her infection.

After the primary outbreak, the virus goes into hiding. It waits for an appropriate trigger, which could be a fever, a systemic infection, a sunburn, stress, a menstrual period, or something that is never identified. When the virus reactivates, a recurrent outbreak occurs, usually at or near the site of the original infection.

Secondary bacterial infection is a common complication of herpes lesions. Vaginally delivered newborns of mothers with active genital herpes may experience blindness or brain damage. Genital herpes has also been statistically connected with higher rates of **cervical cancer,** so infected women are wise to have frequent Pap smears performed. The herpes simplex virus has also been linked to **encephalitis** and **meningitis**.

Herpes simplex lesions usually appear on or around the mouth or genitals, but it is possible for them to appear elsewhere on the body as well. Of special concern to massage therapists is a variety called herpes Whitlow, which is an outbreak of lesions around the nailbeds of the hands. Herpes gladiatorum is a variety of herpes simplex found on the trunk and extremities picked up from athletic mats by wrestlers.

Signs and Symptoms

- Pain or tingling before the lesion appears (prodromic stage)
- Painful, itchy blisters on a red base
- Scabbing after several days
- Whole outbreak may last 2 to 3 weeks

Treatment Options

Prevention is the main thrust for treatment of this condition; this means isolating towels, bedding, and clothing and avoiding sexual contact while lesions are present. Keeping as healthy as possible between outbreaks is an important way to reduce the frequency and severity of herpes episodes.

Medications

A variety of drugs that suppress viral activity and shorten herpes outbreaks are available, but they must be administered at the beginning of the outbreak to be useful. These drugs can also be administered prophylactically to reduce the frequency of herpes simplex outbreaks.

Topical creams for oral herpes can offer viral suppression or pain relief.

Massage Considerations

Risks

- The herpes simplex virus is stable outside of a host. Ideally, clients with active herpes lesions should reschedule their massage. If this is not possible, extra precautions for hygiene should be followed.
- Herpes simplex virus may be communicable during the invisible prodromic phase of infection.
- Herpes lesions contraindicate massage locally. If they are accompanied by fever, malaise, or inflamed lymph nodes, the client may have a secondary infection and should seek medical help.

Benefits

- Clients with a history of herpes but no current lesions or symptoms can enjoy the same benefits from massage as the rest of the population.

Practitioner Advice

- Oral herpes simplex lesions can be itchy and irritating, and it can be difficult to avoid touching the virus-filled blisters. On days when a client has an active herpes lesion, it might be wise to avoid massaging his or her hands.

herpes zoster

Also known as shingles, this condition is a viral infection of the nervous system. The causative agent, varicella zoster, also causes chickenpox. Similar to other members of the herpes virus family, this virus is never fully eradicated from the body. Instead, it goes into a dormant state in the dorsal root ganglia. The virus reactivates when the immune system is weak, and the new infection is usually not chickenpox, but shingles: painful blisters that grow directly on the sensory dendrites of the skin.

The most common complication of herpes zoster is secondary bacterial infection of the blisters. Other complications involve damage to the trigeminal nerve, which can lead to vision problems, hearing loss, and temporary or permanent facial paralysis; this is called **Ramsey-Hunt syndrome**. Herpes zoster occasionally leads to secondary viral and bacterial infections. **Pneumonia**, **encephalitis**, and **meningitis** are all possible complications of this disease.

Signs and Symptoms

- Intense pain before, during, and after blisters erupt
- Pain may persist after lesions heal (postherpetic neuralgia)
- Unilateral presentation of painful blisters in patches along a single dermatome

Treatment Options

Herpes zoster is treated mainly palliatively with a variety of soothing lotions and medications. Chickenpox "booster shots" are now being developed to help prevent herpes zoster outbreaks in adults.

Medications

Antiviral medications can shorten but not prevent herpes zoster. Steroids and analgesics may be used to reduce pain and inflammation.

🖐 Massage Considerations

Risks

- Herpes zoster is extremely painful; clients with acute outbreaks are unlikely to keep massage appointments.
- A mild case that can be covered and kept comfortable is only a local contraindication.

Benefits

- A client with postherpetic neuralgia may find that gentle massage is soothing.
- Clients who have recovered from shingles can enjoy the same benefits of massage as the rest of the population.

heterotopic ossification: see myositis ossificans

hiatal hernia: see hernia

hip replacement: see joint replacement surgery

HIV/AIDS

AIDS (acquired immune deficiency syndrome) is a viral infection with HIV (human immunodeficiency virus) that attacks various agents of the immune system with disastrous results.

HIV enters the body by way of body fluids (blood, semen, vaginal secretions, and breast milk). The first target of HIV is nonspecific macrophages and monocytes. From there, the virus moves up the hierarchy of the immune system to infect the T cells. Without T cells, the entire immune system collapses and leaves the body vulnerable to a wide array of opportunistic diseases.

Early HIV infection can resemble symptoms of **influenza** or **mononucleosis**. Later stages leave a person vulnerable to a number of diseases that are not usually threats to the general population. These include *Pneumocystis jiroveci* pneumonia, **cytomegalovirus** (CMV), Kaposi sarcoma, non-Hodgkin **lymphoma, peripheral neuropathy,** toxoplasmosis, **candidiasis, herpes simplex, herpes zoster, tuberculosis, meningitis, cervical cancer,** and many others.

Signs and Symptoms

- Phase 1: early infection: no symptoms
- Phase 2: fever, malaise, inflamed lymph nodes
- Phase 3: asymptomatic phase
- Phase 4: T-cell counts decrease below $200/mL^3$; indicator diseases develop

Treatment Options

The most successful AIDS treatments to date have targeted the process of viral replication. Although the goal of fully eradicating the virus from infected patients is still a long way off, studies of people who manage to efficiently control their infections will continue to point the way to better treatment options.

Medications

A variety of drugs work to prolong phase 3 of HIV infection. Other medications may be prescribed to help manage some of the side effects of HIV drugs.

Massage Considerations

Risks

- Clients who are HIV positive may be immunocompromised and at risk for picking up minor infectious agents that might be carried by their massage therapists; extra care for good health and hygiene are necessary to keep these clients safe.
- Clients with end-stage AIDS may be quite fragile and unable to adapt to the challenges of rigorous massage.

Benefits

- Clients who are HIV positive but asymptomatic can enjoy the same benefits from massage as the rest of the population.
- Massage improves immune system efficiency and may help increase T-cell counts.
- Clients with end-stage AIDS can benefit from reflexive or energetic work that promotes relaxation and pain relief.

Practitioner Advice

- Practitioners who observe standard precautions for hygiene are not at risk for catching HIV from infected clients. However, some of the secondary infections that may affect clients with AIDS can be spread through casual contact. These include tuberculosis, herpes simplex, and others.

hives

Hives, also called urticaria, are the result of emotional stress or an **allergic reaction**. Histamine release causes a localized inflammatory response, and the edema irritates nerve endings, causing itching.

Hives are closely related to **angioedema** (a very extreme inflammatory response in an isolated area) and **anaphylaxis** (a localized inflammatory response that may become systemic).

Signs and Symptoms

- Begin as small, red wheals
- May join into large, irregular patches
- Patches are itchy and hot
- May last for several hours or days

Medications

Hives are often treated with antihistamines or epinephrine to reduce swelling and itching.

 Massage Considerations

Risks

- Hives contraindicate massage in the acute phase; massage would only bring more blood into an area that is already overactive.
- Use hypoallergenic lubricants for clients with a history of skin allergies.

Benefits

- Massage has no specific benefits for hives.
- Clients with a history of hives and no current symptoms can enjoy the same benefits of massage as the rest of the population.

Hodgkin disease: see lymphoma

Huntington disease

Huntington disease is a condition in which a genetic defect leads to the degeneration of tissue in the brain. It is an incurable, progressive, and ultimately fatal disease.

This condition affects men and women equally and is seen across all parts of the population. It is most frequently diagnosed among adults between 30 and 50 years old, but it has been documented among both older and younger people.

Depression is often a part of the development of Huntington disease. The loss of cognitive function may be confused with **Alzheimer disease**. The development of tics or tremors may be confused with essential **tremor**. All of these disorders need to be investigated before coming to a conclusion about a diagnosis.

Signs and Symptoms

- Movement changes: tics, tremor, dystonia, bruxism (tooth grinding), difficulties with speech and swallowing
- Cognitive changes: memory loss, inability to learn new tasks
- Psychological changes: mood swings, depression, hallucinations, delusions

Treatment Options

Huntington disease is treated symptomatically, depending on which symptoms are most severe.

Medications

Antianxiety medication, antidepressants, tranquilizers, mood stabilizers, or botulinum toxin may be used to manage the symptoms of Huntington disease.

 Massage Considerations

Risks

- A client with Huntington disease may not be able to speak clearly or easily; this makes sensitivity to nonverbal forms of communication especially important.

Benefits

- People with Huntington disease are encouraged to stay as physically active as possible because this appears to delay progression. Massage as a part of a physically active lifestyle can certainly have a role in this strategy.

---

hyperhydrosis

Hyperhydrosis (also spelled hyperhidrosis) is a condition in which the body produces more sweat than necessary for temperature control. Both the apocrine and eccrine sweat glands are affected. The areas most frequently affected are the palms, soles, face, and axillae.

The mechanisms for excessive sweat production are not always clearly understood. Most primary cases of hyperhydrosis appear to be linked to stress, however, which makes it a self-fulfilling prophecy: a person may worry about "clammy palms," which leads to having clammy palms. Although not a threatening condition, hyperhydrosis may interfere with professional and personal relationships.

Hyperhydrosis is usually primary, but it may develop as a complication of an underlying condition such as **hypertension, hyperthyroidism, diabetes mellitus,** or **cancer.**

Signs and Symptoms

- Excessively sweaty palms, feet, face, or axillae
- Symptoms are exacerbated by temperature or stress

Treatment Options

A number of treatment options have been used to treat hyperhydrosis, ranging from antiperspirants to botulinum toxin injections to surgery that severs the sympathetic trunk at the affected levels.

Medications

Anticholinergic medications, sedatives, and tranquilizers can help treat hyperhydrosis, but they have several undesirable side effects.

 Massage Considerations

Risks

- Massage has no specific risks for clients with hyperhydrosis.

Benefits

- Massage has no specific benefits for clients with hyperhydrosis, but it can be a source of positive touch for clients who may feel isolated and self-conscious.

hyperkyphosis: see postural deviations

hyperlordosis: see postural deviations

hypertension

Hypertension is a technical term for high blood pressure. It is defined as blood pressure persistently elevated above 140 mg Hg systolic, or 90 mg Hg diastolic. Pressure inside and outside the arteries increases the risk of damage to the delicate tunica intima. This is often the first step in the development of other more serious forms of cardiovascular disease.

Chronic hypertension has many possible complications, including **edema, atherosclerosis** that develops from damage to the arterial walls, **stroke,** enlarged heart, **heart failure, aneurysm,** vision problems, and **renal failure.**

Signs and Symptoms

- Often no symptoms ("the silent killer")
- Possibly shortness of breath after mild exercise
- Headaches, dizziness
- Swelling of the ankles
- Excessive sweating

Treatment Options

Diet is the first strategy used to manage this condition. An appropriate diet reduces systolic blood pressure readings by anywhere from 6 to 11 points and diastolic blood pressure readings from 3 to 6 points within 2 weeks of initiating the change in eating habits.

Exercise is also crucial for the development of healthy new blood vessels, as well as for weight control. Losing even a small percentage of body weight for obese or overweight patients can have a profound affect on blood pressure and cardiovascular health.

Medications

Antihypertensive medications include digitalis, diuretics, vasodilators, and beta-blockers.

✍ Massage Considerations

Risks

- Clients with hypertension are at risk for several other problems that interfere with fluid management; obtain a whole health history before doing any rigorous circulatory massage.
- Antihypertensive medication and massage together can be a powerful combination. Allow extra transition time at the end of the session for the client to come back to full speed.

Benefits

- Clients who have hypertension but who are physically active can enjoy the same benefits of massage as the rest of the population, with the added bonus that massage can help lower blood pressure.

- Clients who have hypertension and are physically fragile can benefit from the relaxation and parasympathetic balance provided by energetic or reflexive forms of bodywork.

hyperthermia: see heat exhaustion, heat stroke

hyperthyroidism

Hyperthyroidism is a condition in which the thyroid gland produces excessive amounts of thyroid hormones T3 (triiodothyronine) and T4 (thyroxine). Most cases of hyperthyroidism are related to autoimmune attacks against the whole thyroid gland. In these cases, it may also be called Graves disease or diffuse toxic thyroid. More rarely, thyroid hyperactivity may be confined to one or more localized nodes or may be caused by a thyroid infection.

Hyperthyroidism is a potentially dangerous disease, and treatment tends to be aggressive. Consequently, many people who start with hyperthyroidism may develop **hypothyroidism** as a consequence of their treatment.

Signs and Symptoms
- Enlarged thyroid (goiter)
- Anxiety, irritability, insomnia
- Tachycardia (rapid heartbeat)
- Tremor
- Increased perspiration
- Extremely dry skin
- Atrophy of the muscles in the extremities
- Protruding eyes
- Risk of thyroid storm: episodes of hugely increased metabolic activity that can be life threatening

Treatment Options

Hyperthyroidism can be treated in a number of ways, depending on the underlying causes and the severity of the symptoms. Radioactive iodine can be used as a diagnostic tool to measure thyroid activity, but it can also be used to kill off a portion of the thyroid. Antithyroid medication can suppress thyroxine production or interfere with thyroxine activity. As a last resort, surgery may be conducted to remove part of the thyroid. This is avoided if possible because the risk of damage to the parathyroid glands and other structures in the throat is very high.

Medications

People with hyperthyroidism may use beta-blockers to help their control symptoms, or they may use drugs that interfere with the production of T3 and T4. These medications don't eradicate the problem, however, and symptoms recur when the drug regimen stops.

🖐 Massage Considerations

Risks
- Hyperthyroidism sometimes causes pathologically dry skin; this can be a local caution for massage.

Benefits
- If the skin is healthy and the client is comfortable, people with hyperthyroidism can enjoy the same benefits from massage as the rest of the population.
- Clients with hyperthyroidism may especially appreciate the relaxation that massage can help establish.

hypoglycemia

Hypoglycemia occurs when blood glucose levels are abnormally low. The normal range is 60 to 120 mg/dL; hypoglycemia is suspected when blood glucose decreases below 45 mg/dL.

Under normal circumstances, when blood glucose is low, the pancreas releases glucagon to act on the liver to release some sugar. Sometimes the liver may simply not be able to comply, or it responds too slowly. The body, especially the brain, is then in need of fuel and cannot function normally. Mild episodes of hypoglycemia can be annoying, but very extreme episodes can lead to loss of consciousness or even coma.

People with **diabetes** may experience bouts of hypoglycemia when a dose of insulin is not matched by adequate nutrition.

Signs and Symptoms
- Dizziness
- Hunger, nausea
- Headache
- Confusion, inability to concentrate
- Blurred vision
- Sweating and chills
- Shakiness
- Tachycardia (increased heart rate)

Treatment Options
The obvious treatment for hypoglycemia is to eat some easily accessible source of glucose. If episodes are frequent, the person should consult with his or her health care team to explore what factors are contributing to this imbalance.

🖐 Massage Considerations

Risks
- Some research suggests that massage decreases blood sugar, at least temporarily. A client whose blood sugar is unstable might consider keeping a snack close to hand in case he or she experiences a change during or immediately after a massage.

Benefits
- Clients who have occasional hypoglycemic episodes but no current symptoms can enjoy the same benefits from massage as the rest of the population.

hypotension

Hypotension is the condition of having blood pressure that is too low to supply the brain and other tissues with adequate oxygen. It can occur in a variety of circumstances, most having to do with blood pressure regulation systems. If the overall fluid volume or blood volume is low, blood vessels are too dilated, or the heart rate is too slow, the result is hypotension and a high risk of syncope, or fainting.

A person who regularly feels faint may have an underlying condition contributing to this symptom. **Hypoglycemia**, untreated **diabetes mellitus**, and **Addison disease** are all possibilities. Because this condition is often a side effect of medications, any other underlying conditions need to be addressed as well, including **hypertension** and other forms of cardiovascular disease.

Signs and Symptoms

- Dizziness
- Fainting
- Often occurs after exercise or standing up too fast

Treatment Options

Hypotension caused by medicine can often be addressed with adjustments to prescription medication. Other forms of hypotension are treated according to the underlying factors.

Medications

Medications associated with hypotension are the antihypertensive group, including beta-blockers, digitalis, angiotensin-converting enzyme (ACE) inhibitors, and diuretics. Any combination of these medications may have hypotension as a side effect, and adjustments in dosage and combinations may mitigate the problem.

 ## Massage Considerations

Risks

- Massage has no risks for clients with hypotension as long as underlying factors are understood and addressed.
- Clients with hypotension may need help sitting up and more time to transition back into the rest of their day after a massage session.

Benefits

- Massage has no specific benefits for hypotension. Clients with this condition can enjoy the same benefits from massage as the rest of the population.

hypothermia

Hypothermia is a condition in which a person's core temperature decreases below 95°F (35°C). At this point, the ability to create heat internally is lost, and the person needs external help to bring the body temperature back into normal range.

Primary hypothermia is usually brought about by accidental exposure to cold, and secondary hypothermia is brought about by a failure in thermoregulatory function. These phenomena may often overlap, for instance, when a person experiences a trauma such as a head injury or a stroke and then collapses on a cold surface for several hours. Other factors, such as intoxication, can interfere with both the ability to regulate the internal temperature and behavioral responses to cold, increasing the risk of hypothermia.

The people most at risk for life-threatening hypothermia are tiny babies and elderly people. In both these populations, the ability to generate internal heat is limited, and the ability to remove oneself from a cold environment may also be limited.

Persons being treated for hypothermia should also be checked for signs of **frostbite**.

Signs and Symptoms

- Ranges in severity from mild to severe
- Mild confusion
- Loss of fine motor skills
- Apnea (lack of breathing), rigidity

Treatment Options

Hypothermia is treated by heating the injured person. Heating should begin at the core and proceed peripherally. It needs to be done slowly because suddenly dilating blood vessels may lead to circulatory shock. People with mild cases of hypothermia are treated with applications of heated blankets or other tools; people with more severe cases may be treated with the intravenous application of heated fluids.

Massage Considerations

Risks

- A person with acute hypothermia is unlikely to seek massage; if this happens, medical intervention is a more logical choice.

Benefits

- Massage has no specific benefits for hypothermia. Clients who have recovered from this condition can enjoy the same benefits from massage as the rest of the population.

hypothyroidism

The purpose of thyroid hormones T3 (triiodothyronine) and T4 (thyroxine)is to stimulate the conversion of fuel (oxygen and calories) into energy. In hypothyroidism, inadequate amounts of thyroid hormones are produced, so incoming fuel is simply stored instead of used for energy.

Hypothyroidism can develop for a variety of reasons. Hashimoto thyroiditis is an autoimmune attack that suppresses thyroid activity. Many people who undergo treatment for **hyperthyroidism** end up with hypothyroidism. Hypothyroidism can be a birth defect when it is caused by an underdeveloped or missing thyroid gland. Exposure to some medications (especially lithium) or radiation can also suppress thyroid function.

Idiopathic hypothyroidism is the most common form of this disorder, and it is often linked with other chronic conditions, including **chronic fatigue syndrome** and **fibromyalgia**.

Hypothyroidism can also mimic or appear simultaneously with **anemia, candidiasis, sleep disorders, depression**, and other problems related to having low energy and stamina over a long period of time.

It is common for hypothyroid patients to develop **atherosclerosis** because the liver's function to produce the chemicals that expel cholesterol from the body is sluggish. People with high cholesterol levels caused by hypothyroidism do not respond to cholesterol-lowering medications. Fluid retention in the arms and wrists increases the risk of **carpal tunnel syndrome**; fluid retention in the neck along with goiter may cause chronic hoarseness. Very severe cases may cause a patient to become so cold and drowsy that he or she becomes unconscious. This is called myxedema coma, and it is a significant cause of death among elderly patients with hypothyroidism.

Signs and Symptoms

- Weight gain
- Low energy, fatigue, poor stamina

- Sluggish digestion, constipation
- Poor cold tolerance
- Dry, brittle hair
- Heavy menstrual periods
- Possible goiter

Treatment Options

The treatment for hypothyroidism is to supplement thyroid hormones. Hypothyroidism is a progressive disease, and medications must be monitored carefully to ensure that the patient is getting the correct dose.

Alternative methods to boost thyroid function or thyroid hormone uptake, especially acupuncture, reflexology, or acupressure, are successful for some patients with hypothyroidism.

Medications

Hypothyroidism patients often use synthetic or animal-based thyroid supplements to help control their condition. Desiccated animal glands are a useful source, but potency can vary significantly from one batch to another, so many patients find that they have to recalibrate their dosage frequently.

 Massage Considerations

Risks

- Clients with hypothyroidism have a high risk of atherosclerosis and heart disease. These conditions may influence decisions about bodywork, so a full health history is important in these situations.

Benefits

- Massage has no specific benefits for clients with hypothyroidism, but it may improve the quality of life of people who feel chronically drained and lethargic.

ichthyosis

Ichthyosis is a rare disorder in which the skin is pathologically dry. Although it can happen alone, it can also be a symptom of a variety of diseases. When it is a primary disorder, it usually appears on the legs of elderly people, especially in cold weather when the air is very dry; this may also be called xeroderma.

When ichthyosis is a secondary symptom, it can indicate a congenital problem associated with birth defects or certain rare neurologic diseases. Other cases are connected to a variety of diseases, including Hodgkin **lymphoma**, **HIV/AIDS**, **hypothyroidism**, and **Hansen disease**.

Signs and Symptoms

- Dry skin in a distinctive diamond-shaped pattern
- The affected area may be darker than the surrounding skin

Treatment Options

People with ichthyosis need to take special care to preserve the protective coating of sebum on their skin. This is accomplished by bathing less frequently and by applying emollients to the skin while it is still wet. A variety of preparations may be applied to help soften and remove the scales that develop with ichthyosis; these depend on the age of the patient and the cause and severity of the person's disorder.

Medications

Ichthyosis is typically treated with topical ointments or creams to improve the quality and health of the skin. Occasionally, patients may be prescribed oral medications (retinoids) that affect epithelial cell activity.

Massage Considerations

Risks

- Dry skin may crack and bleed; this is at least a local caution.
- Underlying pathologies that may lead to ichthyosis should be understood because some of them may influence decisions about bodywork.

Benefits

- Nonirritating, hypoallergenic lubricants may improve the quality and health of the affected skin.

impetigo

Impetigo is a bacterial infection of the skin. It affects children more often than adults, but anyone can get it. Lesions usually occur around the nose and mouth, sometimes appearing inside the nostrils or ear canals. Although it usually begins somewhere on the head, impetigo can infect the skin anywhere on the body.

Signs and Symptoms

- Rash with small, itchy blisters or pustules filled with clear or murky fluid
- Often occurs where skin is chapped or undergoes a lot of friction
- Blisters are followed by honey-colored crusts

Treatment Options

This is an extremely contagious condition, and because it is both very itchy and most common in children, special precautions are recommended to prevent its spread. The patient must be discouraged from touching or scratching the lesions; impetigo can easily be spread to other parts of the body this way. The lesions must be kept clean and dry, and the crusts must be removed as soon as possible because they harbor bacteria in the moisture underneath. The patient's bedding and towels must be strictly isolated while the infection is present.

Medications

Topical or oral antibiotics are the typical treatment strategy for impetigo.

Massage Considerations

Risks
- Impetigo is highly contagious; it contraindicates massage until the lesions have completely healed.

Benefits
- Massage has no specific benefits for clients with acute impetigo.
- Clients who have recovered from impetigo can enjoy the same benefits from massage as the rest of the population.

Practitioner Advice
- If a client has a child with impetigo at home, the chance is high that the client may be carrying some aggressive bacteria. Consider taking extra precautions about hygiene or encouraging the client to reschedule after the child's infection has cleared.

---

impingement syndrome

Impingement syndrome is an umbrella term for any situation that causes soft tissue to be pinched or obstructed, usually near a joint. It is reported most often in the shoulder (involving the supraspinatus and acromioclavicular joints), but it can also occur at the elbow, knee, and ankle.

Causative factors for impingement syndrome vary by the joint and the person involved. They often begin with a trauma that causes soft tissue inflammation. The accumulation of fluid and scar tissue then presses on the nearby structures, causing pain and loss of range of motion. In some cases, impingement syndrome is brought about by anomalies in the shapes of nearby bones or joints. Left untreated, impingement syndrome may ultimately lead to the tearing or even rupture of affected tendons or ligaments.

Impingement syndrome may be difficult to distinguish from **bursitis** or **tendinopathy**; furthermore, these conditions can be present simultaneously.

People most at risk for most types of impingement syndromes are elderly people, whose tissue tends to be easily injured, and athletes who use repetitive, high-force contractions of specific muscle groups.

Signs and Symptoms
- Pain on active and resistive movement at the affected joint
- Loss of range of motion
- At the glenohumeral joint: asymmetrical scapular winging

Treatment Options

Mild cases of impingement syndrome are treated with physical therapy to re-establish balance in the tensions that surround joints. Surgical intervention usually aims at removing fibrotic material or bone spurs and relieving pressure on the soft tissues.

Medications

Steroid injections may be used to help decrease the local inflammation seen with impingement syndrome. Proliferant therapy can help rebuild frayed tendons or ligaments. Analgesics may be recommended for pain management.

Massage Considerations

Risks

- As long as the therapist works within the client's pain tolerance, massage has no specific risks for impingement syndrome.

Benefits

- Massage may help address muscular imbalances that develop around a joint that is impaired.
- Massage may assist in the speed and quality of healing for clients who are being treated for impingement syndrome.

impotence: see erectile dysfunction

infant torticollis: see torticollis

inflammation

Inflammation is a reaction of injured tissue to defend and protect the body from invasion. This reaction is specifically designed to achieve three basic goals: to dispose of pathogens and cellular debris, prevent the spread of pathogens in the body, and prepare the injured area for healing.

Inflammation occurs in several stages; the length of time each one takes depends on the severity of the injury. The acute phase involves a rapid swing from local vasoconstriction to vasodilation. The activity of mast cells, white blood cells, and platelets helps to isolate the damage and prevent any spread of pathogens deeper into the system.

In the subacute stage, fibroblasts migrate to the injured area to begin to generate the connective tissue that will knit the damaged tissue back together, and slower-moving white blood cells arrive to clean up debris.

In the maturation phase, new scar tissue becomes denser and aligns according to weight-bearing stress. This phase determines how functional scar tissue is where musculoskeletal injuries heal.

Signs and Symptoms

- Pain, heat, redness, swelling
- Loss of function
- Itching, clotting, pus formation
- Enlarged painful area near the lymph nodes if infection is present

Treatment Options

Nondrug interventions for inflammation include RICE therapy (rest, ice, compression, and elevation).

Medications

Anti-inflammatory medications can be steroidal or nonsteroidal. These drugs interfere with the inflammatory process in a variety of ways, and each has potential side effects that can range from stomach irritation to liver failure.

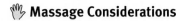 **Massage Considerations**

Risks

- Acute inflammation locally contraindicates circulatory massage, which can make symptoms worse.
- Inflammation caused by acute or untreated infection contraindicates massage.
- Anti-inflammatory drugs can mask pain, so massage in this context must be conservative to avoid the risk of overtreatment.

Benefits

- Reflexive, energetic, or lymphatic modalities can be effective in reducing inflammation as long as no infection is present.
- Inflammation caused by subacute or postacute musculoskeletal injury indicates massage within pain tolerance; this can work to speed the healing process.

---

inflammatory bowel disease: see Crohn disease, ulcerative colitis

---

influenza

Influenza, or flu, is a viral infection of the respiratory tract. The virus invades and attacks mucus-producing cells that line the respiratory tract. The inflammatory response produces fever and a sore throat as leukocytes attack infected mucous membrane cells.

Flu viruses have the ability to mutate as they develop resistance to attack. This makes it impossible for the body to establish permanent immunity; each time it is exposed, the pathogen is different.

Avian flu, or "bird flu," is a variety of virus that spreads easily between birds (including domestic poultry), but so far, it doesn't spread efficiently from bird to human or from human to human. These viruses mutate quickly though, and authorities are preparing in case avian flu is comes a significant health concern in coming years.

Flu can be difficult to differentiate from the **common cold**. One difference is that flu is more likely to progress to **pneumonia** or **acute bronchitis**. This is a particular danger for high-risk populations, including very young and very old people, heavy smokers, people with **diabetes**, people who are immune suppressed, people living in long-term care facilities, and people with chronic lung or heart problems.

Signs and Symptoms

- Range from mild to severe
- Respiratory irritation, runny nose, dry cough
- Fever above 102°F
- Aching muscles and joints; fatigue
- Symptoms lasting up to 2 weeks

Treatment Options

Common sense measures for this viral infection include rest and liquids. Over-the-counter drugs may abate the symptoms but do not speed healing. These medications can be useful; however, if the symptoms are preventing a person from getting the sleep he or she needs to heal.

Medications
Some antiviral medications can help shorten a bout with flu.

 ## Massage Considerations

Risks
- Flu contraindicates massage while it is in early stages.

Benefits
- Massage after the infection has peaked may help speed healing, but symptoms may be exacerbated for a short time. The client should know this risk before proceeding.

Practitioner Advice
- Flu can continue to be communicable for a few days after symptoms begin to subside; this is a risk for massage therapists, who must work hard to stay healthy.

insomnia: see sleep disorders

insulin resistance syndrome: see metabolic syndrome

intermittent claudication: see peripheral artery disease

interstitial cystitis

Interstitial cystitis (IC) occurs when the inner lining of the bladder no longer protects the organ from the acidity of urine. As the problem progresses, the muscular wall of the bladder becomes irritated and then fibrotic and inelastic. Patients find that they have little capacity for storing urine; it is not unusual for them to have to use the bathroom about every 20 minutes.

Many IC patients have symptoms of other chronic pain syndromes, including **fibromyalgia** and **irritable bowel syndrome.**

Signs and Symptoms
- Urinary frequency
- Pain and burning with urination
- Painful intercourse
- May progressively worsen and then stabilize or spontaneously resolve
- May run in cycles of flare-ups and remissions

Treatment Options
Treatment for IC is generally aimed at symptomatic relief and the development of coping skills. The diagnostic tool of bladder distension can often give relief, as can a "distillation" or bladder wash; this is done with dimethyl sulfoxide (DMSO), which can pass into the bladder wall to act as an anti-inflammatory agent and block pain sensations. Exercise, stopping smoking, and dietary changes are also recommended.

Some patients have such severe problems that surgery becomes an option. They may have a new bladder constructed from a segment of the colon, or they may have the bladder removed altogether and replaced with a stoma and external bag.

Medications

Aspirin and other painkillers may be recommended for IC patients. Some other drugs may be used to treat IC, including tranquilizers, antispasmodics, and drugs that promote the regrowth of the bladder lining.

 ## Massage Considerations

Risks
- Massage has no risks for clients with IC as long as they are comfortable on the table.

Benefits
- Many IC patients have other chronic stress-related conditions. Massage may be a useful part of their treatment strategy as long as their need for frequent urination can be met.

iritis, uveitis

Iritis is the inflammation of the iris of the eye. An associated condition, uveitis, refers to inflammation of the iris along with other structures that form the uveal tract of the eye.

Inflammation of the iris or uveal tract can occur as a result of trauma, infection, or autoimmune dysfunction, but it is idiopathic up to 50% of the time. Left untreated, it can lead to adhesions between the lens and the iris and subsequent damage to the optic nerve.

Iritis and uveitis are often complications of underlying autoimmune disorders or infections. Common factors include **lupus, ankylosing spondylitis, sarcoidosis,** and **rheumatoid arthritis**. Infections that may affect the iris include **herpes simplex** and **zoster, syphilis, Lyme disease,** and **tuberculosis**. It is important to distinguish between iritis/uveitis and **conjunctivitis,** which responds to different treatment options.

Signs and Symptoms
- Unilateral eye pain and redness
- Sensitivity to light
- Blurred vision
- Constricted pupil
- Pain with constriction of the other pupil as well
- Abnormal or cloudy aqueous humor fluid

Treatment Options

Dark glasses and warm packs are recommended for iritis or uveitis if they provide some relief. Iritis caused by trauma or infection often clears up within 1 week. Inflammation connected to autoimmune dysfunction may be chronic and recurrent.

Medications

Iritis and uveitis are typically treated with antispasmodics to relax the iris muscle and anti-inflammatory eye drops if no infection is present. Otherwise, antibiotic eye drops may be prescribed.

 ## Massage Considerations

Risks
- Eye inflammation that is not caused by infection is a local caution for massage, but it is important to know whether infection is a factor.

• Eye inflammation that is part of an autoimmune disease process may be connected to other factors that influence choices for bodywork.

Benefits

• Massage has no direct benefits for iritis or uveitis, but it can improve the quality of life for people who live with these conditions.

irritable bowel syndrome

Irritable bowel syndrome (IBS) is a condition in which the bowel is hyperreactive to minor stimuli. In IBS, peristalsis, which should be smooth and rhythmic, becomes uncoordinated and irregular. No injury or structural changes in the digestive tract are observable.

IBS symptoms may mimic several serious digestive system conditions. In particular, **colorectal cancer**, **ulcerative colitis**, and **Crohn disease** must be eliminated as possibilities. Other gastrointestinal tract problems that can look like IBS include parasitic infestations (i.e., *Giardia* infection), food **allergies**, and chronic infections.

IBS frequently appears in conjunction with **fibromyalgia** or **chronic fatigue syndrome**.

Signs and Symptoms

• Abdominal pain, cramps, gas, bloating
• Diarrhea
• Constipation
• Alternating between diarrhea and constipation

Treatment Options

The first treatment for IBS is to consider dietary and stress factors. Nicotine, caffeine, alcohol, and dairy products have been found to be particularly irritating, but no particular food or drink is a definitive trigger for IBS attacks for all patients. Some doctors recommend fiber supplementation; the addition of bulk to the diet can fill the colon more completely and help limit spasms.

IBS is generally considered to be a lifelong condition, so patients are encouraged to find their own best ways to cope through dietary changes, therapy, and relaxation techniques.

Medications

Drug intervention for IBS usually involves antispasmodics, antidiarrheals, antacids, and antidepressants.

 Massage Considerations

Risks

• As long as the client is comfortable, massage carries no risk for IBS patients.

Benefits

• Massage is useful for many IBS patients as long as the individual welcomes touch. It is important to treat these clients very conservatively, especially with any mechanical work around the abdomen, but many of them respond well to the autonomic balancing that bodywork provides.

J

jaundice

Jaundice, from the French *jaune* (yellow), is not a disease in itself but rather a symptom of an underlying liver or gallbladder pathology leading to the accumulation of bilirubin in the blood.

Several types of jaundice have been identified, each categorized by the pathology that created the problem.

- Neonatal jaundice is a condition among newborns involving a liver that is too young to keep up with the normal turnover of red blood cells.
- Hemolytic jaundice is related to any variety of hemolytic **anemia**.
- Hepatic jaundice is related to **malaria, hepatitis, cirrhosis,** or **liver cancer.**
- Extrahepatic jaundice is brought about by an obstruction to bile flow from the liver, as may be seen with **gallstones, pancreatic cancer,** or advanced **pregnancy.**

Signs and Symptoms

- Yellow staining of the skin, mucous membranes, sclera of the eyes
- Dark urine
- Pale feces

Treatment Options

Jaundice is treated according to the underlying cause of liver dysfunction.

Massage Considerations

Risks

- Jaundice accompanies liver dysfunction. Rigorous massage should not be performed until the underlying liver problems have been identified and managed.

Benefits

- Massage has no specific benefits for clients with jaundice. Energetic or reflexive techniques may be welcomed, depending on the client's underlying pathologies.

joint replacement surgery

Joint replacement surgery, or arthroplasty, is a surgical procedure in which damaged bone and cartilage is replaced with artificial surfaces. It is a common intervention for debilitating arthritis of the knee and hip, but it can also be used in joints of the hand, shoulder, and elsewhere.

Specific techniques and materials used in arthroplastic surgery vary depending on the patient's age and activity level. Some prosthetic surfaces are cemented into the affected bones, and other types use porous materials that are eventually infiltrated by new bone growth. These "cementless" prostheses tend to involve a longer recovery period, but they are often more durable than cemented joint replacements.

Joint replacements are usually prescribed to improve the quality of life for people with advanced forms of arthritis. Osteoarthritis is the most common cause of joint damage, but arthroplasty may also be recommended for people with rheumatoid arthritis, lupus, avascular osteonecrosis, and other joint damaging diseases.

Immediate complications related to joint replacement surgery include deep vein thrombosis and pulmonary embolism, allergic reactions to anesthesia and pain medication, and infection of the incision or of the joint itself. Longer-term complications may involve chipping of the cement, receding bone mass away from the prosthesis, or loosening of the joint. These long-term problems may require additional corrective surgery.

Medications

People with new joint replacements may take anticoagulants and antibiotics to reduce their risk of postsurgical complications.

People who have had joint replacements in the past may manage their pain with a variety of nonsteroidal anti-inflammatory drugs.

Massage Considerations

Risks

- Recent surgeries have risks for serious complications, including blood clots and infection. Rigorous massage must be delayed until these risks subside.
- Clients with joint replacements have a more limited range of motion than others, and the consequences of stretching beyond this range are serious. Extra care must be taken when performing stretches or positioning clients to preserve a safe range of motion.

Benefits

- People with new joint replacements are encouraged to become physically active as quickly as possible. Massage within pain tolerance and that doesn't overstress range of motion limitations can have a helpful place in rehabilitation as well.
- Clients with older joint replacements can enjoy the same benefits from massage as the rest of the population, as long as limitations in the range of motion are respected.

jumper's knee: see patellofemoral syndrome

K

keloid scars

Keloid scars are overgrowths of dense connective tissue that develop beyond the borders of an original wound. Keloids are related to an imbalance in the rate of collagen production and collagen destruction during the healing process.

Signs and Symptoms

- Large, discolored, hairless deposits of scar tissue on the surface of the skin
- May develop at the site of any trauma (e.g., acne, piercings, surgical scars)
- Pinkish with a hard, rubbery texture
- Not painful but may occasionally itch or burn

Treatment Options

Keloids can be difficult to treat because they often recur after excision. Some treatment options include steroid injections to reduce collagen deposits, cryotherapy, radiation, and excision followed by high-pressure dressings.

👋 Massage Considerations

Risks
- Massage has no specific risks for keloid scars.

Benefits
- Massage has no specific benefits for keloid scars. Clients with this condition can enjoy the same benefits from bodywork as the rest of the population.

kidney cancer: see renal cancer

kidney cysts: see polycystic kidneys

kidney failure: see renal failure

kidney infection: see pyelonephritis

kidney stones

Also called renal calculi or nephrolithiases, kidney stones are crystals that develop in the renal pelvis. Kidney stones can be composed of several different substances, each one indicative of a different type of metabolic problem. The majority of kidney stones are related to dehydration and problems with calcium metabolism. Other stones may be composed of struvite, cystine, uric acid, or other substances.

Kidney stones can be caused by chronic **pyelonephritis**, and they can also increase the risk of infection. Large stones that disrupt kidney function may also contribute to **renal failure**.

Signs and Symptoms
- Most are silent
- Caused by irritation to the lining of the ureters
- Renal colic: extreme, sharp flank pain with a sudden onset
- Nausea and vomiting may occur
- Fever and chills may occur

Treatment Options

Depending on the size and location of the stone, various treatment options may be pursued. Surgery to remove the stone through a tiny tunnel in the back may be conducted. Uretoscopic stone removal uses a flexible tube to remove the stone from the ureters. Sound waves may be used to break up stones into a size that can be passed safely through the ureters.

People with a history of kidney stones are at increased risk for repeat episodes. Drinking a lot of water and watching the salt and calcium intake can help reduce this risk.

Medications

Several drugs can be prescribed to manage or prevent kidney stones. Diuretics can influence calcium absorption. Some drugs affect uric acid production and excretion, and others affect cystine and struvite production.

Massage Considerations

Risks

- Passing a large kidney stone is extremely painful. A person in this situation needs medical intervention rather than massage.

Benefits

- Clients with a history of kidney stones can enjoy the same benefits from bodywork as the rest of the population. Be sure to encourage drinking a lot of water after the session.

knee replacement: see joint replacement surgery

kyphosis: see postural deviations

L

labyrinthitis: see vertigo

lactose intolerance

Lactose intolerance is a condition that is usually related to a low level of lactase, a digestive enzyme that breaks down lactose into absorbable substances. A strong genetic component is behind most cases of lactose intolerance. Although most humans secrete ample lactase in the first few years of life, not many tend to do so into adulthood. Among Africans, Native Americans, and Asians, rates of lactose intolerance run between 75% and 90%.

Some experts suggest that lactose intolerance leads to bone loss and ultimately an increased risk of osteoporosis. This risk can be avoided if calcium is derived from nondairy sources.

Signs and Symptoms

- Gas, bloating, flatulence, loose stools, and nausea when dairy products are consumed

Treatment Options

A number of options are available to lactose-intolerant people. Introducing dairy foods in small amounts or in forms such as yogurt or hard cheeses may be tolerated well. Simply avoiding dairy products altogether and using other nutritional sources for calcium is another a usable strategy.

Medications

Some people with lactose intolerance supplement lactase enzymes.

Massage Considerations

Risks

- Massage has no specific risks for clients who are lactose intolerant.

Benefits
- Massage has no specific benefits for clients who are lactose intolerant; these clients can enjoy the same benefits from bodywork as the rest of the population.

laryngitis

Laryngitis is inflammation of the larynx, the section of respiratory tract that holds the vocal cords. When these structures are inflamed, they don't vibrate freely. Consequently, the person temporarily loses his or her voice.

Laryngitis is usually a complication of a viral infection (**common cold** or **flu**), but overuse, **allergic reactions**, or **gastroesophageal reflux disease** (GERD) can also inflame the larynx. Rarely, **tuberculosis, syphilis**, fungal infections, or laryngeal cancer can cause symptoms of laryngitis.

Signs and Symptoms
- Hoarseness
- Inflamed lymph nodes
- Usually seen with a cold or the flu

Treatment Options

Viral laryngitis is typically treated with humidifiers, rest, and avoiding cigarette smoke. Otherwise, laryngitis is treated according to the contributing factors.

Medications

If laryngitis is found to be linked to GERD, the patient may be prescribed a proton pump inhibitor. Otherwise, laryngitis is best treated with nonpharmaceutical options.

✋ Massage Considerations

Risks
- People with acute laryngitis are better off resting and recuperating than receiving rigorous massage.

Benefits
- Reflexive or energetic techniques may be supportive for people recovering from laryngitis.
- Clients who have had laryngitis can enjoy the same benefits from massage as the rest of the population.

leaky gut syndrome: see candidiasis

Legg-Calvé-Perthes syndrome: see avascular osteonecrosis

leiomyoma: see fibroid tumors

leprosy: see Hansen disease

leukemia

Leukemia occurs when a mutation in the DNA of one or more stem cells in the bone marrow causes the production of multitudes of nonfunctioning leukocytes. These leukemia cells crowd out the functioning cells in the bone marrow and blood.

Leukemia can be aggressive and quickly progressive, involving the release of immature cells into the circulatory system (acute), or it can be slowly progressive, leading to the release of mature but nonfunctioning cells (chronic).

Unlike many types of cancer, leukemia spreads through the blood rather than the lymph system. It can cause tumors in the lymph nodes (although not as readily as lymphoma), but it also affects the liver, spleen, and central nervous system.

Left untreated, leukemia results in death, usually from excessive bleeding or infection, because platelet and functional white blood cell production are suppressed.

Signs and Symptoms

- Fatigue, low stamina
- Anemia
- Unusual bleeding, bruising
- Chronic infections

Treatment Options

Leukemia treatment depends on what types of cells have been affected, how aggressive the disease is, and what kinds of treatments the patient has already had. Treatment usually begins with chemotherapy. Radiation or surgery may be added, especially if cancerous cells have aggressively invaded any particular organ or location.

Medications

The treatment strategy for leukemia patients often includes chemotherapy.

Massage Considerations

Risks

- Leukemia is spread through the bloodstream, it weakens immunity, and it cause bleeding and bruising; all of these situations contraindicate rigorous massage.

Benefits

- Massage that respects the resilience of the client and the challenges posed by both the cancer and cancer treatments can be supportive to a client who lives with leukemia.
- Leukemia patients who are in remission can enjoy the benefits of massage as long as it stays within their tolerance for challenges to homeostasis.

Lewy body disease

Lewy body disease (LBD), also known as dementia with Lewy bodies (DLB), is a condition in which protein deposits, called Lewy bodies (named after the doctor who first documented them), develop in various parts of the brain from the brain stem up to the cerebral cortex.

The presence of Lewy bodies interferes in the production and reception of several neurotransmitters, especially dopamine and acetylcholine. Consequently, the processes that these neurotransmitters support, including movement, alertness, and cognition, are disrupted.

LBD has much in common with **Alzheimer disease** and **Parkinson disease**. It is distinguished primarily by the experience of well-developed visual and other sense-related hallucinations and by hypersensitivity to central nervous system (CNS) drugs.

Signs and Symptoms

- Progressive dementia
- Fluctuating awareness and alertness
- Visual hallucinations
- Repeated falls
- Fainting
- Delusions
- Disrupted sleep
- Hypersensitivity to CNS drugs

Treatment Options

In addition to drug treatment, physical therapy, massage therapy, aromatherapy, and other interventions may be recommended to improve the function and sense of well-being for patients with LBD.

Medications

Some LBD patients have good success with cholinesterase inhibitors. Other drugs used to treat anxiety, depression, and movement disorders may be recommended for people with LBD, but they are typically given in much smaller doses than for other patients.

🖐 Massage Considerations

Risks

- Clients may become disoriented and uncomfortable; massage therapists must be sensitive to subtle changes in client responses.

Benefits

- Massage may be recommended for people with LBD to help retain motor function and a sense of connectedness to their world.

Practitioner Advice

- Most cases of LBD occur in elderly people. It is important to remember that many other conditions, such as diabetes, osteoporosis, and heart disease, may be present along with LBD. Any of these disorders may require adjustments in how massage is administered.

---

lice

Lice are parasitic animals that feed on human blood. Three major species of lice have been identified—head lice, body lice, and pubic lice—although head lice and body lice appear occasionally to interbreed.

Head Lice

Head lice live in hair on the head and suck blood from the scalp. They lay eggs called nits that are attached to the base of the hair shaft. They can infest any soft, upholstered surface such as furniture, bed linens, or stuffed animals, and they can live for up to 2 weeks off a human host.

Body Lice

Body lice look similar to head lice, but they have different habits. Body lice tend to live in clothing and visit their human hosts for an occasional blood meal. Because regularly washing clothing effectively eradicates body lice, these parasites are usually only seen among transient or homeless populations with limited access to laundering facilities.

Pubic Lice

Pubic lice, also called crab lice, are much smaller than head lice or body lice. They infest any coarse body hair, including pubic hair, axillary hair, or even thick facial hair. Pubic lice are usually spread through intimate contact.

Signs and Symptoms

- Head lice: visible nits glued to the hair shafts
- All lice: itching, sensation of movement on the skin or scalp

Treatment Options

Body lice are treated simply by laundering clothing. Head lice can be treated with applications of pesticidal soap along with manually removing the nits. This must be followed by aggressively cleaning or isolating any other surfaces where lice might collect, including bedding and soft toys. Pubic lice are sensitive to pesticidal soap, and a single application is often sufficient.

🖐 Massage Considerations

Risks
- If a client has signs active lice infestation during an appointment, it is necessary to isolate the linens from the rest of the laundry.

Benefits
- Massage has no specific benefits for people with any kind of lice.
- Clients who have had lice and completed treatment can enjoy the same benefits from bodywork as the rest of the population.

Practitioner Advice
- Parasitic infestation carries a powerful social stigma that is negatively (and inaccurately) associated with poverty and poor hygiene. Remember that *anybody*—including massage therapists—could have this problem.

---

lichen planus

Lichen planus (LP) is an outbreak of flat, itchy lesions on the skin, mucous membranes, or genitals. Most outbreaks of LP are temporary, lasting anywhere from 6 to 18 months.

LP frequently develops concurrently with other disorders. It accompanies a number of autoimmune diseases, including **myasthenia gravis** and **ulcerative colitis**. It is also seen in people with **hepatitis C** and **vitiligo**.

When LP occurs in the mouth, it can closely resemble thrush (**candidiasis**) or other ulcerations. LP in the mouth is also associated with an increased risk of oral **skin cancer,** so patients are counseled to watch it closely; avoid alcohol and tobacco products; and get regular dental care, especially while lesions are present.

Genital LP is associated with a slightly increased risk of vulvar or penile cancer.

Signs and Symptoms

- Itchy, flattened, purplish lesions
- Often on the flexor side of the wrist or medial ankle
- In the mouth: flattened whitened area on the tongue or cheeks
- On the scalp: may cause permanent bald spots
- On the nails: may cause nail loss

Medications

Patients with LP may use topical corticosteroid ointments or oral anti-inflammatory drugs.

Massage Considerations

Risks

- Topical steroid medications can make the skin thin and delicate.
- Massage may make the lesions itchier, so consider these to be a local caution.
- LP resembles both contagious and noncontagious skin diseases; this is another good reason not to work with undiagnosed conditions.

Benefits

- Massage has no specific benefits for clients with LP; as long as adjustments for medications are made, these clients can enjoy the same benefits from massage as the rest of the population.

lipoma

Lipomas are slow-growing, benign fatty tumors. They often develop in the subcutaneous layer of the skin but may also be found throughout the gastrointestinal tract and imbedded in many organs, including the liver, adrenal glands, and breast tissue.

The cause of lipomas is not known. An inherited predisposition may exist because many people report multiple family members with the same condition; however, a specific genetic anomaly has not been identified. Some people find that their lipomas form after a major blow or trauma to the skin.

The main complications associated with lipomas occur when they grow in the digestive tract and they become large enough to obstruct the tract or to bleed. More rarely, lipomas are associated with dysfunction in other organs (notably the adrenal glands and heart). They are not, however, associated with an increased risk of cancer.

Signs and Symptoms

- Painless mass palpable under the skin
- Range in size from tiny to very large
- May not create symptoms unless they are large enough to interfere with function

Treatment Options

Cutaneous lipomas may be surgically removed, either by excision or liposuction. Internal lipomas are typically removed through endoscopic surgery when they interfere with normal function. They do not usually grow back in the same place if the whole tumor is removed.

Medications

Lipomas are not treated with medication.

Massage Considerations

Risks
• Massage carries no risk for a client with lipomas unless the stimulus is somehow irritating to the client.

Benefits
• Massage has no specific benefit for clients with lipomas. These clients can enjoy the same benefits from massage as the rest of the population.

Practitioner Advice
• Clients sometimes hear the word "lipoma" and are alarmed that they might have skin cancer. If a lipoma has been diagnosed by a qualified professional but the client is still concerned, a massage therapist can educate and reassure the client about this benign, noncancerous condition.

---

liver cancer

Primary liver cancer, also called hepatocellular carcinoma, is cancer that originates in the liver. It is distinguished from secondary liver cancer, or metastatic liver disease, which is a result of cancer that originates elsewhere and leads to tumors in the liver.

A history of **hepatitis** B or C, **alcoholism,** and **cirrhosis** are all contributing factors to uncontrolled cellular activity in the liver. This is especially true when a person has any combination of these factors simultaneously. Other risk factors include the presence of a genetic disorder called hemochromatosis, and long-term exposure to a fungus called afloxin B1.

Signs and Symptoms
• Vague abdominal pain that becomes more intense
• Unintended weight loss, food aversion
• Muscle wasting
• Ascites
• Fever
• Abdominal mass
• Jaundice
• Blood test results showing liver dysfunction, hormonal imbalance

Treatment Options

Liver cancer is aggressive and difficult to control, and patients often have underlying liver problems that make them poor candidates for surgery. Furthermore, liver cancer tends not to respond well to chemotherapy or radiation. Consequently, a number of treatment options have been developed to control the growth of the cancer without invasive surgery. These include techniques to burn or freeze tumors through laparoscopic or percutaneous instruments, injections of ethanol to destroy tumor cells, and the use of drugs or implements to block the blood vessels that supply the tumors.

Medications
Liver cancer is not typically treated with medication.

Massage Considerations

Risks
- As with other types of cancer, the risks for working with a client with liver cancer center on the challenges and complications of the cancer and the cancer treatments that the client uses.
- Liver cancer is usually treated with various forms of surgery. Special cautions include surgical and port sites, risk of infection, and positioning for best comfort.

Benefits
- Massage during cancer treatment can help improve sleep, increase appetite, and boost immune system function.
- Massage as a comfort measure can improve the quality of life for person who is approaching death.

lobar sclerosis: see Pick disease

lordosis: see postural deviations

lung cancer
Lung cancer occurs in epithelial cells that are chronically irritated by environmental contaminants. Although cigarette, pipe, and cigar smoke are responsible for 85% to 90% of all cases of lung cancer, other causes have also been identified, including exposure to radon, asbestos, uranium, arsenic, and other carcinogens. These risks are magnified if they occur in conjunction with smoking.

Abnormal cells eventually form tumors in the lungs, but because they have immediate access to both the circulatory and lymph systems, the cells are capable of spreading before tumors are detectable.

Lung tumors can put pressure on other structures, causing problems. **Thoracic outlet syndrome** and **superior vena cava syndrome** are possible complications.

Signs and Symptoms
- Difficult to identify early
- "Smoker's cough" with bloodstained phlegm
- Chest pain, shortness of breath
- Possible mechanical pressure on the brachial plexus, superior vena cava, esophagus, or larynx

Treatment Options
Treatment for lung cancer depends on what kind of cancer is growing and how far it has progressed. Surgery followed by radiation and chemotherapy is the starting point.

Medications

Chemotherapy is part of the standard treatment for lung cancer.

Massage Considerations

Risks

- People undergoing lung cancer treatments are at risk for infection, bleeding, skin damage from radiation, lymphedema, and a number of other complications. All of these conditions have cautions for massage.

Benefits

- Massage can stimulate immune system activity, reduce pain and fatigue, and generally add to the quality of life for patients undergoing very extreme challenges.
- Reflexive or energetic techniques can be comforting and safe for even very fragile cancer patients.

lung collapse: see pneumothorax

lupus

Lupus is an autoimmune attack against various types of tissues in the body. Three varieties of lupus have been identified: drug-induced lupus erythematosus, discoid lupus erythematosus (DLE), and systemic lupus erythematosus (SLE).

Drug-induced lupus is a situation in which rarely prescribed medications create lupus symptoms. These symptoms disappear when the medications are discontinued.

DLE is a chronic skin disease involving scaly red patches with sharp margins that don't itch, or it can create the characteristic malar or "butterfly rash" of redness over the nose and cheeks. The skin can become very thin and delicate, or lesions may become permanently discolored and thickened. If the lesions affect the deep layers of the skin, scar tissue may lead to permanent hair loss. More commonly, acute flare-ups lead to temporary hair loss. About 10% of people with DLE later develop SLE.

SLE is a situation in which antibody attacks are launched against a variety of tissues throughout the body. This can result in **arthritis, anemia, renal failure, deep vein thrombosis, headaches**, psychosis, **seizures, pericarditis, pleurisy,** and **Raynaud syndrome**. Many people with lupus also have **Sjögren syndrome**, either as a complication of lupus or as a free-standing problem.

Signs and Symptoms

- Runs in cycles of flare-ups and remissions
- DLE:
    - Skin symptoms only
    - Malar rash
    - Circular lesions
    - Hair loss
- SLE:
    - Painful arthritis, especially of the hands and feet
    - Headaches and seizures
    - Clotting disorders
    - Raynaud syndrome
    - Inflammation of the serous membranes (pleurisy, pericarditis)
    - Inflammation of the kidneys

Treatment Options

The treatment strategy for lupus is to minimize the negative impact of inflammation during flare-ups. This is usually done with medication.

Medications

Lupus management can include nonsteroidal anti-inflammatory drugs, steroidal anti-inflammatory drugs, antimalarial drugs, and cytotoxic drugs to limit immune system activity.

Massage Considerations

Risks

- Lupus medication has implications for massage; avoid overtreatment with anti-inflammatory drugs and respect immune system impairments seen with cytotoxic drugs.
- During flare, rigorous circulatory massage may be too challenging, especially if the heart, lungs, or kidneys are compromised.

Benefits

- During flare, energetic or reflexive techniques can be soothing and supportive.
- During remissions, any massage that fits within the client's limits of resilience and activity levels can be health promoting.

Lyme disease

Lyme disease is an infection of the spirochetal bacterium *Borrelia burgdorferi*. This pathogen is spread through the bite of two species of ticks, deer ticks (*Ixodes scapularis*) and Western black-legged ticks (*Ixodes pacificus*).

Ticks pick up the spiral-shaped bacteria from the blood of their animal hosts, especially mice. If an infected tick then bites a human, that bacteria may be transmitted to the human host. The bacterial invasion can cause several different reactions, depending on the severity and the stage of the infection.

Lyme disease can be difficult to diagnose because it mimics several other disorders, including **rheumatoid arthritis, Bell palsy, fibromyalgia, chronic fatigue syndrome, flu,** and **mononucleosis.** Furthermore, other tick-borne infections (**ehrlichiosis** and babesiosis) may create similar symptoms, but they don't respond to the same treatment protocols.

Signs and Symptoms

- Early localized disease:
    "Bull's eye rash"
    High fever
    Headache
    Malaise
- Early disseminated disease:
    Irregular heart beat
    Headache
    Bell palsy
    Numbness
    Memory loss
- Late stage:
    Joint inflammation, especially at knee, shoulder, or elbow

Treatment Options

Lyme disease is typically treated with medication.

Medications

Lyme disease is treatable with antibiotics, but the course of medication may be longer than for other bacterial infections.

 Massage Considerations

Risks

- Lyme disease can cause arthritis, numbness, and circulatory problems. All of these have implications for massage, so it is important to obtain a thorough health history.
- Joint pain with Lyme disease can be intermittent. Acute joint inflammation contraindicates rigorous massage.

Benefits

- Massage within pain tolerance and with respect for resilience and activity levels can be supportive for clients with Lyme disease to maintain flexibility and deal with some of the other complications of this infection.

Practitioner Advice

- Massage therapists are in a unique position to see ticks where our clients might miss them. Ticks are most likely to latch onto the skin at the popliteal fossa, the axilla, in or around the ear, and anywhere on the scalp or hairline.
- If a massage therapist finds a tick on a client's body, the client should be informed. If both the therapist and client consent, the tick should be removed with tweezers squeezed as close to the skin as possible; the tick should be pulled directly upward, not twisted out. The area should be disinfected, and the tick should be put into a plastic bag and frozen to take to the doctor in case symptoms develop. If any mouthparts are left in the host, a doctor should be consulted immediately, regardless of whether symptoms develop.
- The Centers for Disease Control and Prevention (CDC) warns that any liquid expressed from a tick could carry bacteria; the person removing a tick should avoid coming into direct contact with it. The CDC further advises that exposing the tick to toxins or a hot match may cause the animal to regurgitate into the host, increasing the risk of infection.

lymphangitis/lymphadenitis

Lymphangitis is an infection with inflammation in the lymphangions (the lymphatic capillaries), and lymphadenitis is an infection with inflammation of the lymph nodes. These are usually complications of infections that develop somewhere on the skin. **Erysipelas**, **herpes simplex**, or **fungal infections** such as athlete's foot are common triggers.

If some bacteria get past the filtering action of the lymph nodes, the infection may enter the bloodstream. Then the situation changes to **septicemia**, or blood poisoning, which is life threatening. This is why medical intervention is advisable at the earliest possible opportunity.

Signs and Symptoms

- Signs of infection at a skin lesion: pain, heat, redness, swelling
- A scarlet track running toward the nearest lymph nodes
- Swollen lymph nodes, fever, malaise
- Fast onset

Treatment Options

Lymphatic infections are treated with medication.

Medications

Aggressive antibiotic therapy is used for lymphangitis/lymphadenitis to reduce the risk of septicemia.

Massage Considerations

Risks

- Acute infections contraindicate massage. Fortunately, the symptoms of lymphatic infections are generally extreme enough that clients are likely to cancel massage appointments.

Benefits

- Massage has no specific benefits for people with lymph system infections.
- Clients who have fully recovered from lymphangitis or lymphadenitis can enjoy the same benefits from massage as the rest of the population.

Practitioner Advice

- Lymphatic infections are risks for massage therapists with open hangnails or other portals of entry on their hands. These conditions show why practicing good hygiene, covering skin lesions, and maintaining excellent baseline health are important for people in this profession.

lymphedema

Lymphedema is an accumulation of fluid and proteins in the interstitial spaces, usually of an arm or leg. Primary lymphedema occurs with a congenital malformation of lymph vessels or nodes. Secondary lymphedema, the most common variety, usually develops because cancer, surgery, radiation, scarring from infection, trauma, or parasites impede the lymph system from processing the many liters of fluid it is designed to filter every day.

The main difference between regular **edema** and lymphedema is the presence of proteins in the interstitial spaces. These accumulate when the forces that cause fluid accumulation outweigh the forces that allow fluid to flow back into circulatory capillaries. Interstitial proteins cause fluid retention through osmotic pressure.

Several vicious cycles contribute to lymphedema and its complications. Retention of fluid can mechanically collapse nearby lymph capillaries, impeding the movement of fluid out of the area. Excessive interstitial fluid presses cells far from supplying capillaries, which makes the exchange of nutrients and wastes sluggish and inefficient. The risk of cellular damage, skin breakdown, and subsequent infection is high, and bacteria thrive in the protein-rich interstitial fluid of people with lymphedema. After this condition has developed, it can be managed, but it will probably never be completely resolved.

In industrialized countries, lymphedema is usually associated with cancer or cancer treatment (surgery to remove lymph nodes or scarring from radiation damage). **Breast cancer** affects nodes in the axilla, and **prostate, testicular, uterine, ovarian,** and **cervical cancer** can affect the inguinal nodes. In developing countries, parasitic worms (filariasis) may invade the inguinal lymph nodes, causing lymphedema in the leg.

Signs and Symptoms

- Appears in the extremities, ranging from mild to severe
- Pain

- Feeling of fullness or heaviness
- Loss of range of motion
- Mild: soft skin, pitting edema
- Moderate: firm swelling not alleviated with elevation
- Severe: grossly enlarged limb, impaired circulation, risk of ulcers, infection

Treatment Options

Very precise skin care is the first defense against an episode of lymphedema; guarding against infections and minor injuries is important to limit inflammation and the direction of excessive blood flow into the affected limb.

If an episode has developed, compression mechanisms (including bandages, special clothing, and pumps) are used to help prevent long-term damage from weakened, stretched-out tissues. Manual lymph drainage or lymph drainage techniques are forms of massage that are well accepted in lymphedema management because they help reroute lymph from the affected limb to a different set of lymph nodes.

Medications

Antibiotics are used if lymphedema progresses to bacterial infection.

Massage Considerations

Risks
- Lymphedema contraindicates rigorous circulatory massage, which can exacerbate the situation.

Benefits
- Lymph drainage modalities can be extremely helpful to prevent or treat episodes of lymphedema.

lymphoma

Lymphoma is any type of cancer of the lymph nodes. Lymphoma is usually discussed as Hodgkin lymphoma and non-Hodgkin lymphoma, which includes many subtypes of the disease.

This disease begins with a mutation of the DNA of the affected cells in the lymph nodes, which includes some types of T cells, B cells, or natural killer cells. The mutated cells begin to replicate, producing massive numbers of nonfunctioning lymphocytes. This causes the lymph nodes to enlarge, initiating the other symptoms associated with lymphoma, including anemia, night sweats, itchy skin, and fatigue.

The incidence of lymphoma is higher among **HIV**-positive patients than it is among the general population. Epstein-Barr virus, which is associated with **mononucleosis**, has been linked to Burkitt lymphoma. Human T-cell lymphotropic virus is associated with T-cell lymphoma. And having the *Helicobacter pylori* bacterium (also associated with peptic **ulcers**) increases the risk of developing lymphoma that originates in the stomach wall.

Signs and Symptoms

- Painless enlargement of the lymph nodes, especially at the neck, axilla, inguinal area
- Anemia
- Fatigue

- Unintended weight loss, loss of appetite
- Night sweats
- Itchy skin
- Late stage: decreased immunity

Treatment Options

Chemotherapy and radiation are the usual choices treatment choices for lymphoma, but some other options are finding success, including allogenic and autologous bone marrow transplants and radioimmunotherapy (a process in which special antibodies that have been treated with radioactive iodine are injected into the body, where they attack and destroy cancer cells).

Medications

Chemotherapy is usually included in lymphoma treatment.

Massage Considerations

Risks

- Active lymphoma contraindicates rigorous circulatory massage because of the challenges of fluid management.
- Lymphoma treatments carry several cautions for massage, including toxicity and impaired immunity.

Benefits

- Gentle massage for lymphoma patients, as for other cancer patients, has several benefits, including better sleep, increased immune system activity, better appetite, and overall improvement in the quality of life.

macular degeneration

Age-related macular degeneration (AMD) is a condition in which the macula (the part of the retina devoted to central vision) deteriorates, usually because of problems with nutrient and waste exchange in the eye.

Dry macular degeneration is the most common form of AMD, accounting for 85% to 90% of all cases. In this situation, wastes accumulate in the retina, showing as small yellowish spots in the eye called drusen. Wastes interfere in macular function, and central vision is gradually but painlessly lost over a period of many years.

Wet macular degeneration accounts for 10% of AMD diagnoses but 90% of AMD-related blindness. In this case, tissue behind the macula develops excessive new blood vessels. These can mechanically distort the macula, or the new capillaries can leak or bleed. Either way, wet macular degeneration tends progress more rapidly and has a higher risk of causing significant and debilitating vision loss.

Signs and Symptoms

- Loss of central vision; peripheral vision stays intact
- Colors fade
- Straight lines appear wavy

Treatment Options

Treatment options for AMD are limited. Some laser surgery techniques for wet AMD have been developed, but they are only appropriate for a small percentage of patients, and the benefits of the surgery are often short lived. No options have yet been established for dry AMD, but several are in development.

Medications

Macular degeneration is not treated with medication except for some locally applied medications in treatments for wet AMD.

🖐 Massage Considerations

Risks
- Massage has no specific risks for macular degeneration.

Benefits
- Massage has no specific benefits for macular degeneration. Clients with this condition can enjoy the same benefits from massage as the rest of the population.

mad cow disease: see Creutzfeldt-Jakob disease

major depressive disorder: see depression

malaria

Malaria (named for "bad air") is a protozoan infestation first of liver cells and then of red blood cells. The protozoa are transmitted by *Anopheles* mosquitoes. Introduced into the bloodstream, the parasites congregate in the liver, where they may incubate or remain dormant for days, weeks, or longer. They then destroy infected hepatocytes and move back into the bloodstream, where they invade erythrocytes. Infected erythrocytes eventually rupture. Toxins released from this cellular destruction lead to the symptoms of malaria.

Complications of severe malaria include **jaundice** (related to long-term liver damage), **anemia** from destroyed erythrocytes, splenomegaly or splenic rupture, **renal failure**, **seizures**, coma, and possibly death. The most common form of malaria is also the most dangerous.

Signs and Symptoms
- May be silent in the early stages
- Runs in cycles of flare and remission
- Fever, chills, muscle aches, fatigue, nausea, vomiting, diarrhea
- Complications can be life threatening

Treatment Options

Treatment of malaria begins with prevention. This can include mosquito abatement programs, mosquito repellants with DEET, and sleeping nets treated with mosquito repellant. Other treatment options are based on medications.

Medications

Antimalarial drugs can be used as prophylactics to reduce the risk of infection or to treat an infection already underway. A vaccine to prevent malaria is in development.

Massage Considerations

Risks

- Although the chance that a massage therapist working in the United States might have a client with malaria is small, it is important to remember that this disease alters liver and kidney function and impairs fluid flow, contraindicating rigorous circulatory massage.

Benefits

- Clients with a history of malaria may have permanent damage to the liver and other tissues. Energetic or reflexive work may be supportive for these clients.
- Clients with a history of malaria and no long-term effects can enjoy the same benefits from massage as the rest of the population.

malignant melanoma: see skin cancer

manic depression: see depression

Marfan syndrome

Marfan syndrome is the result of a genetic mutation that leads to the production of dysfunctional fibrillin, a key connective tissue fiber. Consequently, certain connective tissues throughout the body may be weak or otherwise dysfunctional. The musculoskeletal system, the heart and aorta, and the eyes are at highest risk for problems related to Marfan syndrome. These issues include **osteoarthritis**, **postural deviations**, aortic **aneurysm**, detached retina, and other complications.

This is an autosomal defect, which means it is not gender specific. Although Marfan syndrome is usually passed from parent to child, about 25% of all cases are suspected to be spontaneous mutations of otherwise healthy genes.

Signs and Symptoms

- Abnormally long fingers and toes
- Ligament laxity
- Distortion of the thorax: flattened or protruding sternum
- High risk for osteoarthritis, scoliosis, joint injuries
- High risk for weak heart valves, aortic aneurysm
- High risk for myopia, dislocated lens, detached retina

Treatment Options

Only the symptoms of Marfan syndrome can be treated; no therapy can reverse the action of mutated genes.

Surgical interventions are not always necessary, but when the curve of scoliosis or the shape of the thorax interferes with normal breathing, this may be corrected. Similarly, if early-stage aneurysm or mitral valve prolapse is identified, these situations can be surgically addressed.

Medications

Beta-blockers are frequently prescribed to Marfan syndrome patients to reduce the work of the aorta. Prophylactic antibiotics are recommended when even distant procedures are performed because heart valves are highly susceptible to infection.

🖐 Massage Considerations

Risks

- Clients with Marfan syndrome have weak connective tissue and are often advised to avoid contact sports and activities that put these systems at risk for injury. Modalities should be chosen to avoid challenging the cardiovascular system and ligament laxity.

Benefits

- Carefully performed massage can improve breathing and chest restriction for clients with Marfan syndrome.
- Other goals can include promoting relaxation and parasympathetic balance without taxing the circulatory system.

---

mastoiditis

Mastoiditis is an infection and inflammation of the hollow air cells of the mastoid bone. It is usually a complication of **otitis** media or a middle ear infection.

Several causative agents for mastoiditis have been identified, including *Streptococcus pneumoniae* (a drug-resistant form of this bacterium may be responsible for increasingly stubborn and aggressive ear infections and complications), group A streptococcus bacteria, and *Haemophilus influenzae*. When any of these bacteria causes a middle ear infection, a contiguous connection with the hollow areas in the mastoid bone presents the possibility that the infection could move into this bone. Necrosis of healthy tissue and abscesses may result.

Complications of untreated mastoiditis and middle ear infections may include permanent hearing loss, **Bell palsy**, and **meningitis**.

Signs and Symptoms

- Fever, malaise
- Swelling, redness, tenderness behind the ear, especially in conjunction with an ear infection

Treatment Options

If antibiotics are insufficient, surgery to remove the infected areas of the bone may be recommended.

Medications

Antibiotics are the first recourse in treating mastoiditis.

🖐 Massage Considerations

Risks

- Acute infection, especially with fever, systemically contraindicates massage.

Benefits
- Massage has no specific benefits for clients with mastoiditis.
- Clients who have recovered from mastoiditis can enjoy the same benefits from massage as the rest of the population.

Practitioner Advice
- Clients who have had surgery to remove part of the mastoid process may have anomalies in the shape of the skull and attachments of the local muscles.

medial tibial stress syndrome: see shin splints

Ménière disease

Ménière disease is an idiopathic condition of the inner ear that affects hearing and balance. The cause of the disease is unknown and may include different factors for individual cases, including a genetic predisposition, food sensitivities, viral infection, excessive endolymph that may contaminate perilymph, or a history of injury or trauma to the inner ear.

Signs and Symptoms
- Episodes of spinning vertigo, tinnitus, distorted hearing
- Episodes preceded by sensation of fullness or blockage in the ear
- Episodes increase in frequency and severity
- Begins unilaterally; may spread to affect both ears
- Cold sweats, nausea, vomiting with vertigo
- "Brain fog": confusion, short-term memory loss, poor concentration
- Eventual permanent hearing loss
- Some predictable triggers: stress, change in air pressure, chocolate, caffeine, smoking, high-salt diet

Treatment Options

Ménière disease is not curable, but some symptoms can be treated. Adherence to a low-salt diet reduces the frequency and severity of episodes for many patients. Stopping smoking and avoiding loud noises and other triggers are other important measures used to control this condition.

Some surgical interventions have been developed for this condition, but they are reserved for patients whose hearing is already irretrievably damaged. A labyrinthectomy essentially "disconnects" the inner ear, resulting in total hearing loss on the affected side, along with a reduction in vertigo and tinnitus. If the patient goes on to develop Ménière disease in the other ear, however, surgery is no longer an option because it will interfere with hearing and all balance-regulating mechanisms.

Medications

Diuretics and antianxiety medications can address some of the symptoms of Ménière disease.

Massage Considerations

Risks
- Some Ménière disease patients find that their symptoms are exacerbated when their heads are in certain positions or when they lower or raise themselves from a table in certain ways.

As long as these positions are avoided, massage has no specific risks for people with Ménière disease.

Benefits
- Some people report that craniosacral therapy may reduce Ménière disease symptoms in some clients.
- As long as the client's position on the table doesn't exacerbate the symptoms, people with Ménière disease can enjoy the same benefits from massage as the rest of the population.

meningitis

Meningitis is an infection and inflammation of the meninges, specifically the pia mater and arachnoid layers of connective tissue membrane that surround the brain and spinal cord. It is usually caused by bacterial or viral infection.

Meningitis can be contagious, although not all the people exposed to meningitis-causing pathogens contract the disease. A high percentage of exposed people experience no symptoms or only experience symptoms of a **cold** or mild **flu**. Only about one of every 1,000 people exposed to meningitis develop the disease.

Meningitis can cause permanent central nervous system damage if the infection is severe. **Paralysis**, deafness, and mental disability are possible complications, especially in infections of infants.

Signs and Symptoms
- Very high fever and chills
- Deep red, purplish rash
- Extreme headache, irritability
- Aversion to light
- Stiff neck
- Drowsiness
- Impaired speech
- In very extreme cases: nausea, vomiting, delirium, convulsions, coma

Treatment Options
Treatment for meningitis depends on the causative factors. Viral meningitis is generally treated with supportive therapy, including rest, fluids, and good nutrition while the patient's immune system fights back.

Most people emerge from meningitis infections with no lasting damage.

Medications
If a bacterial infection is identified, antibiotics are administered immediately.

🖐 Massage Considerations

Risks
- Acute meningitis systemically contraindicates massage.

Benefits
- Clients who are recovering from meningitis may benefit from the relaxation and immune support offered by gentle, reflexive, or energetic modalities.

- Clients who have fully recovered from meningitis with no lasting effects can enjoy the same benefits from massage as the rest of the population.

meniscus tear

The menisci (Greek for "little moons") are crescent-shaped, specialized cartilages located on the superior aspect of the tibial plateau. The knee has medial and lateral menisci. The menisci have several functions, including distributing the pressure of the femur across the top of the tibia, stabilizing anterior–posterior movement of the femur, manufacturing joint fluid, and providing proprioception for movement at the knee.

Menisci blend into the synovial capsule of the knee at the peripheral edges. This portion of the cartilage is vascularized enough to be called the "red zone." The center of the cartilage is removed from blood supply and is called the "white zone." Areas where the two zones blend are called the "red–white zone." Injuries to different areas of the menisci have different chances for healing, depending on the level of vascularization.

The menisci slide back and forth on the tibia to help track the femur correctly. The posterior horn of the medial meniscus is the least moveable area and is consequently most vulnerable to injury. Meniscus injuries can include small tears, chips, or whole detachments where the central part of the cartilage essentially flips back into the joint space.

The most typical meniscus injury in a young person occurs when the knee is in flexion and a rotational force is put upon it, as during a quick turn or pivot. In older patients, meniscus tears may have a gradual onset and get progressively worse without any specific trauma.

Signs and Symptoms
- Significant swelling and pain at the joint line of the knee
- Clicking, catching, locking, and feeling that the knee may "give way"

Treatment Options

Treatment options for meniscus injuries vary according to the size and location of the injury. Small lesions, especially in older, nonathletic people, may not be treated surgically at all. Tears that occur in the red zone or the red–white zone may be repaired with a prognosis for full or nearly full recovery. For tears in the white zone, loose material may be surgically removed, but long-term results show a significant increase in the risk of osteoarthritis at the knee. Physical therapy, along with an adjusted exercise regimen, is nearly always a part of meniscus injury recovery.

Medications

A person with a new or recently treated meniscus tear is likely to be taking analgesics, anti-inflammatory drugs, or both to help manage some of the symptoms of this injury.

Massage Considerations

Risks
- New and inflamed meniscus tears locally contraindicate rigorous massage and stretching.

Benefits
- Massage can't directly access structures inside the knee capsule, but lymphatic techniques can help manage some of the inflammation that may contribute to pain and dysfunction.

- Clients recovering from meniscus injuries can benefit from the muscular support massage can offer to strengthen tissues outside the knee capsule.

menopause/perimenopause

Menopause refers to the moment the ovaries permanently stop secreting enough hormones to initiate a menstrual cycle. The time leading up to this event is called perimenopause, and many of the symptoms associated with declining hormone secretion occur during this period. Menopause itself is not absolutely identified until menstruation has completely stopped for a full year.

It is important to emphasize that the symptoms of perimenopause can be uncomfortable and inconvenient, but this process is not a disease; rather, it is a natural part of the aging process.

Signs and Symptoms

- Hot flashes
- Night sweats
- Insomnia
- Mood swings
- Decreased sex drive
- Vaginal dryness
- Confusion, short-term memory loss, poor concentration
- Symptoms abate when hormone secretions stabilize

Treatment Options

A variety of nondrug treatments, including dietary adjustments, exercise, yoga, meditation, and other health-promoting activities, can be used for the symptoms of perimenopause. Many women use medical interventions as well, at least until their hormonal secretions stabilize.

Medications

Symptoms of perimenopause have traditionally been treated with hormone replacement therapy (using various forms of estrogen and progesterone to replace low secretion rates). Recent findings show that this strategy has more risks than previously understood, so new emphasis is being placed on finding the smallest possible dose for the shortest possible period to improve mood and function.

Massage Considerations

Risks

- Massage has no specific risks for women undergoing perimenopause.
- Postmenopausal women are more likely to have osteoporosis and heart disease than the rest of the population, so these issues need to be addressed.

Benefits

- Because massage involves supportive, nurturing, informed touch, it can reinforce the positive aspects of women's physical experience and help them through what can be a difficult time.

metabolic syndrome

Metabolic syndrome is a collection of physical signs and symptoms that individually increase the risk for certain diseases, but when seen together, increase that risk to near certainty.

The five main features of metabolic syndrome include high triglycerides, low high-density lipoproteins, hypertension, central obesity, and high fasting blood glucose levels. Other possible features of metabolic syndrome include a high risk of blood clotting, high levels of C-reactive protein (an indicator of inflammation), and polycystic ovary disease in women.

These factors are not particularly alarming when they appear alone, but in combination, they set the stage for an extremely elevated risk of type 2 **diabetes, atherosclerosis, heart attack, heart failure, aneurysm,** and **stroke.**

Signs and Symptoms

- Central obesity ("apple" rather than "pear" shape)
- Disruptions in cholesterol
- Hypertension
- High blood glucose, insulin resistance

Treatment Options

Short-term goals for metabolic syndrome include managing hypertension, lowering blood glucose, and correcting cholesterol levels with medical intervention.

Long-term goals include increasing physical activity and losing weight. Limiting alcohol use and quitting smoking are other important steps.

Medications

People with metabolic syndrome may regulate their blood sugar levels with drugs that influence insulin production or sensitivity and with statins to regulate their cholesterol levels. Antihypertensive drugs may include beta-blockers, diuretics, angiotensin-converting enzyme (ACE) inhibitors, and digitalis.

Massage Considerations

Risks
- If a client with metabolic syndrome is physically active, massage may have no specific risks.
- If a client with metabolic syndrome is severely limited by stamina or cardiovascular weakness, any bodywork must be adapted to stay within the client's tolerance.

Benefits
- Noncirculatory types of massage can promote relaxation and parasympathetic balance without challenging the cardiovascular system of clients with metabolic syndrome.

methicillin-resistant *Staphylococcus aureus* infection

Methicillin-resistant *Staphylococcus aureus* (MRSA) is a drug-resistant bacterial infection of the lungs, urinary tract, or skin.

MRSA was first identified as nosocomial infections (hospital-based pathogen) in the 1950s. In these settings, as well as nursing homes, dialysis centers, and other health care facilities, the bacteria are usually associated with surgical wounds, urinary tract infections, pneumonia, and septicemia.

In 1998, MRSA began to be recognized in community settings, notably athletic facilities and prisons. These infections are typically related to skin-to-skin contact, cuts and abrasions, and contaminated surfaces.

MRSA infections are particularly dangerous to people who are otherwise immunosuppressed. The risk of the infection complicating to **septicemia** is high for these populations.

Signs and Symptoms

- Skin infections resembling boils or spider bites
- Fever, fatigue, pain
- Unresponsive to methicillin, penicillin, oxacillin, and amoxicillin

Treatment Options

MRSA infections are treated with appropriate medication.

Prevention of MRSA infection is an important emphasis for athletic and other settings where infection is possible. Preventive measures include washing and carefully covering all open sores, avoiding picking at or touching open sores, not sharing any personal items such as towels and razors, and disinfecting all surfaces.

Medications

Treatment for MRSA infection requires high doses of powerful antibiotics. These may have to be administered intravenously if the infection has spread into the lymph or circulatory system. Lesions may be lanced and drained. Pain is usually managed with nonsteroidal anti-inflammatory drugs. MRSA infections can recur if antibiotic treatment is not completed.

🤚 Massage Considerations

Risks

- Acute infections, especially with fever, systemically contraindicate massage.
- A client with an undiagnosed "spider bite" should be treated by a doctor before receiving massage.
- MRSA is communicable through contaminated surfaces; take extra hygiene precautions if exposure is suspected.

Benefits

- Massage has no specific benefits for clients with active MRSA infections.
- Clients who have fully recovered from MRSA infection can enjoy the same benefits from massage as the rest of the population.

miliaria rubra

Also known as "prickly heat," miliaria rubra is a condition involving blocked sweat ducts in the skin.

Hot, humid weather is the leading factor behind prickly heat. Sweating, especially in combination with mechanical occlusions such as clothing, bandages, and synthetic fabrics, may lead to excessive numbers of normal skin-dwelling bacteria. The sticky waste products of these bacteria then clog sweat ducts. Sweat accumulates behind the blockages, and itchy red pustules develop.

Miliaria rubra carries the risk of two complications: the risk of **heat exhaustion** because of the lack of sweating in affected areas and the risk of secondary infection in the form of **impetigo** or abscesses.

Signs and Symptoms
- Small, hot, red bumps
- May be in a pattern of the hair follicles
- Often at the skin folds and sites of friction
- Itchy, prickly sensation
- Persists for several weeks

Treatment Options
Miliaria rubra is prevented by avoiding excessive sweating and friction, especially in hot, humid climates.

Lanolin or calamine lotions may be recommended for comfort and to improve skin function.

Medications
Prophylactic antibiotics can reduce the initial symptoms, but antibiotics begun after the onset of symptoms are usually not effective at shortening the duration of the rash.

🖐 Massage Considerations

Risks
- Massage can make itching worse in affected areas; consider this condition a local contraindication.
- Clients with a history of this condition may need to use hypoallergenic lubricants and to remove any oil or lotion as soon after a massage as possible.

Benefits
- Massage has no specific benefits for clients with miliaria rubra.
- As long as their symptoms are not exacerbated, clients with this condition can enjoy the same benefits from bodywork as the rest of the population.

miscarriage: see abortion, elective and spontaneous

---

mites

Tiny mites called *Sarcoptes scabiei* are the cause of skin lesions called scabies. The female mites burrow under the skin in warm, moist spots, where they drink blood, defecate, urinate, and lay eggs so the next generation can carry on. The mites' waste is highly irritating, which causes an itchy allergic reaction in most hosts. If scratching damages the skin, the risk of secondary infection is high.

Mites spread readily through close personal contact or through contact with an infested person's clothing or linens. However, they only live a few hours without contact with a host.

Signs and Symptoms

- Reddish or grayish tracks in infested areas: groin, axilla, under the breasts, waist line, palmar surface of the hand
- Irritated blisters or pustules
- Risk of secondary bacterial infection
- Itching that gets progressively worse over time

Treatment Options

Mites are treated by bathing with pesticidal soap. This treatment can damage the skin, so it must be used carefully. The mites die within several hours of being separated from human contact, so washing and then isolating bedding, towels, and clothing for that length of time help prevent further outbreaks. It is not necessary to fumigate the home because scabies mites don't stray far from their hosts.

Medications

Mites are not treated with medication other than pesticidal soap.

Massage Considerations

Risks

- If a massage therapist thinks he or she might have been exposed to mites by accident, the client's linens should be isolated from the rest of the laundry, and the therapist should see a doctor right away. Scabies lesions sometimes don't show up for 4 weeks or more; it takes that long to build up enough toxins to be irritating. But the therapist is may be contagious the whole time, and anyone he or she works with could also become infested.

Benefits

- Massage has no specific benefits for clients who have mites.
- Clients who have recovered from mite infestations can enjoy the same benefits from bodywork as the rest of the population.

mixed connective tissue disease

Mixed connective tissue disease (MCTD) is a condition in which the signs and symptoms of several autoimmune disorders coexist and overlap in one person, although the severity tends to be less extreme than is usually seen with any single autoimmune disorder. Overlapping symptoms of MCTD usually include aspects of **lupus** and **scleroderma**. Symptoms of **rheumatoid arthritis**, **Raynaud syndrome**, and **Sjögren syndrome** may also be present.

Complications of MCTD include skin ulcers and **gangrene**, pulmonary hypertension and effusion, myocarditis, and **vasculitis**.

Signs and Symptoms

- Vary according to combinations of factors
- Joint pain, fatigue
- Painful nodules on the hands and elbows
- Sluggish digestion
- Raynaud phenomenon, swollen fingers, signs of scleroderma
- Shortness of breath with pulmonary hypertension, pleural effusion
- Discolored skin, ulcerations, infection, risk of gangrene with vasculitis
- Possibility of renal failure

Treatment Options

Plasmapheresis may be used to remove dysfunctional antibodies from the blood of people with MCTD. Patients are usually counseled to avoid excessive sun exposure, which tends to exacerbate symptoms.

Medications

Medication options for MCTD treat the symptoms, including topical steroids for skin lesions, anti-inflammatory drugs to manage joint and muscle pain, and blood pressure medication to relieve symptoms of vasculitis.

 Massage Considerations

Risks

- MCTD may affect lung and kidney function; these problems have implications for massage.
- MCTD may cause ulcerations and a risk of infection on the skin.
- Any massage or bodywork for a client with MCTD must be designed to stay within the person's activity levels and capacity for adaptation.

Benefits

- Massage has no specific benefits for MCTD, but gentle work may help ease joint pain, improve digestion, and promote parasympathetic effect.

---

moles

Moles (or nevi) are benign neoplasms (areas where melanocytes replicate onsite without invading the surrounding tissues). The melanocytes produce excessive melanin (the coloring agent for skin).

Risk factors for moles' becoming **skin cancer** are determined by when they appear (anything that appears after age 20 years is suspect), how big they are (anything bigger than 6 mm bears watching), and whether any of them stand out as different from other nearby moles.

Signs and Symptoms

- Small areas of darkened skin
- Symmetrical, unicolored

Treatment Options

Suspicious-looking moles that appear after age 20 years or that change over time are typically removed for examination.

Medications

Moles are not treated with medication.

 Massage Considerations

Risks

- Massage has no specific risk for clients with moles.

Benefits
- Massage has no specific benefits for clients with moles. These clients can enjoy the same benefits from massage as the rest of the population.

Practitioner Advice
- Massage therapists may be able to see moles that clients don't know they have; this can be valuable information to share.

---

molluscum contagiosum

Molluscum contagiosum is a relatively benign viral infection of the skin with the molluscum contagiosum virus, a member of the poxvirus family. It affects two major groups: young children and sexually active adults with infected partners.

Molluscum contagiosum is usually a self-limiting infection, and lesions typically disappear several months to a few years after they appear. In the meantime, they are contagious, and touching a lesion and then touching some other part of the body can spread them.

When molluscum contagiosum appears as a sexually transmitted disease, patients are encouraged to test for other STDs, including **chlamydia**, **gonorrhea**, and **genital warts**. It is important to note, however, that the viruses that cause genital warts are not related to the pathogen that causes molluscum contagiosum.

When molluscum contagiosum accompanies **HIV/AIDS** or other immunosuppressing disorders, the lesions tend to be larger, more aggressive, and longer lasting.

Signs and Symptoms
- Small, round, slightly itchy, wartlike lesions
- Pink, yellow, brown, flesh colored lesions
- May have a small dimple in the middle
- In young children: frequently found on the chest, arms, legs, face
- As sexually transmitted infection: found on the groin and genitals

Treatment Options
Because this is a contagious condition, people with molluscum contagiosum are usually counseled to have the lesions removed. This is accomplished with a variety of topical chemical applications, lasers, or cryotherapy.

Medications
Molluscum contagiosum may be treated with topical applications to help remove the lesions.

✋ Massage Considerations

Risks
- Molluscum contagiosum can spread from one part of the body to another and from one person to another. It at least locally contraindicates direct, hands-on massage or bodywork, although contact through a sheet or clothing may be safe.
- Clients with this condition would do well to treat it before receiving massage.

Benefits
- Massage has no specific benefits for clients with molluscum contagiosum.
- Clients with a history of molluscum contagiosum but no current symptoms can enjoy the same benefits from massage as the rest of the population.

mononucleosis

Mononucleosis ("mono") is a viral infection of the salivary glands and throat, which then moves into the lymphatic system by way of B cells. The causative agent in about 90% of all cases is the Epstein-Barr virus, a member of the herpes family. Another pathogen that may cause mononucleosis is cytomegalovirus, another member of herpesviridiae.

Incubation of a mononucleosis infection can last up to 60 days, during which time it is highly contagious but not strongly symptomatic. It is spread most efficiently through direct oral contact, which is why it is sometimes called the "kissing disease." After an initial infection, the virus goes dormant, but it may become active later without distinguishable symptoms. It is contagious during these recurrences.

Mononucleosis carries a risk of some complications. Strep throat is a common secondary infection, but more serious complications include central nervous system infections, damage to the heart, and problems with breathing because of dangerously inflamed lymph nodes.

Splenomegaly (enlargement of the spleen because it is filtering out damaged blood cells) occurs in about half of mononucleosis patients; if the spleen is damaged during this time, it could rupture. About 20% of patients also experience **hepatitis.** A small percentage of mononucleosis patients develop a splotchy, measles-like rash, especially if they are concurrently taking amoxicillin or ampicillin (two penicillin-family antibiotics that are prescribed for strep throat).

Signs and Symptoms

- In young patients: may be silent
- Prodrome: general fatigue, malaise
- Fever of 102°F to 104°F
- Sore throat
- Swollen, painful lymph nodes
- May take several months to recuperate

Treatment Options

Mononucleosis does not respond to antiviral medications. The typical approach is to treat the symptoms and wait for it to be over. Mononucleosis patients in recovery need to curtail activities that exhaust them and to avoid situations that could put them at risk for damaging the spleen.

Medications

Acetaminophen may be recommended for fever, but other medications tend to be ineffective for mononucleosis.

Massage Considerations

Risks

- Acute mononucleosis contraindicates massage.
- During recovery from mononucleosis, the lymph nodes and spleen may be congested and not fully functional. This may limit the applicability of circulatory and lymphatic techniques.

Benefits

- Energetic or reflexive massage that supports healing properties without taxing the lymph or immune systems may be a valuable addition to the lengthy healing process for clients with mononucleosis.

- Clients who have fully recovered from mononucleosis can enjoy the same benefits from massage as the rest of the population.

Morton neuroma

Morton neuroma is a condition in which the perineurium (the connective tissue wrapping around a section of peripheral nerve fibers) becomes enlarged. This usually occurs between the third and fourth metatarsal heads. When the perineurium grows, the foot bones and supportive ligaments directly press on the nerve, leading to symptoms on the plantar surface of the foot.

Morton neuroma is a common source of foot pain but not the only source. For the best possible outcome, it is important to differentiate Morton neuroma from any of the several other foot injuries that can create similar symptoms. Other possibilities include osteonecrosis of the metatarsal heads, stress **fractures**, **ganglion cysts**, **hammertoes**, intermetatarsal **bursitis**, and extensor tendon **tenosynovitis**. Perhaps the most commonly missed possibility is synovitis at the metatarsal–phalangeal joint.

Signs and Symptoms

- Dull ache in the foot that intensifies to a sharp, burning pain on the plantar aspect
- Exacerbated by foot compression, percussive activities
- Pain that lasts for minutes to hours
- Usually relieved with release of pressure and massage
- Recurring episodes

Treatment Options

Conservative treatment for Morton neuroma begins with changing footwear to flat, wide, padded shoes (i.e., athletic shoes). Orthotics or gel packs may be suggested to redistribute weight as it is transferred through the foot. Cryotherapy and deep massage are often used to reduce symptoms in the short term.

Surgery for Morton neuroma essentially severs the nerve at the metatarsal head. This is sometimes curative, but complications include the risk of a new neuroma at the nerve stump.

Medications

If less invasive interventions are not sufficient, cortisol injections may help shrink the connective tissue wrapping that compresses the nerves.

 Massage Considerations

Risks
- Excessive pressure or manipulation of the foot may elicit or exacerbate pain. Otherwise, massage has no specific risks for clients with Morton neuroma.

Benefits
- Carefully applied deep massage to the intrinsic muscles and ligaments of the foot, along with a change in footwear and increased awareness of optimal alignment, may ease Morton neuroma symptoms.

motor neurone disease: see amyotrophic lateral sclerosis

mucormycosis: see zygomycosis

multiple-chemical sensitivity syndrome

Multiple-chemical sensitivity syndrome (MCSS) is also called "idiopathic environmental intolerance." This condition is acquired after documentable exposure to a triggering substance. Symptoms affect multiple body systems; their severity occurs in relation to measurable (but not usually toxic) levels of chemical triggers. Chemically unrelated substances may trigger symptoms, and symptoms leave no objective evidence of permanent organ damage.

MCSS shows a lot of overlap with **fibromyalgia** and **chronic fatigue syndrome**, which can cloud the diagnostic process.

Signs and Symptoms

- Vary widely
- Chronic headaches
- Joint pain
- Cognitive difficulties
- Weakness
- Dizziness
- Heat intolerance
- Presence of a progressively growing group of triggers

Treatment Options

Mainstream and complementary practitioners may recommend gentle detoxification programs combined with avoidance of known triggers. This is a challenge for patients who are sensitive to plastics (including the plastic bottles that hold filtered water); pesticides, hormones, and fertilizers found in most foods; synthetic fabrics; the chemicals used to treat building materials; any kind of air pollution; and possibly the heavy metal amalgams that may be part of patients' dental work.

Acupuncture, dietary adjustments, and careful exercise regimens may be recommended to help restore lost balance and resilience in overtaxed systems. Ultimately, the most realistic goal of a person with MCSS may be to manage his or her condition rather than to "get over it."

Medications

MCSS is not treated with medication.

Massage Considerations

Risks

- Massage facilities hold many potential risks for people with MCSS. Detergents or bleach used to launder massage linens may be a trigger, as may be candles, scents, essential oils, incense, or the perfume worn by a previous client. All lubricants need to be evaluated carefully, not only for allergenic ingredients but also for the risk of contamination from pesticides or the plastic bottles in which it may be stored.

Benefits

- If environmental irritants can be controlled, massage may be a supportive, strengthening, and preciously rare time for a person to feel that his or her body is a good place in which to live.

multiple sclerosis

Multiple sclerosis (MS) is a condition characterized by inflammation and degeneration of myelin sheaths in the central nervous system (CNS). As the myelin is replaced with scar tissue, the electrical impulses meant to tie the whole system together literally short circuit. This results in transient or permanent motor and sensory paralysis.

Many experts consider MS to be an autoimmune disease. It often works in cycles of inflammatory flare followed by periods of remission. If the inflammation during a flare penetrates through the myelin sheath to affect the neurons, damage may be permanent.

Part of getting a definitive diagnosis for MS involves ruling out other disorders that create similar symptoms. This is a long list, including **Lyme disease**, **fibromyalgia**, **chronic fatigue syndrome**, **HIV/AIDS**, other autoimmune diseases, vascular problems in the CNS, and many others.

The progression of this disease is highly unpredictable. Some of the basic patterns are:
- Relapse/remitting (R/R): Definite periods of flare-ups are followed by long periods of remission. It may be years between episodes.
- Primary progressive (PP): Patients show a steady decline in function; flare-ups are frequent.
- Benign MS: The patient has only one flare-up in his or her lifetime.
- Malignant MS: This is a rapidly progressive form of the disease, with little respite (if any) between flare-ups.

Other presentations of MS are combinations of R/R or PP patterns.

Signs and Symptoms

- Gradual or sudden onset of muscle weakness
- Spasms
- Changes in sensation: numbness, paresthesia
- Optic neuritis
- Urinary incontinence
- Sexual dysfunction
- Digestive upset
- Fatigue
- Depression
- Cognitive changes: short-term memory loss, poor concentration, confusion

Treatment Options

Nondrug interventions for people with MS include mild exercise and physical or occupational therapy designed to maintain strength and function as long as possible. Eating well and getting adequate amounts of high-quality sleep are important for maintaining health and prolonging remissions. Stress management techniques, including massage, are often recommended for the same reasons.

Medications

Steroidal anti-inflammatory drugs may be used to control flares, but their side effects are severe, so they are usually a temporary measure. Interferon-betas may be injected; these may limit immune system activity and prolong remission.

Massage Considerations

Risks

- MS during a flare contraindicates rigorous massage that may present too much challenge for adaptation.

- Many MS patients find that overstimulation can trigger painful muscle spasms. This can be avoided with slow strokes that can be easily predicted and anticipated.
- Many MS patients don't tolerate rapid changes in temperature, and heat may lead to muscle spasms.
- Numbness is a local contraindication for any massage that has the goal of changing the quality of the tissue.

Benefits
- If sensation is present, massage can be useful as an agent against stress (which seems to trigger relapses), depression, and spasticity, and it can help maintain the health and mobility of the tissues.
- In areas where sensation is impaired, light effleurage or energetic strokes are more appropriate.

multiple system atrophy

Multiple system atrophy (MSA) is a progressive central nervous system disorder that has several different presentations. This pattern of signs and symptoms was first known as Shy-Drager syndrome. More recently, this term has been applied to one pattern of a larger disorder that is now called MSA.

Three main versions of MSA have been identified, although patients may display any of these features in varying combinations. These include Shy-Drager syndrome, striatonigral degeneration, and olivopontocerebellar atrophy.

Signs and Symptoms
- Shy-Drager syndrome
    - Orthostatic hypotension with lightheadedness
    - Fatigue
    - Blurred vision
    - Poor coordination (ataxia)
    - Urinary incontinence
    - Constipation
    - Central sleep apnea
    - Loss of language skills
    - Muscle wasting
- Striatonigral degeneration
    - Tremor
    - Rigidity
    - Hypokinesia or bradykinesia (difficulties in initiating movement)
- Olivopontocerebellar atrophy
    - Dysfunction in balance, coordination
    - Dysfunction with muscle tone
    - Speech and language dysfunction

Treatment Options

MSA is treated by its symptoms. If language or swallowing reflexes degenerate, a speech language pathologist may be able to help preserve function.

Medications

MSA may be treated with drugs for Parkinson disease, including dopamine agonists. Other medications can treat orthostatic hypotension, incontinence, constipation, and impotence.

Massage Considerations

Risks

- Clients with MSA may have movement disorders, urinary incontinence, and problems with speech. Any of these disorders may require adjustments in how massage is performed.
- Clients who have hypotension and poor reflexes may need assistance getting on and off the table.

Benefits

- Massage may help reduce the stiffness and rigidity seen in some MSA patients. This may assist in slowing the progression of the disease.

---

mumps

Mumps is a viral infection of the salivary glands and other tissues.

Mumps is easily transmissible through the saliva and mucous secretions. It incubates for 12 to 24 days before symptoms develop, but it is communicable starting around day 4 of the infection. Around 20% of people with mumps don't develop significant symptoms, but they are still capable of transmitting the virus to others.

Mumps usually infects the salivary glands but may infect other tissues as well, including the ovaries, testes, pancreas, and central nervous system. The risk of complications from this infection led to the development of the mumps vaccine, which is typically given as part of the "MMR" (measles, mumps, rubella) series in childhood.

Mumps complications are potentially dangerous. The older the person is when he or she is infected, the greater the risk of serious complications. These include **pancreatitis**, spontaneous **abortion** for pregnant women, orchitis (swelling of the testicles) for men, **encephalitis**, **meningitis**, and hearing loss.

Signs and Symptoms

- Low fever, malaise
- Inflammation of the parotid salivary glands
- Possible inflammation of other glands or tissues

Treatment Options

Mumps is a highly preventable infection with the use of the mumps vaccine.

After an infection has become established, the only treatment is supportive therapy in the form of compresses to relieve the pain of swollen glands, good nutrition, and plenty of rest.

Medications

Mumps infections are not treated with medication.

 Massage Considerations

Risks

- Acute infection contraindicates rigorous massage.

Benefits

- Clients who have fully recovered from mumps can enjoy the same benefits from massage as the rest of the population.

muscular dystrophy

Muscular dystrophy (MD) is a group of several closely related diseases involving genetic anomalies and the metabolism of fuel for energy in muscle tissue. These mutated genes lead to degeneration and wasting of muscle tissue. Eventually, the connective tissue shrinks, pulling bony attachments closer together in permanent contractures. It usually begins in the skeletal muscle but can ultimately affect the breathing muscles and the heart.

MD can progress to affect the spine, joints, heart, and lungs. Most people with Duchenne MD die at a young age of cardiac or respiratory failure.

MD is occasionally (but not always) accompanied by mental disability. Other conditions that accompany these diseases include contractures and **postural deviations** that develop as the skeletal muscles tighten and pull on the spine and rib cage.

All varieties of MD are X-linked inherited diseases (the affected gene is carried by the mother but is only passed on to her sons). It is possible for a female to have MD, but both her father and mother would have to carry the mutated genes.

Signs and Symptoms

- Duchenne and Becker MD
    Development of problems with walking in toddlerhood
    Leg pain
    Waddling gait, constant plantarflexion
    Pseudohypertrophy of the calf muscles
- Myotonic MD
    Myotonia: stiffness or spasm occurring after muscular contraction
- Facioscapulohumeral MD
    Affects the muscles of the face, shoulder, and upper arm
- Limb-girdle MD
    Affects the shoulders, upper arms, pelvis
- Emery-Dreifuss MD
    Contractures of the Achilles tendon, elbow, and spine
- Oculopharyngeal MD
    Affects the eyes and pharynx muscles

Treatment Options

MD has no cure; treatment focuses on enhancing coping skills. Some interventions aim to prolong the use of the muscles and limbs, and surgery is sometimes recommended to release tight tendons or straighten a distorted spine.

Medications

Prednisone is a steroidal anti-inflammatory drug that can temporarily preserve function, but the side effects of long-term use are serious.

🤚 Massage Considerations

Risks

- Massage has no specific risks for MD patients as long as they can adapt to the changes that massage brings about.

Benefits
- This is a disorder of muscle function, but sensation is intact. Massage can be used along with physical therapy to slow the progression of contractures and improve the general quality of life.

myalgic encephalomyelitis: see chronic fatigue syndrome

myasthenia gravis

Myasthenia gravis (MG) is an autoimmune disease that involves the degeneration or destruction of specific receptor sites at neuromuscular junctions. Acetylcholine receptors are impaired or completely disabled in MG patients. This means that muscle cells can't be stimulated by their motor neurons. MG is a progressive condition, but it is usually manageable.

Signs and Symptoms
- Weakness, fatigability in the affected muscles
- Usually begins at the eyes or lower facial muscles: flattened smile, ptosis (drooping eyelids), difficulty with eating and speech
- Exacerbated by repetitive activity, overexertion, heat, some medications
- Progression may level off after a few years
- Progression may later resume to affect the muscles of the trunk

Treatment Options

Treatment of MG usually has two goals: to boost nerve transmission and to suppress immune system activity at the neuromuscular junctions. In the event of a MG crisis (a sudden onset that threatens the patient's ability to breathe), plasmapheresis may be used to remove antibodies from the blood.

Medications

Medication for MG includes drugs that limit the normal destruction of acetylcholine by local enzymes and steroids that suppress immune system activity.

Massage Considerations

Risks
- Excessive heat may aggravate MG symptoms.

Benefits
- Massage may help preserve stamina and muscle function.

myeloma

Myeloma (literally, "marrow tumor") is a blood cancer involving a genetic mutation in maturing B cells found in the bone marrow. This causes the B cells to proliferate into tumors, secrete cytokines that stimulate osteoclast activity, and produce faulty antibodies.

Myeloma tumors typically grow in the spine, pelvis, ribs, or skull. They can interfere with blood production, leading to **anemia**, poor clotting, and reduced resistance to infection. Faulty antibodies produced by myeloma cells can break into fragments called Bence Jones proteins. These can accumulate in the kidneys, leading to a risk of **renal failure**.

Myeloma can occur in only one location (solitary myeloma), in several bone sites at once (multiple myeloma), or outside bone tissue (extramedullary plasmacytoma).

Signs and Symptoms
- Silent in the early stages
- Bone pain, fractures
- Kidney dysfunction
- Amyloidosis (accumulation of inflammatory proteins) in the heart and lungs

Treatment Options
Myeloma is often resistant to treatment. Chemotherapy and stem cell transplantation are often suggested.

Medications
Myeloma may be treated with chemotherapy.

Massage Considerations

Risks
- Myeloma can involve bone fragility and a risk of fractures.
- As with other types of cancer, the challenges of treatment require adaptations in bodywork modalities.

Benefits
- Gentle massage may help ease pain, mitigate the side effects of medication, and improve the quality of life for clients with myeloma.

myocardial infarction: see heart attack

myofascial pain syndrome

Myofascial pain syndrome (MPS) involves an accumulation of many active, painful trigger points. Trigger points begin with sustained, involuntary contraction of an isolated group of sarcomeres (the overlapping units of myofibrils that create the striations associated with skeletal muscles). When a microscopic contraction pulls on the rest of the myofiber, it creates a taut band. This gives rise to two simultaneous problems: an increased need for fuel and a decreased supply of blood because of local ischemia. This situation is sometimes called an adenosine triphosphate (ATP) energy crisis. Chemicals that increase sensitivity and pain are released, including prostaglandins, bradykinin, serotonin, substance P, and others, generating pain. In response to pain, the muscle attempts to tighten further, causing more secretion of acetylcholine. Poor local circulation limits the availability of acetylcholine-neutralizing enzymes and inhibits the movement of calcium back into channels in the cell membrane. The consequence is a tiny and involuntary but prolonged and painful contraction of one part of a muscle cell.

Prolonged immersion in pain-causing chemicals carries a toll on local sensory neurons. Some research suggests that the neurons become locally demyelinated, which may contribute to the unique referred pain pattern seen with trigger points.

MPS is often discussed as a condition related to **fibromyalgia**, but it is important to delineate between the trigger points seen with MPS and the tender points seen with fibromyalgia; digital pressure can relieve trigger points but exacerbates tender points. The issue is further confused by the fact that tender points and trigger points can exist simultaneously.

Signs and Symptoms

- Occurs in discrete regions rather than throughout the body
- Hypertonic knots or taut bands in the soft tissue
- Pressure may elicit a twitch response
- Trigger points refer pain to distant areas

Treatment Options

MPS is treated by eradicating trigger points. This is accomplished in a number of different ways, including topical application of an aerosol vapocoolant, local injections of anesthetics, dry needling, and massage. All of these approaches work to interrupt the ATP energy crisis, allowing the tight fibers to relax while the muscle is stretched.

Because MPS often develops out of chronic overuse or poor ergonomics, the patient's movement and work habits are often examined so perpetuating factors may be eliminated.

Medications

MPS is not usually treated with medication.

Massage Considerations

Risks

- Massage has no specific risks for clients with MPS.

Benefits

- Massage can substantially increase the local circulation to help resolve active trigger points. This can be done through static or pulsing pressure on the trigger point.
- Massage can help clear metabolic wastes out of areas where trigger points have been active.
- Massage can help increase awareness about postural or movement patterns that contribute to trigger point irritation.

---

myositis ossificans

Myositis ossificans, also called heterotopic ossification, is the development of calcifications in soft tissue areas. Typically, it begins with a trauma and intermuscular bleeding or **hematoma**. The blood pools between layers of muscles, where it quickly coagulates. The liquid disperses, leaving behind a calcium/iron formation that looks and feels like a bone fragment.

Eventually, the body recognizes that the calcium deposits don't belong there, and it breaks down and reabsorbs the bony growth. This can take months or years, but the lesion spontaneously resolves in most people.

This condition is a particular risk for people with **spinal cord injuries** who use wheelchairs. Areas where blood can thicken and clot have a tendency to form painful calcium deposits.

Signs and Symptoms

- Usually affects large muscles, especially the quadriceps femoris and biceps brachii
- Acute stage: the area feels bruised

- Subacute stage: the area feels hard and locally tender
- Postacute stage: no pain, but dense bony deposits are present in the soft tissues

Treatment Options

Treatment for myositis ossificans tends to be conservative. To limit further bleeding, patients are recommended to rest and isolate the injured area in the acute stage. In the subacute stage, passive stretching is used to restore range of motion, followed by exercises to restore normal muscle strength.

If a calcified mass interferes with muscle or tendon function, it can be surgically removed. This kind of surgery is avoided whenever possible, however, because this condition tends to resolve without intervention.

Medications

Myositis ossificans is not usually treated with medication.

🖐 Massage Considerations

Risks
- Myositis ossificans locally contraindicates massage, which may increase bleeding and injury of damaged tissues.

Benefits
- Massage with caution around the borders of the lesion, along with stretching and exercise, may help speed the process by which these bony deposits can be broken down and reabsorbed by the body.

myotonic muscular dystrophy: see muscular dystrophy

N

narcolepsy: see sleep disorders

nasal polyps

Nasal polyps are benign growths that extend from the nasal mucosa or within the nasal sinuses. The process by which they begin is not well understood, but they are associated with long-term inflammation and irritation of the nasal passages, as seen with allergic rhinitis, bronchial asthma, fungal infections of the sinuses, and chronic sinusitis. They can grow in clusters or as one large polyp.

Nasal polyps are linked to chronic systemic inflammation and have a genetic predisposition. They are frequently seen in children with **cystic fibrosis**. People with polyps should be evaluated for cystic fibrosis and **asthma**.

Untreated polyps may cause **sleep apnea** because they interfere with breathing. They may also increase the risk of infectious **sinusitis**. In rare circumstances, very large polyps may exert pressure on the craniofacial bones and cause distortions in the shape of the face.

Signs and Symptoms

- Difficulty breathing through the nose
- Impaired sense of smell
- Chronic sinus drainage, stuffy nose, headache
- Frequent sinus infections

Treatment Options

Surgery to remove polyps is conducted when medications no longer work, but patients often find that this is not a permanent solution.

Medications

Nasal polyps can be treated with topical or oral steroidal anti-inflammatory drugs. Antihistamines and decongestants are usually discouraged.

Massage Considerations

Risks

- Clients may not be comfortable lying flat.
- Screen for the risk of sinus or respiratory infections.
- If clients use anti-inflammatory drugs, make appropriate adjustments.

Benefits

- Careful massage of the face with comfortable positioning may promote healthy sinus drainage and clearing.

necrotizing fasciitis: see cellulitis

nephrolithiases: see kidney stones

neuroma: see Morton neuroma

nosebleed

Epistaxis is the medical term for nosebleed. Nosebleeds typically occur when a network of blood vessels in the highly vascularized nasal sinuses ruptures. Nosebleeds occur most frequently in the winter, when people are likely to be in warm, dry, heated air and when the risk of respiratory infection and irritation is high.

In older adults, epistaxis is frequently related to underlying conditions that may include bleeding disorders, a risk of cancer, **hypertension**, and **atherosclerosis**. Also, mature people who take anticoagulant medications may have an increased risk for nosebleed.

Signs and Symptoms

- Bleeding from the nose
- Usually resolves within a few minutes
- If episodes are frequent and persistent, medical intervention may be necessary

Treatment Options

Most nosebleeds can be treated at home by pinching the soft tissues of the nose and pressing them back toward the face for 5 minutes or more. Applying ice to the face or the back of the neck may be helpful. Frequent and extreme nosebleeds may be treated with cauterization or applying topical medications inside the nose.

Medications

If a nosebleed can't be controlled with basic measures, a doctor may pack the patient's nose with topical medication to promote vasoconstriction.

Massage Considerations

Risks

- In the absence of underlying pathology, massage has no specific risks for clients with nosebleeds.
- Mature clients who get frequent nosebleeds should find out the cause.
- A nosebleed during a massage requires stopping the session until the bleeding is resolved.

Benefits

- Massage has no specific benefits for clients who have nosebleeds.
- Clients who have occasional nosebleeds with no underlying pathology can enjoy the same benefits from massage as the rest of the population.

nummular eczema: see dermatitis/eczema

nystagmus

Nystagmus is a rhythmic oscillation of the eyes. This condition is congenital (a person is born with abnormalities in the visual pathway) or acquired (problems with vestibular input develop later in life).

Any damage or problem in the complex connections between the eyes and the central nervous system can create a type of nystagmus. Many different forms of this condition have been identified, each with a specific pattern of movement.

When nystagmus is acquired, it can be a sign of another problem, such as **multiple sclerosis** or brain tumors.

Nystagmus is frequently accompanied by **vertigo, tremor** of the head, and **torticollis.**

Signs and Symptoms

- Ocular oscillations
- Horizontal or vertical plane; torsion or rotary form
- Usually bilateral, although one side may be more extreme than the other

Treatment Options

Some medications make nystagmus worse; the first step in treatment is to eliminate or replace these medications. Corrective lenses or glasses with prisms can help control some symptoms. If a specific and operable lesion is found in the brain, surgery may be conducted to correct it.

Medications

Injections with botulinum toxin can be effective if the problem is motor control of the extraocular muscles.

Massage Considerations

Risks

- Nystagmus has no specific risks for massage.
- Vertigo symptoms may be exacerbated when a client sits up; the therapist should allow extra time for this transition.

Benefits

- Clients with nystagmus can enjoy the same benefits from massage as the rest of the population.

O

obesity

Obesity is the state of storing excessive body fat. Although several methods of measuring body fat exist, the most commonly accepted one that accommodates for variations in height and build is body mass index (BMI).

The BMI formula is weight (in pounds) multiplied by 703; this number is divided by height (in inches) squared. A person is considered overweight with a BMI between 25 and 29.9. Obesity is diagnosed at a BMI between 30 and 39.9. Severe obesity is diagnosed at any BMI over 40.

The list of weight-related disorders that accompanies obesity is long and includes some life–threatening conditions. **Metabolic syndrome** is a collection of signs that point to a risk of type 2 **diabetes, atherosclerosis**, and heart disease. Obesity also significantly increases the risk for **stroke, sleep apnea, osteoarthritis, gallstones**, fatty liver and **cirrhosis, gastroesophageal reflux disease** (and consequently **esophageal cancer**), stress incontinence, menstrual irregularities, and infertility.

Signs and Symptoms

- Excessive fat storage in relation to height and build

Treatment Options

Treatment for obesity begins with an assessment of risk and the development of management techniques. Behavioral therapies can support people making new and difficult decisions about eating. The goal is for people to increase their exercise while decreasing their caloric intake.

If changes to diet and exercise are unsuccessful, other treatment options may be pursued, including various types of medication and bariatric surgery.

Medications

Some medications work to suppress appetite or boost metabolism, but they don't tend to work without a careful eating and exercise plan.

🖐 Massage Considerations

Risks
• Massage therapists must screen obese clients for cardiovascular disease, diabetes, and arthritis and must make appropriate adjustments in goals and modalities.

Benefits
• Massage is a supportive, affirming, nonjudgmental activity for people who live in a society that, regardless of how common this condition is, tends to judge and punish them for taking up too much space.

obsessive–compulsive disorder: see anxiety disorders

oculopharyngeal muscular dystrophy: see muscular dystrophy

onychomycosis: see fungal infections

open wounds and sores

Skin can be damaged in many ways, and each injury has its own technical term. Some common skin lesions include lacerations (rips and tears), incisions (cuts), excoriations (scratches), fissures (cracks), papules (firm, raised areas, such as pimples), vesicles (blisters), pustules (vesicles filled with pus, such as whiteheads), punctures (any kind of hole), avulsions (something has been ripped off, such as a finger or an ear), abrasions (scrapes), and ulcers (sores with dead tissue that don't go through a normal healing process).

When skin injuries lead to an excessive accumulation of scar tissue, the resulting lesion is called a **keloid** scar.

Signs and Symptoms
• See descriptions above

Treatment Options
Skin injuries can be treated with antiseptic or antibiotic cream; various types of bandages; or if necessary, sutures or other interventions to hold the edges of the wound together for best healing.

Medications
Besides making sure wounds are kept as clean as possible and applying antiseptic chemicals, most sores are not treated with medication.

🖐 Massage Considerations

Risks
• Open wounds at least locally contraindicate massage. The contraindication is systemic if the skin damage is caused by an underlying disorder that could be exacerbated by massage.

Benefits
- Massage around the perimeter of a noninfected lesion may stimulate circulation, help speed healing, and minimize scar tissue.

optic neuritis

Optic neuritis is inflammation of the optic nerve. It is usually unilateral. It can occur as the result of a viral infection (e.g., measles or chickenpox) or as part of an autoimmune attack on the myelin sheaths around the nerve fibers (as seen with **multiple sclerosis**).

Signs and Symptoms
- Loss of vision that may last for several weeks
- Sudden onset of blurriness
- Problems with color differentiation
- Eye pain

Treatment Options

Optic neuritis is typically treated with medication. If a person has repeated episodes, he or she may be tested for multiple sclerosis.

Medications

Steroidal anti-inflammatory drugs can shorten episodes of optic neuritis.

Massage Considerations

Risks
- Massage has no specific risks for optic neuritis.
- Clients with this condition may also have multiple sclerosis; this condition has some implications for massage.
- Massage therapists may need to make adjustments in modalities for clients who use steroidal anti-inflammatory drugs.

Benefits
- Clients with a history of optic neuritis can enjoy the same benefits from massage as the rest of the population.

Osgood-Schlatter disease

Osgood-Schlatter disease (OSD) is a condition involving irritation and inflammation at the site of the quadriceps attachment on the tibial tuberosity. It occurs when the quadriceps muscles are vigorously used in combination with rapid growth of the leg bones.

When an athletic child has a growth spurt, the leg bones can grow faster than the muscles and fascia that cross the knee. The quadriceps tendon can pull away from the bone, causing a type of **tendinopathy**. In extreme cases, the tibial tuberosity itself can become damaged or even avulsed. It is common for OSD patients to develop a large, permanent spur at the quadriceps insertion. OSD is usually unilateral, but a small number of athletes can develop inflammation of both knees.

Signs and Symptoms

- Occurs mostly in athletic teenagers
- Acute stage: knee is hot, swollen, painful at the tibial tuberosity
- Subacute stage: the tibial tuberosity is enlarged

Treatment Options

Treatment for OSD focuses on reducing pain and limiting damage to the quadriceps attachment at the tibia. Hydrotherapy and careful stretching are often sufficient to manage the symptoms. Patients with more severe cases may require casting and physical therapy or even surgery to remove bone chips if the tibia fractures at the site of the tension.

Medications

People with acute OSD may use analgesics to help manage inflammatory pain.

Massage Considerations

Risks

- Acute OSD locally contraindicates massage.

Benefits

- Lymphatic work may help reduce inflammation when OSD is very painful.
- In subacute OSD, massage with stretching can address quadriceps tension that may irritate the tibial tuberosity.
- Clients with a history of OSD and a permanently enlarged tibial tuberosity can enjoy all the benefits from massage as the rest of the population.

---

osteoarthritis

Also called degenerative joint disease, osteoarthritis (OA) is a condition in which the synovial joints, especially weight-bearing joints, are irritated, inflamed, and eventually deformed, typically as a result of long-term wear and tear.

OA usually begins with damage to the articular cartilage inside the joint capsule. When one surface is no longer smooth, the contacting surfaces are also damaged. Eventually, the bones may adapt by becoming thickened at the condyles and growing osteophytes or bone spurs at the sites of most stress. Muscles that cross the arthritic joint tend to become hypertonic as they try to stabilize a painful area. Ultimately, atrophy may develop through lack of use.

Contributing factors for OA include loose ligaments and joint instability, repetitive pounding stress, hormonal and nutritional imbalance, dehydration, and being overweight or **obese**. The joints most at risk for this condition are the knees and hips.

OA is the leading factor behind most **joint replacement surgeries**.

Signs and Symptoms

- Pain and stiffness at the affected joints
- Acutely hot inflammation is rare
- Increased pain with changes in external air pressure
- At the knee or hip: can interfere with the ability to walk

Treatment Options

The goals of treatment for OA are to reduce pain and inflammation and limit or reverse the damage incurred to the joint structures. These goals are accomplished in a number of different ways, depending on how advanced the condition is.

Exercise within pain tolerance is recommended to reduce weight and maintain joint function. Nutritional supplements to help regenerate new cartilage are useful for some people. A last-ditch option for many OA patients is joint replacement surgery.

Medications

Symptoms of OA can be treated with nonsteroidal anti-inflammatory drugs of various kinds.

Massage Considerations

Risks
- If inflammation is acute, OA locally contraindicates massage.

Benefits
- Massage can decrease tension in the muscles that cross arthritic joints.
- Careful joint mobilization and stretching may help preserve function.

---

osteogenesis imperfecta

Osteogenesis imperfecta (OI) is a genetic disorder in which collagen that provides the framework for bones and other connective tissues is incorrectly formed or is not present in sufficient amounts. This leads to bones that fracture with little or no stress. A common term for OI is "brittle bone disease."

OI occurs in four basic types ranging from mild to extremely severe. OI patients have a high risk for **osteoporosis** and bone **fractures,** and they often experience problems with lung function and **postural deviations**.

Signs and Symptoms
- Spontaneous fractures that occur in infancy and early childhood
- Bluish or grayish sclera of the eye
- Ligament laxity
- Brittle teeth

Treatment Options

This genetic disorder cannot be corrected. Treatment options are designed to protect the patient from further fractures. Gentle exercise to maintain bone density is recommended, and exercise in water (swimming or water aerobics) is often a safe option. Surgery to insert rods into the long bones for extra support is sometimes conducted, as well as surgery to correct scoliosis if necessary.

Medications

OI may be treated with hormone supplements that promote osteoblast activity and increase bone density.

Massage Considerations

Risks
- Clients with OI have pathologically brittle bones; avoid percussion and all modalities that put traction or other force on bones.

Benefits
- Clients with mild forms of OI, especially if they are physically active, are safe for massage.
- Clients who have more severe OI may benefit from energetic or reflexive work for relaxation and pain relief without risks to their bones.

osteomalacia

Osteomalacia, or "soft bones," is a metabolic disorder involving a deficiency of available calcium or phosphorus, leading to poor mineralization of bones and a risk of fractures. When osteomalacia occurs in children, it is also called rickets.

Causes of osteomalacia vary and can include vitamin D deficiency, reactions to anticonvulsant medication or dialysis, chronic **renal failure**, **hyperthyroidism**, excessive use of antacids, toxicity with fluoride or aluminum, or liver disease.

It is important to test for osteomalacia when an adult develops signs of fatigue and bone pain because this condition strongly resembles **osteoporosis**, and it requires different treatment for the best possible outcome.

Signs and Symptoms
- Fatigue, malaise
- Bone pain
- Muscle weakness
- In children: bowed legs; irregular growth plates, especially in the femur

Treatment Options
Treatment for osteomalacia depends on the precipitating factors. Options range from vitamin D supplements to chelation of the blood to remove toxins that contribute to bone problems.

Medications
Osteomalacia patients may take calcium and vitamin D supplements in an effort to boost their bone density.

 Massage Considerations

Risks
- Osteomalacia leads to brittle bones and a risk of fracture. Modalities that exert pressure or traction on the bones should be avoided.
- Osteomalacia may be linked to renal failure or hyperthyroidism. Both of these conditions influence decisions about massage.

Benefits
- If they do not have an underlying disorder, clients with osteomalacia can enjoy the same benefits from carefully administered massage as the rest of the population.

osteomyelitis

Osteomyelitis is the presence of infectious agents in bone tissue. The affected area can spread through the periosteum, bone cortex, cancellous bone, or marrow. Bacteria are the usual agents, but fungal infections can also be present.

Osteomyelitis can occur as a complication from another infection somewhere else in the body or through direct contact between bones and infectious agents during severe trauma or surgery. When children develop this infection, it is usually in the long bones; adults typically develop the infection in the vertebrae or pelvic bones.

Factors that increase the risk of osteomyelitis include having **diabetes** (especially with puncture wounds of the foot), **sickle cell disease**, **alcoholism**, **AIDS**, or recent orthopedic surgery.

Unsuccessfully treated osteomyelitis may lead to spinal cord compression if it affects the vertebrae or **amputation** if it develops in the extremities.

Mastoiditis is a specific type of bone infection related to ear infections (**otitis**).

Signs and Symptoms
- Can be acute or chronic
- Acute: pain at the infection site, fever, malaise, fatigue, local edema, erythema
- Chronic: pain at the infection site, resistance to treatment, drainage of pus from the skin
- Elevated C-reactive protein, erythrocyte sedimentation rate

Treatment Options
In addition to antibiotics, surgical debridement (removal of permanently damaged bone) is a key part of osteomyelitis treatment.

Medications
Osteomyelitis is treated with oral or intravenous antibiotics. Affected bone may also be implanted with antibiotic-treated beads.

Massage Considerations
Risks
- Acute infection contraindicates massage.
- Clients with chronic osteomyelitis should avoid rigorous massage until the infection has begun to respond to treatment.

Benefits
- Reflexive or energetic techniques that help boost immune system function and reduce pain are the best options for clients with osteomyelitis until the infection has completely resolved.
- Clients who have fully recovered from osteomyelitis can enjoy the same benefits from massage as the rest of the population.

osteonecrosis: see avascular osteonecrosis

osteoporosis

Osteoporosis means "porous bones." In this condition, calcium is pulled off the bones faster than it is replaced, leaving the bones thinned, brittle, and prone to injury.

Calcium is consumed in nearly every chemical reaction that results in muscle contraction, blood clotting, and nerve transmission. Calcium ions also help maintain the proper pH balance in the blood. When less calcium enters the body through nutrition than is needed on a daily basis, it is drawn off the bones. Spongy bone is more metabolically active than dense bone, so the femoral neck and vertebral bodies are the most vulnerable to bone thinning.

Complications of osteoporosis mostly involve pathologically weak bones. Thinned vertebrae lead to a loss of height and the characteristic rounded "widow's hump" of **hyperkyphosis**. Chronic and acute back pain appear in this stage as the vertebrae continue to degenerate. People with osteoporosis are also prone to other fractures with little or no cause; these are called spontaneous or pathologic **fractures**.

One condition that can contribute to osteoporosis is **hyperthyroidism**. If this is condition is treated, the bone loss it causes may be reversible.

Signs and Symptoms
- Often silent until advanced
- Spontaneous fractures, usually of the femoral head or vertebral bodies

Treatment Options

Diet and exercise are important parts of the treatment strategy for osteoporosis. Dietary adjustments focus on taking in calcium in an easily absorbable form. Exercise programs take advantage of the fact that bone remodels according to the stresses placed on it. For people with osteoporosis, gentle weight training or walking is more beneficial for bone density than low-impact exercises, such as swimming or cycling.

Medications

Pharmacologic interventions for osteoporosis include drugs that inhibit resorption of calcium (bisphosphonates, calcitonin, and estrogen analogues) and medications that promote new bone formation (parathyroid hormone analogues).

🖐 Massage Considerations

Risks
- Clients with osteoporosis can't tolerate excessive pressure or percussion.
- Elderly clients with osteoporosis may have several other conditions at the same time; some of these conditions may have implications for massage as well.

Benefits
- Massage does not reverse osteoporosis, but it can improve pain and mobility, increasing the quality of life of clients with the condition.

Practitioner Advice
- Clients with osteoporosis and hyperkyphosis may need extra cushioning support to be comfortable on the table.

otitis

Otitis is the medical term for ear infections. These can take place in three forms: outer ear infections (otitis externa), middle ear infections (otitis media), and inner ear infections (otitis interna).

Children are at highest risk for most ear infections, but adults can get them, too, usually as a complication of a **cold**, sore throat (**pharyngitis**), or **flu**. Most ear infections get better without other complications, but chronic conditions that occur while a young child is developing skills can interfere with speech and language development.

Otitis Externa

Otitis externa is an infection of the outer ear involving the pinna and canal outside the eardrum. Infections there are often related to aggressive removal of cerumen (earwax), which is a naturally protective substance. Abrasions to the skin may become infected with local bacteria, fungi, or *Candida* spp. Otitis externa can become serious when the infection reaches the local lymph nodes or bones.

Otitis Media

Otitis media, also called "swimmer's ear," is an infection or inflammation in the middle ear (the air space deep to the eardrum). In this space, the tiny ear bones (the malleus, incus, and stapes) transfer sound waves from the eardrum to the nerves in the inner ear; these vibrations are then translated into sound perception in the brain. When this space is filled with pus or water, the bones can't vibrate freely, and sound perception is suppressed.

Otitis Interna

Otitis interna is a rare situation in which infection or inflammation affects the cochlea (the section of the ear that holds the organs for sound and balance). This can lead to disabling **vertigo**.

Signs and Symptoms

- Pain, fever, irritability
- Drainage from the ear
- Loss of hearing
- Loss of balance

Treatment Options

Outer ear infections can be prevented with good ear care. Mixtures with vinegar or alcohol are sometimes recommended to loosen excessive earwax. Chronic repeating middle ear infections may be treated with the insertion of small metal or plastic tubes through the eardrum; this equalizes air pressure on either side of the eardrum and reduces the risk and frequency of further infections for the 6 to 12 months that the tubes stay in place.

Medications

Middle ear infections have traditionally been treated with antibiotics, but the research on the benefits of this (versus waiting until the infection naturally subsides) is inconclusive.

 Massage Considerations

Risks

- Acute infection with fever and malaise contraindicates circulatory massage.

Benefits
- Massage is unlikely to speed the recovery time of clients with otitis.
- Gentle modalities may be welcome for their soothing effect on a child in distress because of otitis.
- Clients who have fully recovered from any form of otitis can enjoy the same benefits from massage as the rest of the population.

---

ovarian cancer

Ovarian cancer is the growth of malignant tumors on the ovaries, usually starting in the epithelial cells.

Epithelial tumors of the ovaries fall into several different categories, each with different growth patterns and prognoses. Some of these tumors are slow growing and may never become malignant. But many types of epithelial ovarian tumors aggressively invade not only the ovaries but other pelvic and abdominal organs as well. These tumors are life threatening, not only because they are so prone to metastasis but also because they create few (if any) noticeable symptoms in their early stages. Early symptoms can mimic **ovarian cysts**, delaying a timely diagnosis and reducing the chance of a successful treatment outcome.

Risk factors for ovarian cancer include familial history (the first-degree female relatives of a woman with ovarian cancer have a 50% chance of developing the disease); reproductive history (it is most common in women who have never had children or who have taken fertility drugs); health history (women who have the breast cancer genes *BRCA1* or *BRCA2* or who have had **breast** or **colorectal cancer** have an increased risk); hormone replacement therapy used for **menopause;** and some toxic exposures, including radiation, asbestos, and talcum powder.

Signs and Symptoms
- May be silent or very subtle
- Sense of heaviness in the pelvis
- Abdominal discomfort: bloating, nausea, diarrhea, constipation
- Change in the menstrual cycle, vaginal bleeding
- Weight gain or loss
- Abdominal mass, increased girth in the abdomen, ascites

Treatment Options

Ovarian cancer is generally treated with surgery and chemotherapy. Surgery is done to remove the ovaries (oophorectomy) and sometimes the uterine tubes and uterus as well.

Medications

Chemotherapy for ovarian cancer can be conducted orally at home or intravenously in a hospital. One method delivers the cytotoxic drugs directly into the peritoneum, where they can have immediate access to malignant tumors.

Massage Considerations

Risks
- Risks related to ovarian cancer include abdominal massage that may disrupt active growths and massage anywhere else that the cancer may have metastasized.
- Risks related to ovarian cancer treatment include complications of chemotherapy and surgery that require adjustments in bodywork modalities.

Benefits
- As with other kinds of cancer, massage may improve the tolerance of cancer treatment by supporting immune system activity, promoting sleep and appetite, reducing pain and anxiety, and generally improving the quality of life of clients undergoing a tremendous challenge.

ovarian cysts

Ovarian cysts are fluid- or blood-filled cysts that develop on the ovaries. Some of these cysts can interfere with ovarian function, and some can be an indicator of a risk of ovarian cancer.

The most common types of ovarian cysts are follicular cysts and corpus luteum cysts. Follicular cysts occur when the follicle that holds a mature egg doesn't rupture completely, and a blister forms at the site. Corpus luteum cysts form when a blister grows over the site after an egg was released. Corpus luteum cysts can delay subsequent ovulations and produce pregnancylike symptoms (nausea, vomiting, breast tenderness) until they spontaneously resolve, usually within 1 or 2 months.

A third type of ovarian cyst is related to a condition called **polycystic ovary disease**. This condition involves enlarged ovaries with multiple small cysts. The interference in hormone secretion that this condition creates can lead to **obesity,** loss of the menstrual cycle, **acne,** and hirsutism (increased body hair).

Other types of ovarian cysts include cystadenomas (these are usually benign epithelial tumors, but they do carry a risk of becoming malignant) and dermoid cysts or teratomas, which contain primitive cells that may develop into hair, teeth, and other tissues. Some cysts may be related to **endometriosis,** or they may be varieties of precancerous growths that may develop into **ovarian cancer.**

Signs and Symptoms

- May be silent unless irritated
- May cause a constant dull ache in the lower abdomen on the affected side
- When enlarged: firm, painless swelling in the pelvis
- Possible pain with intercourse
- Possible low back or leg pain from pressure on the lumbosacral plexus nerves

Treatment Options

Ovarian cysts that don't spontaneously resolve may be aspirated, but more often, surgery is performed to remove them. The affected ovary is usually removed, too. In some cases, a complete removal of the ovaries and uterus is recommended because some types of cysts tend to recur and can develop into cancer.

Medications

Follicular and corpus luteum cysts are often treated with oral contraceptives, which alter hormonal secretions and allow the cysts to recede completely or shrink to a size that is easily removed.

Massage Considerations

Risks
- Ovarian cysts contraindicate deep abdominal massage; not only are they vulnerable to rupture, but they displace pelvic organs, putting other structures at risk for injury.

Benefits
- Soft abdominal massage can be very soothing for women with diagnosed ovarian cysts.
- Elsewhere on the body, clients with ovarian cysts can enjoy the same benefits from massage as the rest of the population.

Paget disease

Paget disease is a condition in which normal bone is reabsorbed and replaced with disorganized fibrous connective tissue, which never completely calcifies. This leaves the affected bones weak, distorted, and vulnerable to fracture.

Typically, this disease occurs in two stages. In the vascular stage, bone is replaced with jumbled, chaotic fibrous tissue, which is supplied by vast numbers of new blood vessels. Then in the sclerotic stage, the new material becomes brittle rather than strong. The bones most often affected by this disease are the spine, skull, pelvis, femur, and lower leg.

Paget disease is associated with an increased risk of bone **fractures**. **Heart failure** is another risk because the deposits are highly invested with new blood vessels, which puts a great load on the cardiovascular system. If the bony deformation affects the cranial bones, pressure on the brain may lead to **headaches** or vision or hearing loss. About 1% of Paget disease patients develop a rare form of bone cancer.

Signs and Symptoms
- Often completely silent until advanced
- Deep bone pain
- Palpable heat at the affected bones
- Hearing or vision loss, headaches, pinched nerves
- Bowing in the femur or lower legs

Treatment Options
To maintain function and healthy bone mass as long as possible, careful exercise is the first recommendation for people with Paget disease.

Medications
Aspirin and anti-inflammatory drugs may be suggested for pain relief. Calcitonin analogues or bisphosphonates may be prescribed to inhibit osteoclast activity.

Massage Considerations

Risks
- Fragile, brittle bones contraindicate deep pressure and percussion.
- A compromised cardiovascular system may not be able to adapt to the changes that massage brings about.

Benefits
- Massage that adapts for bone and cardiovascular health may relieve pain and support the ability of clients with Paget disease to do recommended exercise and physical therapy.

palmar fasciitis: see Dupuytren contracture

pancreatic cancer

Pancreatic cancer begins as the mutation of genes that trigger uncontrolled growth of cells in the pancreas. When tumors arise in the exocrine ducts, they are referred to as adenocarcinomas. When they grow in the islet cells, they are called neuroendocrine tumors. In either case, the tumors tend to grow quickly and invade nearby tissues simply by spreading outward. The duodenum, stomach, and peritoneal wall are often affected by these local extensions. When cells invade the abdominal lymph system, the liver is often the first site of metastasis.

A history of type 2 **diabetes** or chronic **pancreatitis** may increase the risk of developing pancreatic cancer.

Signs and Symptoms
- Abdominal discomfort, loss of appetite, unintended weight loss
- Jaundice if a tumor obstructs the common bile duct
- Pruritus, rashes with liver congestion
- Indigestion, ascites, hepatomegaly
- Dysregulation of blood glucose

Treatment Options

If pancreatic cancer is found while it is operable, surgery is conducted as quickly as possible. Combinations of radiation and chemotherapy can slow the progress of the disease and may shrink tumors to an operable size.

Ultimately, the treatment options for pancreatic cancer probably include hospice care for the dying person. At this point, any comfort measures are appropriate and welcomed.

Medications

Chemotherapy and drugs for pain relief are the main pharmacologic interventions for pancreatic cancer.

Massage Considerations

Risks
- This is a painful condition; abdominal massage and client positioning must be adjusted for the challenges of pancreatic cancer.
- Chemotherapy, surgery, and radiation carry other cautions for massage, specifically in relation to infection risk, side effects, and general fragility.

Benefits
- Massage reduces pain and anxiety, improves sleep and appetite, and helps patients better tolerate cancer treatments.
- Massage may be a wonderful comfort measure for clients facing the end of life.

pancreatitis

Pancreatitis is inflammation of the pancreas that is often caused by a blockage of the pancreatic ducts. If these ducts are blocked or if the gland develops cysts or abscesses, the digestive enzymes it produces may destroy the pancreas tissue itself; this is called autodigestion.

Acute pancreatitis can be related to blunt trauma, congenital malformation, infection, **gallstones**, **cystic fibrosis**, and exposure to toxins. In acute pancreatitis, the pancreatic duct is blocked, and secretions cannot empty into the small intestine. If the underlying cause of acute pancreatitis is resolved, this condition may be short lived, and most patients fully recover.

Chronic pancreatitis involves long-term wear and tear that leads to permanent damage to the delicate epithelial tissue of the gland. Chronic pancreatitis is almost always related to **alcoholism**, although other factors, including heredity and autoimmune dysfunction, may also contribute. The pain associated with chronic pancreatitis can be so persistent and extreme that **chemical dependency** on narcotic painkillers is a significant risk for these patients.

Signs and Symptoms
- Upper abdominal pain that may refer to the back
- Unintended weight loss
- Blood glucose dysregulation
- Jaundice if the common bile duct is blocked

Treatment Options
Pancreatitis is treated according to the cause. If it is related to gallstones, they are removed so the ducts can flow freely. If abscesses form, they are drained or removed. If tissue has died because of autodigestion, it is also removed. The pancreatic duct may be surgically reopened, or a stent may be inserted.

Medications
Pancreatitis is treated with supplements of digestive enzymes and painkillers.

Massage Considerations

Risks
- Acute pancreatitis contraindicates massage until the symptoms have fully resolved.
- Clients with chronic pancreatitis may require some adjustments in positioning. Deep abdominal massage is contraindicated for these clients.

Benefits
- Massage has no specific benefits for acute or chronic pancreatitis other than relief from pain and anxiety.
- Clients with a history of pancreatitis and no current symptoms can enjoy the same benefits from massage as the rest of the population.

panic disorder: see anxiety disorders

panniculitis

Panniculitis is the inflammation of subcutaneous fat tissue. It is often discussed as lobular or septal panniculitis, referring to whether the inflammation affects the lobes of fat cells or the connective tissue septae that divide them.

When blood supply to fat deposits is interrupted, the cells may break down or become inflamed. Acute panniculitis, which is often caused by cold or trauma, may also be called nodular fat necrosis. Chronic situations are usually complications of underlying disorders that affect the blood vessels.

Panniculitis is often a complication of a primary problem that involves arterial or venous blood flow. **Lupus**, **scleroderma**, **polyarteritis nodosa**, **lymphoma**, and **pancreatitis** are sometimes involved.

Signs and Symptoms

- Development of a single or multiple palpable fatty nodules in the subdermis
- The nodes may be tender or discolored with a thick texture
- The nodes may seep oily fluid
- The nodes typically last several weeks and then disappear

Treatment Options

Treatment for panniculitis depends on the underlying contributing factors. Rest and elevation are recommended for lesions caused by trauma. Compression stockings may be recommended for other cases. Surgery is conducted to remove ulcerated or necrotic lesions.

Medications

Some panniculitis patients can be treated with steroidal anti-inflammatory drugs.

Massage Considerations

Risks

- Panniculitis related to systemic disease and impaired immunity contraindicates rigorous massage.
- Panniculitis related to cold or trauma may be just a local caution.

Benefits

- Massage may assist circulatory turnover in areas that have been impaired. This is appropriate only when underlying diseases or conditions have been addressed and as long as the therapist works within the client's pain tolerance.

---

paralysis

Paralysis is a condition in which neurologic function to some part of the body is interrupted. Motor paralysis involves damage to the motor pathway in the central nervous system (CNS) (upper motor neurons) or the peripheral nervous system (lower motor neurons).

Damage to the upper motor neurons shows as spastic paralysis, in which one set of muscles—usually the flexors—is in continual contraction while the antagonists release. Flaccid paralysis, on the other hand, reflects damage to the lower motor neurons in the peripheral nervous system. Hemiplegia and diplegia indicate a problem in the brain, and paraplegia or quadriplegia show spinal cord damage.

Paralysis can occur in a range of severity, depending on how much nerve tissue has been damaged. Paresis, or weakness, may be a sign of relatively minor damage, and full spasticity or flaccidity show more severe problems. In addition, CNS injuries lead to muscle contractures that may progress as the patient's posture and movement patterns adapt to new limitations.

Many conditions and types of trauma can lead to paralysis. CNS damage can be associated with **traumatic brain injury, stroke,** tumor, **multiple sclerosis, cerebral palsy, spinal cord injury,** bone spurs, **rheumatoid arthritis, amyotrophic lateral sclerosis,** and some rare metabolic disorders. Peripheral nerve injuries may be caused by **Bell palsy, carpal tunnel syndrome, thoracic outlet syndrome, Guillain-Barré syndrome, diabetes,** and exposure to some toxins.

When spinal cord injuries occur in the low back, they may affect both the spinal cord itself and the peripheral nerve roots of the cauda equina, leading to symptoms of both upper and lower motor neuron damage.

Signs and Symptoms
- Spastic paralysis
    Hypertonicity
    Clonus
    Painful muscle spasms
    Loss of function
- Flaccid paralysis
    Weakness
    Hypotonicity
    In the vagus nerve: poor digestive motility

Treatment Options
Paralysis is treated according to its cause. Physical therapy to improve strength, resilience, and mobility is usually recommended. Surgeries to release contracted tendons or move functioning muscle attachments may be conducted.

Medications
Some medications, including Botox, can interfere with CNS motor impulses to improve function.

🖐 Massage Considerations

Risks
- Clients with paralysis may have a loss of sensation. This contraindicates rigorous massage that intends to change the quality of tissue because clients cannot give feedback about pain or overtreatment.
- Clients with spastic paralysis have muscles that are hypertonic, stiff, and brittle. These muscles are vulnerable to injury.

Benefits
- Massage with exercises and stretching can work with postural reflexes to maintain function and slow or prevent the progression of paralysis.
- Given with respect for changes in sensation and other functional limitations, massage can dramatically improve the quality of life for clients with paralysis.

Parkinson disease

Parkinson disease is a movement disorder involving a reduction in dopamine production in the basal ganglia of the brain. This leads to difficulty with motor control; the balance between the prime movers and antagonist muscles is lost, coordination degenerates, and controlled movement becomes very difficult.

It is not clear what initiates the changes seen in patients with Parkinson disease. Environmental agents, genetic abnormalities, exposure to certain drugs, and repeated head trauma have been listed among the possible factors.

Signs and Symptoms

- General achiness, weakness, fatigue
- Resting tremor
- Bradykinesia (difficulty initiating movement)
- Rigidity, poor postural reflexes
- Tightening of the facial muscles and voice
- Shuffling gait, risk of falling
- Poor-quality sleep
- Depression, mental degeneration

Treatment Options

Parkinson disease is usually treated with medication. If medication isn't sufficient and the patient is a good candidate, deep brain stimulation (a device that can limit tremors is implanted in the thalamus) and other surgical interventions may be tried.

Medications

The loss of dopamine production in Parkinson disease can be addressed with a synthetic precursor of dopamine that can cross the blood–brain barrier, but it is usually a temporary solution. Many patients acquire resistance to the drug, and it has a number of troubling side effects, including hallucinations and dementia. Some dopamine agonists can be substituted when it becomes necessary, or it can be prescribed with other drugs that mediate the side effects.

Massage Considerations

Risks

- Clients with Parkinson disease have difficulty with movement and may need help getting on and off the massage table.

Benefits

- The rigidity of the flexor muscles seen in people with Parkinson disease is not the same as spasticity seen in those other central nervous system disorders, and it can be at least temporarily relieved with massage.
- Massage can help relieve anxiety and depression.
- Massage can improve the quality of sleep for Parkinson disease patients, which can be an important intervention that substantially improves the quality of life.

paronychia

Paronychia refers to an infection of the skin around the nail fold. It may be either chronic or acute, and the causative pathogen varies for the different types.

Acute paronychia is often preceded by trauma to the nail or fingertip. Damaged tissue allows nearby bacteria to create a local infection. Varieties of *Staphylococcus* and *Streptococcus* bacteria are common factors in these situations.

Chronic paronychia may have a slower onset or may occur in episodes connected with long-term or frequent immersions in water. The causative factor in these cases is usually *Candida albicans*, the same yeast seen with systemic **candidiasis**. Chronic paronychia is also common in people who have **psoriasis**.

Signs and Symptoms

- Acute paronychia
    Swollen, painful, red area
    Pus under the skin around the nailbed
- Chronic paronychia
    Swollen, tender nail folds
    Thickened, discolored nail plates
    The cuticles may separate from the nail plate, leading to a high risk for infection

Treatment Options

Treatment for paronychia depends on whether it is chronic or acute and what the causative factor is. When it is caught early, acute paronychia be treated with warm water soaks, oral antibiotics, and draining the abscess if necessary.

Chronic paronychia is treated by keeping the area as dry as possible and using topical or oral antifungal medication.

Acute or chronic paronychia may be treated with surgery if other interventions are unsuccessful.

Medications

Medical intervention for paronychia includes oral antibiotics or antifungal medication as appropriate for the type of infection.

Massage Considerations

Risks

- Acute and chronic paronychia locally contraindicate massage, which could potentially introduce new pathogens into a compromised area.

Benefits

- Massage has no specific benefits for clients with paronychia.
- If the infection is controlled and not acute, clients with paronychia can enjoy the same benefits from massage as the rest of the population.

Practitioner Advice

- With frequent immersions in water and exposure to pathogens on other people's skin, massage therapists are at risk for paronychia. This risk can be reduced with careful skin care, including controlling hangnails and covering any visible lesions, especially around the fingernails.

patellofemoral syndrome

Patellofemoral syndrome (PFS) is a condition in which the patellar cartilage becomes damaged as it contacts the femoral cartilage. Overuse or uneven tension that pulls the patella to one side or the other may contribute to the damage.

PFS, which is also called "jumper's knee," can be a precursor of **osteoarthritis** at the knee. It may be confused with patellar tendinitis. This is an important distinction because although PFS involves damage inside the joint capsule that may be irreversible, patellar tendinitis is much more treatable and has a more promising prognosis.

Signs and Symptoms

- Pain at the anterior aspect of the knee
- Stiffness after immobility
- Crepitus: grinding, crackling noise in the knee during movement

Treatment Options

This condition is irritated by percussive exercise. If any activity becomes prohibitive, it can probably be replaced with something gentler, such as swimming, walking, cycling, or skating. Patients may have to experiment to find the exercise activities that work best.

Physical therapy for PFS often includes exercises to strengthen and balance tension in the muscles that cross the knee and influence knee alignment. The quadriceps, hamstrings, tensor fascia latae, and deep lateral rotators are often addressed in the challenge to improve alignment and stop the progression of damage that PFS can cause.

Medications

Clients with knee pain may use nonsteroidal anti-inflammatory drugs to help manage their symptoms.

Massage Considerations

Risks

- Massage carries no risks for PFS except for the unusual circumstance in which the knee is hot, painful, and inflamed.

Benefits

- Massage can reduce the stiffness and chronic pain experienced in muscle–tendon units that cross the knee joint, but it cannot assist in rebuilding worn-out patellar cartilage.
- Massage may help with muscle tension and alignment problems that contribute to PFS.
- Clients with PFS can enjoy the same benefits from massage as the rest of the population.

pellagra

Pellagra is a nutritional deficiency related to the B vitamin niacin and the amino acid tryptophan. When these nutrients are in short supply or when other disorders interfere with their uptake, symptoms of pellagra develop.

Niacin is an important nutrient for many functions, but it is especially involved in regulating the inflammatory response. A niacin deficiency leads to inflamed patches on the skin and mucous membranes of the gastrointestinal tract. Tryptophan has an important role in central nervous system (CNS) function, and without it and niacin, significant deterioration of the CNS occurs.

People in the United States today are unlikely to develop primary pellagra, but secondary pellagra develops when other disorders interfere with niacin and tryptophan uptake. Some predisposing conditions include chronic diarrhea, **ulcerative colitis**, **Crohn disease**, dialysis, and **alcoholism**.

Signs and Symptoms
- Diarrhea
- Dermatitis: red, itchy, scaly patches on the dorsum of the hands and feet and around the neck; malar rash
- Dementia

Treatment Options
Pellagra is treated with nutritional supplements.

Medications
Pellagra is not treated with medication.

Massage Considerations

Risks
- Massage therapists in the United States are most likely to see pellagra as a complication of an underlying disorder. Cautions surrounding these primary problems must be addressed as part of deciding whether massage is appropriate.
- The rash seen with pellagra is painful and can involve blisters and compromised skin; this is at least a local contraindication for massage.

Benefits
- Massage has no specific benefits for clients with pellagra.

---

pelvic inflammatory disease

Pelvic inflammatory disease (PID) refers to infections anywhere in the upper reproductive tract of women. Infection of the uterus (endometritis), infection of the uterine tubes (salpingitis), or abscesses on the ovaries all fall under the umbrella term of PID.

PID is usually the result of a bacterial infection that begins in the vagina and then spreads to the uterus, uterine tubes, and ovaries and into the pelvic cavity. These infections are often complications of a sexually transmitted disease; **chlamydia** or **gonorrhea** are the most common agents. It can also be a complication of an incomplete elective or spontaneous **abortion**.

Complications of PID are potentially quite serious. Infection in the peritoneal cavity can become **peritonitis**. Chronic inflammation can cause scarring of the uterine tubes, leading to infertility or a high risk of ectopic **pregnancy**. And many women diagnosed with PID experience chronic pelvic pain that outlasts the infection by many years.

Signs and Symptoms
- May be acute or chronic
- Acute
    Abdominal and low back pain
    Fever, chills
    Nausea, vomiting
    Painful intercourse
    Vaginal discharge
    Heavy, irregular menstruation

- Chronic
    Mild abdominal pain
    Backache
    Heavy menstruation
    Painful intercourse
    General lethargy

Treatment Options

PID is treatable with rest, cessation of sexual activity for several weeks, and antibiotics.

Medications

Most PID infections clear up with oral or intravenous antibiotics. It is important to treat the patient's sex partners as well to prevent reinfection with the same pathogens.

Massage Considerations

Risks
- Acute PID systemically contraindicates massage until the client has completed her course of antibiotics.
- Clients with chronic PID should also be treated with antibiotics before receiving massage, but they may be able to tolerate some gentle work.

Benefits
- Energetic or reflexive massage modalities can be a calming, supportive intervention for clients who are working to overcome a chronic infection.
- Clients who have completely treatment for PID and have no lasting symptoms can enjoy the same benefits from massage as the rest of the population.

pericarditis

Pericarditis is inflammation of the double-walled serous membrane that surrounds the heart. Excess pericardial fluid may also accumulate when the membrane walls are inflamed.

Pericarditis can develop under several circumstances, including infection, autoimmune disease, or kidney problems or as a complication of trauma or a **heart attack**.

Infectious pericarditis is usually a complication of a viral disease. Coxsackie virus, **mumps**, **mononucleosis**, **flu**, and **polio** can all cause inflammation of the pericardium. Bacterial pericarditis is rare but may occur as a part of an active **tuberculosis** infection. Fungal pericarditis develops most often as a complication of a fungal infection in the lungs (**aspergillosis**) or as a postoperative complication of cardiac surgery.

Uremic pericarditis develops when **renal failure** leads to excessive uric acid in the blood. This can lead to inflammation of the pericardial sac, which, in a vicious circle, interferes with heart function, exacerbating renal problems.

Several autoimmune diseases, including **lupus**, **scleroderma**, **rheumatoid arthritis**, and **polyarteritis nodosa**, can cause inflammation of the pericardium.

In most cases, an episode of pericarditis lasts several days or weeks but then subsides with no further incidents. When the inflammation is long lasting and severe, as may be seen in people with autoimmune diseases, the pericardium may become thickened and inelastic. This can interfere with the strength of the heart beat and ultimately lead to **heart failure**.

Signs and Symptoms

- Sharp, piercing, stabbing sensation in the chest
- Possible fever, malaise
- Symptoms are worse while supine and are relieved when sitting

Treatment Options

The treatment of pericarditis depends on the underlying cause. Extensive damage to the pericardial sac may require surgery to repair the affected areas. Dialysis to assist damaged kidneys may be used to treat uremic pericarditis. Other treatments include medications.

Medications

Chemotherapy or immunosuppressant drugs are sometimes used when pericarditis is related to autoimmune dysfunction. Otherwise, painkillers and rest are the best options for short-term bouts of pericarditis.

 Massage Considerations

Risks

- Any massage that challenges the circulatory system or heart function should be delayed until all signs of pericarditis have passed.

Benefits

- Massage has no specific benefits for clients with pericarditis.
- Energetic or reflexive massage may offer general support, pain relief, and anxiety reduction for clients with pericarditis.
- Clients who have had pericarditis but who have no lingering symptoms or problems can enjoy the same benefits from massage as the rest of the population.

periodic limb movement disorder: see sleep disorders

periostitis: see shin splints

---

peripheral artery disease

Peripheral artery disease (PAD), also called intermittent claudication, is a condition in which single or multiple arterial blockages develop in the legs. These don't necessarily limit adequate blood supply during rest, but during exercise, the muscle demands for oxygen and nutrition quickly outpace the blood flow that blocked arteries can supply.

PAD is most common among men older than age 50 years. The biggest risk factor for dangerous consequences (i.e., the need for amputation because blood flow is permanently blocked) is smoking.

PAD may mimic several sources of lower leg pain; it is important to rule out these conditions to achieve effective treatment. **Osteoarthritis** at the knee, **deep vein thrombosis**, chronic compartment syndrome (a type of **shin splints**), **complex regional pain syndrome**, entrapment of the popliteal artery, and **peripheral neuropathy** can all create transient leg pain.

As a complication of **atherosclerosis**, PAD occurs in conjunction with other cardiovascular conditions, as well as **diabetes**.

Signs and Symptoms
- Predictable lower leg pain with exercise
- Pain subsides with rest
- Suppressed pulse on the affected side
- Possible atrophy of the calf muscles

Treatment Options
This condition is typically treated with mild exercise. Patients are instructed to walk to the point at which pain begins, rest until pain subsides, and then walk again. The goal is to increase the collateral blood supply to the affected muscles. Other underlying conditions must also be controlled, which may call for treatment of diabetes and the use of anticoagulant medication.

Medications
Underlying conditions that lead to PAD may call for medications, including diabetes drugs, antiplatelet or anticoagulant drugs, and drugs to manage heart disease.

Massage Considerations

Risks
- Clients with PAD probably have other cardiovascular conditions that may impact decisions about massage; obtain a complete health history for best results.

Benefits
- Massage that is within the typical challenges of a client's daily activities is safe and appropriate for people with PAD as long as their other cardiovascular risks have been addressed.

---

peripheral neuropathy

Peripheral neuropathy (PN) is a situation in which peripheral nerves, either singly or in groups, are damaged through lack of circulation, chemical imbalance, trauma, or other factors.

PN occurs most frequently as a complication of **diabetes** mellitus, **alcoholism**, or **HIV/AIDS**. **Lupus** and **scleroderma** can also involve peripheral neuritis. Shingles (**herpes zoster**) and postherpetic neuralgia are types of PN. More rarely, this condition develops because of certain vitamin deficiencies (especially B_{12}) or exposure to toxic substances.

Mechanical pressure on nerves can also cause PN. Examples of this kind of problem include **carpal tunnel syndrome; disc disease; double-crush syndrome; trigeminal neuralgia;** and any kind of trauma, tumors, or bone spurs that might result in nerve pressure.

Signs and Symptoms
- Burning pain, tingling in the hands or feet
- Gradually spreads proximally toward the trunk
- Hypersensitivity followed by numbness
- Specific muscle weakness, atrophy when motor neurons are affected (including digestive problems with the vagus nerve)

Treatment Options
Treatment for PN depends entirely on the underlying pathology that is causing the nerve damage. Topical ointments with pepper (capsaicin) sometimes offer some relief. Other

therapies include transcutaneous electrical nerve stimulation, biofeedback, acupuncture, relaxation techniques, and massage to improve circulation in the affected extremities.

Medications

Chronic pain is often treated with tricyclic antidepressants or antiseizure medications.

 ## Massage Considerations

Risks

- PN is usually a complication of an underlying disorder; these issues must be addressed in making decisions about massage or bodywork.
- Numbness, reduced sensation, and pain are all cautions for massage, either because the client cannot give informed feedback about comfort or because massage may be irritating.

Benefits

- If massage can soothe irritable nerves and improve circulation without exacerbating symptoms, it may be an appropriate choice.

---

peritonitis

Peritonitis is an infection that has become established in the peritoneal space, where it is dark, moist, and about 100°F, a perfect growth medium for pathogens. Furthermore, some key immune devices are absent; white blood cells have no direct access, nor do any corrosive fluids such as digestive juices that might impede bacterial expansion.

Peritonitis can be a spontaneous event, as in stagnant abdominal distention (ascites) seen with **cirrhosis** or tumors that block fluid flow. More often, peritonitis is a complication of an infection such as **appendicitis** or **pelvic inflammatory disease**. Problems that compromise the walls of the digestive tract (**ulcers, ulcerative colitis, Crohn disease, diverticular disease**) may also increase the risk of peritonitis if the gastrointestinal tract is perforated and intestinal contents spill into the peritoneum.

Signs and Symptoms

- Diffuse abdominal pain; may localize at the site of infection
- Nausea, vomiting, dehydration
- Reduced urine output
- Difficulty passing gas, bowel movements
- Abdominal swelling, intestinal paralysis

Treatment Options

Treatment for peritonitis varies according to its cause and severity. At the very least, antibiotics are needed. Emergency situations require abdominal surgery to remove or repair the ruptured organ and to wash out the peritoneal cavity as fully as possible. When peritonitis is caught early, it usually responds well to treatment, but if it is left too long, it can be deadly.

Medications

Peritonitis is treated with orally or intravenously administered antibiotics.

 ## Massage Considerations

Risks

- Acute peritonitis systemically contraindicates massage.

Benefits
- Massage has no specific benefits for clients with peritonitis.
- Clients with a history of this condition but no current symptoms can enjoy the same benefits from massage as the rest of the population.

pertussis

Pertussis, also called whooping cough, is a bacterial infection of the upper respiratory tract.

Pertussis can lead to some severe and dangerous complications for young children, including middle ear infections (**otitis** media), **pneumonia**, **seizures**, **apnea**, and brain damage.

Among teens and adults, pertussis is annoying but seldom dangerous. The coughing can be so severe, however, that bruised or broken ribs (**fractures**) or **hernias** may occur.

Signs and Symptoms
- Low fever, malaise, sneezing, coughing
- Cough that persists for weeks and becomes increasingly severe
- Cough that leaves the patient breathless
- Cough that has the characteristic "whoop" sound in young children

Treatment Options

Pertussis is preventable through vaccination, but recent findings show that the coverage from a childhood inoculation may not last into adulthood.

When this infection occurs in young children, it is especially important to keep the breathing passageways open, so a hospital stay may be recommended.

Medications

Antibiotics shorten the duration of whooping cough but not cure the disease. Cough suppressants tend not to be useful for pertussis.

Massage Considerations

Risks
- Acute pertussis contraindicates massage; the client is fighting an aggressive bacterial infection, and the therapist's own protection from a childhood vaccine may not provide coverage into adulthood.

Benefits
- Massage has no specific benefits for clients with pertussis.
- Clients who have fully recovered from whooping cough can enjoy the same benefits from massage as the rest of the population.

pharyngitis

Pharyngitis is the technical term for sore throat, which is inflammation of the pharynx from infection or other causes.

Viral infections related to the **common cold** or the **flu** are the most common sources of pharyngitis. Bacterial infections, including "strep throat," account for a smaller number of cases, although the statistics vary greatly.

Both viral and bacterial agents of pharyngitis are communicable through nasal secretions. These can be spread as airborne pathogens (e.g., sneezing) or through contaminated hands touching surfaces that are then touched by other people.

Other causes of sore throat include pollutants, dry air, **gastroesophageal reflux disease**, cigarette smoke, **allergic reactions**, and foreign bodies.

Strep throat is associated with a risk of some minor and some severe complications, ranging from **sinusitis** or ear infections (**otitis**) to **glomerulonephritis** and **rheumatic fever**. The risk of these complications has led to aggressive treatment with antibiotics for sore throats.

Signs and Symptoms

- Sore throat that may be bright red
- Runny nose, red eyes with a viral infection

Treatment Options

Viral infections of the pharynx clear up without intervention in about 10 days. They don't respond to antibiotics and are best treated with rest, fluids, and humidified air. Bacterial infections do respond to antibiotics, but an accurate culture must be obtained so the right antibiotic can be used.

Medications

Antibiotics are used for bacterial throat infections, but care must be taken to choose the right class of drugs.

Massage Considerations

Risks

- Acute throat infections systemically contraindicate rigorous circulatory massage.

Benefits

- Reflexive or energetic techniques support immune system activity, improve the quality of sleep, and possibly help speed healing when a client is recovering from pharyngitis as long as the client is no longer contagious.

Practitioner Advice

- Some infections remain potentially contagious after the symptoms begin to subside; extra hygiene precautions are appropriate during this time.

phobias: see anxiety disorders

Pick disease

Pick disease, also called lobar sclerosis, is a progressive, dementing disease that primarily affects personality and language.

In this condition, swellings called "Pick bodies" appear on neurons in the frontal and anterior portions of the temporal lobes. Personality changes with declining function follow. People with Pick disease may experience some memory loss, but they are more likely to exhibit indifference to things that once interested them and inappropriate behavior as their centers of judgment degenerate.

Pick disease resembles **Alzheimer disease** (AD) in many ways, but it has some key differences. First, the average age of onset for Pick disease is 40 to 60 years old; it is older for AD. Pick disease affects women more often than men; AD is the opposite. The leading signs of Pick disease are personality changes and progressive apathy; for AD, the leading sign is memory loss. Whereas Pick disease tends to be localized to the frontal and temporal lobes, AD affects more of the brain. Finally, the neurochemical changes that occur in the brain are different for Pick disease and AD, although they are only observable in autopsy.

Signs and Symptoms

- Changes in personality
- Progressive apathy
- Poor judgment
- Loss of language
- Rigidity and tremor with progression to the motor centers of the brain

Treatment Options

Pick disease is treated with the same drugs used for AD to prolong function and reduce symptoms. Assistance for living and support for caregivers are the other major interventions.

Medications

Medications for Pick disease include cholinesterase inhibitors and antianxiety medications.

🖐 Massage Considerations

Risks

- Clients with Pick disease may not communicate verbally; massage therapists must be sensitive to their nonverbal signals about comfort and pain.

Benefits

- Massage can't improve the course of Pick disease, but it may be able to ease anxiety and provide a calming, grounding experience.

---

pinworms

Pinworms are small parasites (about $1/2$ inch or smaller) that infest the digestive tract and cause itching around the anus.

Children are the most common hosts of pinworms. Tiny eggs on contaminated surfaces (including the fingers and fingernails) enter the mouth and are swallowed. The worms hatch in the intestine and migrate to the colon. Females emerge from the anus to lay eggs on nearby skin, which causes significant itching. When the host scratches and then spreads the eggs to other surfaces, the cycle begins again.

Eggs left in sheets or on surfaces can survive for up to 2 weeks. They don't tolerate direct sunlight, however, so people with an infestation are counseled do their laundry frequently and to open the window shades and blinds in their bedrooms.

Signs and Symptoms

- Intense itching around the anus, especially at night
- Worms or eggs may be caught in tape applied to the anus at night

Treatment Options

Pinworms are treated with medication.

Medications

Oral antiparasite medication is used to eradicate pinworms. One dose with a follow-up 2 weeks later is usually sufficient.

Massage Considerations

Risks

- Because massage therapists don't work closely around the anus, the risk of catching or spreading pinworms from this site is negligible. However, the eggs may be spread with the infected person's hands or left in linens, which are more reasons to be conscientious about practicing standard hygienic precautions.

Benefits

- Massage has no specific benefits for clients with pinworms.
- Clients who have had pinworms can enjoy the same benefits from massage as the rest of the population.

pinkeye: see conjunctivitis

piriformis syndrome

Piriformis syndrome is a condition in which the piriformis, one of the deep lateral rotators, puts excessive pressure on the sciatic nerve, leading to symptoms that radiate down the length of the nerve.

The piriformis muscle can irritate the sciatic nerve by pressing on it as it goes through the sciatic notch of the ischium, but in some people, the sciatic nerve actually bisects the piriformis muscle. These people probably have an increased risk for sciatic pain from muscle tightness than the general population.

Although some experts discuss piriformis syndrome as one type of **sciatica**, others delineate sciatica as irritation to the nerve roots of the sciatic nerve and piriformis syndrome as occurring in a distal location.

When a person has sciatic pain, it is important to get a clear diagnosis to design the best possible treatment program. Other problems that can mimic sciatic pain include sacroiliac joint irritation, **disc disease**, hamstring **tendinopathy**, and other adhesions within the deep lateral rotators.

Signs and Symptoms

- Pain that radiates from the buttock to the back of the thigh and down the leg
- Paresthesia (tingling, reduced sensation)
- May be exacerbated by sitting, climbing, walking, running

Treatment Options

Piriformis syndrome often responds well to noninvasive options; careful stretching and exercise, along with alignment adjustments in posture and the feet, may make significant improvements. Activities that exacerbate symptoms may have to be replaced with others, at least until the irritation subsides. Surgery to take pressure off the sciatic nerve may be conducted as a last resort.

Medications
Steroid injections may be recommended if other interventions don't relieve pain.

Massage Considerations
Risks
- Deep work around the piriformis without regard for pain tolerance or uncomfortable positioning may exacerbate symptoms.

Benefits
- Techniques that aim to reduce tightness, improve alignment, and promote bilateral balance in the deep lateral rotators can be very helpful in reducing sciatic pain caused by piriformis tightness.

---

pityriasis rosea

Pityriasis rosea is an idiopathic rash that appears on the skin, lasts for several weeks, and then disappears, usually never to be seen again. Leading theories suggest a viral cause, but no specific pathogen has been identified. It does not appear to be highly contagious.

Pityriasis rosea is easy to identify by its appearance, but many doctors suggest a blood test to rule out secondary **syphilis**, which can have a similar presentation.

Signs and Symptoms
- Usually begins with one large lesion, a "herald patch"
- Many lesions appear on the trunk, skin folds, extremities
- Lesions are round or oval, red, itchy
- Lesions have clearly defined borders and a crinkly texture
- Lesions may last 5 to 10 weeks
- Discoloration can persist after the rash subsides

Treatment Options
Moderate exposure to ultraviolet radiation is sometimes recommended to help clear up the lesions.

Medications
Topical or oral steroids may be prescribed to control itching, but these don't cure or shorten the pityriasis outbreak.

Massage Considerations
Risks
- Heat may exacerbate the symptoms.
- Massage directly on the rash may make the lesions itchier; consider these a local contraindication.
- Clients who take steroidal anti-inflammatory drugs may have altered reactions to massage.

Benefits
- Massage has no specific benefits for clients with pityriasis rosea.
- Clients who have recovered from pityriasis rosea can enjoy the same benefits from massage as the rest of the population.

plantar fasciitis

Plantar fasciitis (PF) is a condition involving pain, inflammation, and poor healing of the plantar fascia, which stretches from the calcaneus to the metatarsals on the plantar surface of the foot.

The pain that accompanies PF occurs when the foot has been immobile for several hours and then used. The fibers of the fascia begin to knit together during rest and are retorn each time the foot goes into even gentle weight-bearing dorsiflexion.

Causes of PF have to do with overuse or alignment stresses. Being overweight can predispose people to PF, as can wearing shoes without good arch and lateral support. Flat or pronated feet are also associated with this problem. Very tight calf muscles are also contributing factors, especially for runners.

PF occasionally develops as a complication of other problems in the feet, notably **gout** or **rheumatoid arthritis**.

Signs and Symptoms
- Acute foot pain on the first steps after rest, especially first thing in the morning
- Pain returns with prolonged standing or walking
- Sharp "bruised" feeling, often just anterior to the calcaneus on the plantar surface

Treatment Options

The most important thing to do for PF is to relieve the tensions that cause the plantar fascia to be reinjured every morning when the foot first hits the floor. This can be accomplished with heat and massage, shoe inserts, and a splint that keeps the foot in passive dorsiflexion during sleep so the fibers can heal in a stretched position.

No single treatment is universally effective; each patient must experiment with the treatments that meet his or her own needs. It takes patience to overcome this stubborn injury; even the most successful treatment options often take up to 12 weeks to completely resolve injuries.

Medications

Medical interventions for PF include oral and topical nonsteroidal anti-inflammatory drugs and corticosteroid injections.

Massage Considerations

Risks
- Acute inflammation contraindicates deep massage; however, inflammation that is hot and swollen is rare with PF.

Benefits
- Massage is often recommend for patients with PF because it can help the disorganized collagen in the plantar fascia to heal efficiently and to relax the tight calf muscles that constantly pull on the feet.

pleurisy

Pleurisy, also called pleuritis, is inflammation and irritation of the pleurae (the double-walled serous membranes that wrap around the lungs).

Under normal circumstances, the pleurae are smooth and lubricated with a small amount of fluid to eliminate friction between surfaces in the thoracic cavity. Pleurisy develops when an underlying disorder creates inflammation and the two layers of the pleurae begin to rub against each other instead of sliding smoothly over each other.

Pleurisy can be dry or can accompany pleural effusion (an accumulation of fluid between the visceral and parietal layers of the pleurae). In the short term, pleural effusion can help relieve the pain associated with pleurisy because the fluid acts as a lubricant. But ultimately, pleural effusion can interfere with breathing, or the fluid can become dangerously infected in a condition called empyema.

Pleurisy is a complication of some other disorder. Most causes of pleurisy affect the lungs directly, but some of them can create inflammation indirectly through changes in systemic inflammatory chemicals. A short list of possible causes of pleurisy includes **flu, pneumonia, lupus, rheumatoid arthritis, sarcoidosis, tuberculosis,** pulmonary **embolism, lung cancer, pancreatitis,** asbestosis, **pneumothorax,** and chest trauma.

Signs and Symptoms
- Depends on the underlying causes
- Sharp pain with breathing, especially deep breathing
- Dry cough, fever
- Breath sounds are audible through a stethoscope

Treatment Options
Pleurisy is treated by dealing with the underlying disorder first. If significant pleural effusion is present, the fluid is drained.

Medications
Nonsteroidal anti-inflammatory drugs and cough suppressants are the typical medications used for pleurisy.

🖐 Massage Considerations

Risks
- Decisions about working with a client with pleurisy depend on what underlying disorder created the problem. In situations in which the infection has subsided but pleural irritation persists, massage carries no significant risk.

Benefits
- Massage has no specific benefits for clients with pleurisy, but if underlying contraindications are ruled out, massage can improve sleep and boost immune system function, which may contribute to a shorter healing process.

pneumonia

Pneumonia is a general term for inflammation of the lungs that is usually caused by pathogenic invasion. Infectious agents that cause pneumonia include bacteria

(*Staphylococcus*, *Streptococcus*, tuberculosis, and others), viruses (often flu or syncytial virus), fungi, protozoa, and mycoplasma.

The lungs are on the receiving end of any contaminants that enter the respiratory system. When an infection strikes there, the tiny, vulnerable alveoli fill up with dead white blood cells, mucus, and fluid backed up from the capillaries. Eventually, diffusion is impaired, abscesses may form, and capillary damage may occur, allowing red blood cells into the alveoli and eventually into the sputum.

Edema associated with pneumonia is not always limited to the alveoli. In extreme cases, fluid may be found between the visceral and parietal layers of the pleurae. This can lead to **pleurisy,** which is scarring and limitation of movement between the pleurae during breathing.

Pneumonia is nearly always a complication of another disorder that weakens the immune system or impairs the breathing process. People who have had a **stroke, heart failure, alcoholism,** or cancer die of pneumonia more often than any other disease. People who are bedridden or survivors of **spinal cord injury** are also susceptible because their cough reflex is often impaired, so they cannot expel mucus easily. Having a pre-existing chest problem, such as the **flu, bronchitis, emphysema,** or **asthma,** is an open invitation for pneumonia. And finally, being immunosuppressed because of tissue transplants, **AIDS, leukemia,** or use of steroids or cytotoxic drugs makes people particularly vulnerable to pneumonia.

Signs and Symptoms
- Vary widely in severity
- Cough with thick, colored sputum
- High fever up to 104°F, chills
- Delirium
- Chest pain, shortness of breath, cyanosis
- Muscle aches

Treatment Options
Symptomatic relief and supportive therapy include breathing humidified air, drinking ample fluids, and supplementing oxygen if necessary.

Medications
Bacterial and mycoplasma pneumonias generally respond well to antibiotics, but viral infections do not respond to these medications.

Massage Considerations
Risks
- Acute pneumonia contraindicates Swedish massage and rigorous circulatory massage.
- Clients recovering from pneumonia may not be comfortable lying flat on a table for a full session.

Benefits
- Reflexive and energetic modalities may be supportive for clients with pneumonia, with care to limit communicability.
- Tapotement or other percussion on the back and chest may help in the expulsion of material after the infection has subsided.
- Clients who have fully recovered from pneumonia can enjoy the same benefits from massage as the rest of the population.

pneumothorax

Pneumothorax is a situation in which air flows into the pleural space, leading to a partial or full collapse of the lung. This can occur in several ways.

Primary spontaneous pneumothorax occurs mostly in tall men between 20 and 40 years old. It is most likely to happen with external air pressure changes, as in an airplane or while scuba diving. It is usually a minor problem that resolves without interference, but the recurrence rate is high.

Secondary spontaneous pneumothorax is related to other lung diseases that create weak areas in the lung that rupture. **Emphysema, cystic fibrosis, sarcoidosis, lung cancer**, and some types of **pneumonia** are conditions that increase the risk of secondary spontaneous pneumothorax.

Tension pneumothorax is a medical emergency in which a penetrating injury essentially creates a one-way valve for air to flow into the pleural space, leading to full lung collapse. Mechanical pressure of the collapsed lung on the heart, along with interference in venous return in the pulmonary circuit, leads to cardiovascular collapse and shock.

Other types of pneumothorax include complications from rib **fractures**, surgery, damage from mechanical ventilators, and other factors.

Signs and Symptoms

- Chest pain
- Dry cough
- Shortness of breath
- May lead to shock or cardiac arrest if severe

Treatment Options

Small pneumothoraxes are usually left untreated because the air pocket in the pleural space is typically reabsorbed within a few days or weeks. The risk of recurrence is fairly high, however, so people who have had multiple episodes may consider surgery to correct the weakened area of the lung.

If the pneumothorax is larger, a tube is inserted through the chest into the air pocket to vacuum out the air, allowing the lung to reinflate.

Medications

Pneumothorax is not treated with medication except to address the underlying causative factors.

✍ Massage Considerations

Risks

- Clients with a tendency for spontaneous pneumothorax might want to discuss massage with their primary care providers; direct pressure or percussion on the trunk or abdomen may interfere with a normal recovery.

Benefits

- Massage has no specific benefits for clients with current pneumothorax.
- Clients who have completely recovered from pneumothorax can enjoy the same benefits from massage as the rest of the population.

poison ivy, poison oak, poison sumac

Poison ivy, poison oak, and poison sumac are all plants that have a chemical in their sap called urushiol. Urushiol is a highly allergenic substance in leaves, stems, and roots that causes a reaction on the skin involving inflammation, itchiness, and blisters. This is a type of allergic contact **dermatitis** that develops about 12 to 48 hours after contact. Up to 85% of the population has an allergic reaction to urushiol.

Poison ivy, poison oak, and poison sumac reactions occur in three ways: through direct contact, indirect contact, and as an airborne substance. When a person comes in direct contact with plant sap, the rash has a streaked appearance indicating where the leaves were brushed. Indirect contact occurs after touching something else that carries the sap, such as yard care equipment, camping gear, or a pet that has run through the woods. The sap doesn't evaporate or lose its potency for many months, which means that even equipment not used since the previous season may be a source of the allergen. Finally, burning the plants releases urushiol into the air. It continues to be a potent allergen even as airborne molecules.

Open or weeping blisters and repeated scratching increase the risk of secondary bacterial infections as a complication of this rash. Occasionally, a rash can lead to a very extreme **allergic reaction** in the shape of **angioedema** or **anaphylaxis**.

Signs and Symptoms

- Red, itchy rash
- Blisters followed by crusts
- Can take up to 10 days to heal
- Thin, delicate skin is more reactive than thicker skin

Treatment Options

If a person knows that he or she has been exposed to urushiol, the areas should be washed in cold running water, and exposed clothing should be laundered as soon as possible. A cool shower or a lukewarm bath with baking soda or oatmeal is often recommended. It is important to avoid heat, which exacerbates inflammation. Hypoallergenic moisturizers may also help relieve itching and help heal itchy, blistered skin.

Medications

Poison ivy and similar allergic reactions are treated with oral antihistamines and oral or topical steroids to control inflammation and itching.

Massage Considerations

Risks

- If a client receives massage before he or she is aware of urushiol exposure, it is possible to spread the allergen further on the client and to the massage therapist.
- After the rash has emerged, it locally contraindicates any massage that might exacerbate itching or put compromised skin at risk for secondary infection.

Benefits

- Massage has no specific benefits for urushiol exposure.
- If the exposure is small and covered or if the client has completely recovered, clients who have had poison ivy, poison oak, or poison sumac can enjoy the same benefits from massage as the rest of the population.

polio

Poliomyelitis is a viral disease that targets the intestinal mucosa first and the anterior horn nerve cells later.

The polio virus usually enters the body through the mouth; contaminated water is the usual medium. The virus gets past the acidic environment of the stomach and sets up an infection in the intestine. New virus is expelled in fecal matter, possibly to contaminate water elsewhere.

For 99% of people exposed to the polio virus, this is the end of their infection. But in about 1% of people who are exposed, the virus travels into the central nervous system, where it targets and destroys nerve cells in the anterior horns of the spinal cord. This impedes motor messages leaving the spinal cord, which in turn leads to rapid deterioration, atrophy of muscles, and motor **paralysis**.

The paralysis caused by polio is motor only; sensation is still present. And because the motor nerves tend to overlap each other in the extremities, some muscle fibers may still function, even though a whole level of motor neurons may have been damaged. Furthermore, anterior horn cells that survive the initial attack can create new nerve connections to help re-establish motor control during recovery. Unfortunately, these cells can become overtaxed later in life, leading to **postpolio syndrome**.

The most serious form of this disease, bulbar polio, attacks not only the anterior horn cells of the spinal column but the nuclei of some cranial nerves as well. Patients with this kind of damage risk death from respiratory or **heart failure**.

Signs and Symptoms

- Primary stage: nausea, diarrhea, fever, headache
- Later: motor paralysis

Treatment Options

Two stable, inexpensive vaccines have been developed that can prevent polio. It is important to take the complete vaccine series, however, because weakened polio virus may survive an incomplete vaccination process. Aggressive vaccination programs have made polio all but extinct in most of the world, but it is still present in areas where the vaccines have not been successfully administered.

Moist heat applications, physical therapy, and massage have been used to treat polio survivors after the initial infection has subsided. Together, hydrotherapy and massage can help limit contractures and keep functioning muscle fibers healthy and well nourished.

Medications

After this viral infection has started, polio is typically not treated with medications.

✋ Massage Considerations

Risks

- Acute infection of any kind contraindicates rigorous circulatory massage.

Benefits

- Because sensation is intact, clients who have had polio and some loss of muscle function can give accurate feedback about their pain and comfort. This makes this condition appropriate for any kind of bodywork that improves function.

polyarteritis nodosa

Polyarteritis nodosa (PAN) is an idiopathic condition involving inflammation and microaneurysms in small- and medium-sized arteries throughout the body. When arteries become damaged, the tissues they supply are deprived of oxygen. PAN can affect any tissue in the body, but it most commonly creates problems in the skin of the legs, nerves of the extremities, and blood supply to the kidneys and brain.

PAN shows some indications of being an autoimmune disorder, but it is not yet well understood. Some people develop symptoms of PAN after exposure to **hepatitis** B or C, but most PAN patients do not have this history.

PAN is a type of **vasculitis**. Complications of untreated PAN are very severe and must be treated aggressively. They can include **peripheral neuropathy, renal failure, hypertension, heart attack, pericarditis, heart failure, stroke, deep vein thrombosis, aneurysm,** scleritis, and tender nodules in the skin.

Signs and Symptoms

- Vary, depending on the individual
- Fever, malaise
- Weight loss
- Muscle aches, headache, abdominal pain
- Complications, as described above

Treatment Options

PAN is typically treated with medication.

Medications

Oral steroidal anti-inflammatory drugs are the treatment of choice for PAN. This intervention extends life expectancy by a significant margin. When PAN accompanies hepatitis B or C, interferon and other antiviral medications may also be prescribed.

Massage Considerations

Risks

- PAN contraindicates rigorous circulatory massage because the cardiovascular system is severely compromised.

Benefits

- Clients with PAN may benefit from the parasympathetic, pain-relieving, and immunosupportive aspects of energetic or reflexive modalities as long as they are conducted where the skin is healthy and intact.

polycystic kidney disease

Polycystic kidney disease (PKD) is a condition in which fluid-filled cysts grow on and in the kidneys. Eventually, these cysts impair kidney function to the extent that the person needs dialysis or a kidney transplant.

Autosomal dominant PKD and autosomal recessive PKD are both inherited conditions. Acquired cystic kidney disease is a condition in which the kidneys develop multiple cysts as a result of long-term kidney problems. People who have been on dialysis for 5 years or more have a high risk of developing acquired cystic kidney disease.

Because the kidneys are responsible for so many tasks, losing kidney function opens the door to many other serious problems, including **kidney stones, urinary tract infection, hypertension**, cerebral **aneurysm**, and **renal failure**.

Furthermore, the genetic anomaly associated with PKD is also involved in other tissue problems, including **diverticular disease**, mitral valve prolapse, liver and pancreatic cysts, and inguinal or umbilical **hernias**.

Signs and Symptoms

- Often subtle in the early stages
- Backaches, side aches, headaches
- Obvious or hidden hematuria
- Complications of kidney dysfunction: kidney stones, urinary tract infection, hypertension

Treatment Options

The most important part of management for PKD—which as a genetic disorder, cannot be cured—is to control the blood pressure. This can be accomplished through diet and exercise along with use of blood pressure medications.

Surgery may be conducted to shrink the external cysts and reduce kidney pain, but this does not slow the progression of the disease or prevent eventual renal failure. Ultimately, most PKD patients use dialysis and hope for a successful kidney transplant.

Medications

Medication used to treat PKD can include antihypertensive drugs, antibiotics for infections, and analgesics for other body pain. Patients who undergo kidney transplants must also take immunosuppressant drugs to avoid rejecting the foreign tissue.

 Massage Considerations

Risks

- PKD contraindicates rigorous circulatory massage that focuses on moving a lot of fluid through a compromised system.

Benefits

- Energetic or reflexive techniques that promote a decrease in blood pressure and general relaxation may be helpful and supportive for clients with PKD.

---

polycystic ovary syndrome

Polycystic ovary syndrome (PCOS) is a collection of signs and symptoms that have to do with ovarian dysfunction and a number of other endocrine and metabolic problems.

Normal ovaries produce a variety of hormones that work with the pituitary hormones to establish the menstrual cycle. In PCOS, testosterone and luteinizing hormone levels are high, and follicle-stimulating hormone levels are low. Consequently, ovulation becomes irregular and infrequent. Menstruation is likewise irregular, and the endometrium may undergo potentially cancerous changes.

PCOS is closely linked to high insulin levels. One theory holds that hyperinsulinemia (brought about by insulin resistance) contributes to excessive testosterone production. This also points to links between PCOS and **metabolic syndrome** and **obesity**.

Ultimately, between several hormonal imbalances and menstrual disruption, the ovaries become enlarged, with hypertrophy of the stromal (connective tissue support) tissues. The follicles that should release ripened eggs are blocked and grow into multiple fluid-filled cysts.

PCOS resembles some other disorders that should be ruled out before treatment is begun. A pituitary tumor or other types of **ovarian cysts** can bring about similar signs and symptoms. Obviously, these conditions need to be investigated before a treatment protocol is begun.

Signs and Symptoms

- Irregular menstruation
- Infertility
- Obesity
- Excessive body and facial hair; loss of head hair
- Acne

Treatment Options

PCOS is treated mainly by managing the symptoms and other disorders. Controlling insulin is an important step. This is usually done through diet and exercise along with medication to control blood sugar and the menstrual cycle. Surgery may be conducted laparoscopically to "drill" the ovaries, a procedure that is thought to destroy testosterone-producing cells and thereby reduce symptoms.

Medications

PCOS may be treated with insulin-lowering drugs and birth control pills.

Massage Considerations

Risks

- Women with PCOS may have risks related to diabetes and cardiovascular health; these must be screened to make the best decisions about massage.
- Deep abdominal work in the pelvic bowl may pin or irritate enlarged ovaries.

Benefits

- Massage won't resolve PCOS, but it can soothe and support clients with this condition.

Practitioner Advice

- Women with PCOS may have ovaries that are enlarged and found higher in the pelvic cavity that normal. Massage of the psoas or iliacus muscles may endanger these delicate structures.
- Clients with a history of ovarian cysts or other pelvic disruptions (e.g., endometriosis) should receive this type of bodywork from the side or some other position so their ovaries are not at risk of being impinged or bruised.

---

polycythemia

Polycythemia (also called polycythemia vera) is a condition in which the bone marrow produces too many blood cells, especially erythrocytes.

Most cases of polycythemia are idiopathic. The condition occasionally arises as a complication of another disorder, usually a lung problem that stimulates the production of more blood cells to carry more oxygen.

The presence of too many blood cells can lead to serious problems. People with polycythemia are at risk for spontaneous bleeding and bruising and for **thrombosis,** which could lead to pulmonary **embolism, heart attack,** or **stroke.**

Signs and Symptoms

- Headache, dizziness, visual disruptions
- Numbness, tingling
- Itchy rashes on the skin
- Painful cyanosis of the extremities
- In extreme cases: enlarged liver and spleen, ascites, backache, shortness of breath, blood in the stool

Treatment Options

No permanent treatment for polycythemia has been developed. Regular phlebotomy (drawing blood) is a simple intervention that is sufficient for many people. Typically, 2 units of blood are drawn at a time, and the procedure is repeated every few months.

Polycythemia is a potentially life-threatening disease, so it is important to treat it consistently and thoroughly.

Medications

Chemotherapy, immune therapy, or radioactive drugs may be recommended to slow down bone marrow activity.

🖐 Massage Considerations

Risks

- Massage influences fluid flow; some patients with polycythemia may not tolerate rigorous circulatory work well.
- Massage modalities must be carefully gauged to fit within the challenges of the client's activities of daily living.

Benefits

- Massage has no specific benefits for clients with polycythemia.
- If modalities are within the client's ability to adapt, clients with polycythemia can enjoy the same benefits from massage as the rest of the population.

polymyalgia rheumatica

Polymyalgia rheumatica (PMR) is a poorly understood condition that affects mostly women older than age 50 years. As its name implies, it involves multiple sites of joint and muscle pain, often concentrated around the neck, trunk, shoulder, upper arms, hips, and thighs. In a typical case, a person has a sudden onset of significant pain and stiffness in these areas that persists for up to 2 years and then spontaneously resolves.

Although a precise cause for PMR has not been found, it seems clear that a genetic predisposition plays a part. Patients also often have elevated inflammatory markers, which point to immune system hyperactivity.

PMR is usually a self-limiting condition, but a small percentage of patients develop a type of **vasculitis** called temporal arteritis or giant cell arteritis. This condition can lead to permanent blood vessel damage and vision loss, so it must be treated aggressively.

Signs and Symptoms

- Sudden onset of pain and stiffness in the trunk, proximal limbs
- Usually bilateral
- Joints and bursae may be inflamed; no joint erosion
- May show low fever, weight loss, fatigue, depression

Treatment Options

PMR is treated with medication.

Medications

The treatment for PMR is steroidal anti-inflammatory drugs. Although these drugs can be extremely useful, they have a number of serious side effects, including bone thinning, blood glucose disruption, and others, so doctors usually aim to find the lowest possible dose for the shortest possible duration to achieve the best results.

Massage Considerations

Risks

- Clients with PMR are generally inflamed, and rigorous massage may add to that activity.
- Steroidal anti-inflammatory drugs may mask pain signals, alter tissue responses, and increase the risk of other complications.

Benefits

- Massage that respects how anti-inflammatory drugs may alter tissue response may be able to address some of the pain and stiffness seen in people with PMR.

postherpetic neuralgia: see herpes zoster

postoperative situations

The term "postoperative situations" encompasses any situation in which a person is recovering from closed or open surgery. Closed surgery is conducted with tiny incisions into the abdomen or by accessing other areas through the blood vessels or gastrointestinal tract. Open surgery involves large incisions to provide access to a part of the body. The risks associated with closed surgery are generally less dangerous than those seen with open surgery.

Complications related to surgery include infection (and hospital-acquired infections such as **methicillin-resistant *Staphylococcus aureus* infection** or ***Clostridium difficile* infection** tend to be aggressive and difficult to fight off) and the risk of blood clots and pulmonary **embolism**. Organ transplant recipients are additionally challenged by a lifetime commitment to immunosuppressant drugs, which makes them vulnerable to other infections.

Signs and Symptoms

- Depend on the type of surgery: incisions can range from tiny to large

Treatment Options

Postoperative recovery often includes promoting movement and ambulation as soon as possible to reduce the risk of blood clots and speed healing. Other postoperative care varies depending on the nature of the surgery.

Medications

Clients who have had surgery may take a wide range of medication, including various forms of analgesics, blood thinners, antibiotics, and immunosuppressant drugs.

Massage Considerations

Risks

- Incompletely healed wounds are potential sites for infections; these are at least a local contraindication.
- Bedridden clients may have a risk for thrombophlebitis.
- Immediately after surgery, patients may take a variety of medications that influence choices for massage and bodywork.

Benefits

- Reflexive or energetic techniques can improve sleep, reduce anxiety, and generally support the health of clients who are too fragile to receive more rigorous types of bodywork.
- Carefully applied massage can speed healing and improve the quality of scar tissue around surgical scars.
- Clients who have completely healed from surgery and are free of complications can enjoy the same benefits from massage as the rest of the population.

postpartum depression: see depression

postpolio syndrome

Postpolio syndrome (PPS) is a progressive muscular weakness that develops anywhere from 10 to 40 years after an initial infection with the **polio** virus.

PPS is the result of normal aging combined with the loss of a percentage of the anterior horn cells from the initial polio attack. The surviving cells, despite or because of whatever new synapses they were able to make in the recovery process, become severely overtaxed, and progressive muscular weakness and pain result.

PPS may resemble **osteoarthritis, fibromyalgia,** and other chronic pain disorders. It is useful to obtain an accurate diagnosis so the person can work to slow the progress of the degeneration and maintain function as fully as possible.

Signs and Symptoms

- Develops many years after the initial infection
- Cycles of degeneration alternating with stable periods
- Sudden onset of fatigue, achiness, weakness
- Breathing difficulty (dyspnea), trouble swallowing (dysphagia)
- Sleep disturbances

Treatment Options

PPS is treated by reducing muscular and neurologic stress, including having braces adjusted, changing activity levels, and participating in exercise programs that encourage the use of muscles not supplied by the damaged nerves. People with PPS need to avoid excessive use of their affected muscles because exercise to these damaged tissues can cause permanent damage to the working fibers.

Medications

Advanced, severe PPS are sometimes treated with a cholinesterase inhibitor that improves communication between the muscles and nerves.

 ## Massage Considerations

Risks

• Massage has no specific risks for clients with PPS as long as bodywork does not exacerbate symptoms.

Benefits

• Massage may help improve muscular nutrition and metabolic turnover.
• Massage may assist in promoting efficient movement and muscle contractions.

posttraumatic stress disorder: see anxiety disorders

postural deviations

Postural deviations occur when the natural curvatures of the neck, thorax, and low back are overdeveloped. Hyperkyphosis ("humpback"), hyperlordosis ("swayback"), and scoliosis ("S," "C," or "reverse-C" curve) are the specific postural deviations addressed here.

Exaggerated spinal curvatures develop in all directions and often incorporate spinal rotations as well. Thus, scoliosis is usually not merely a left–right aberration but involves a spiral twisting of the vertebral column. Similar lateral imbalances can be observed with most cases of hyperlordosis and hyperkyphosis.

It is important to note the difference between functional problems with postural deviations and structural problems. When soft tissues (muscles, tendons, ligaments) pull bones out of the best alignment, it is a functional problem, and it is generally treatable. But if the bones are constantly pulled in one direction or another, they eventually change shape to adapt to those stressors. Furthermore, some congenital and metabolic problems involve bony malformations. In these cases, the condition is a structural dysfunction and is much harder to reverse.

Underlying disorders, especially central nervous system problems that lead to **paralysis**, may bring about some cases of postural deviations. **Spina bifida** and **cerebral palsy** may cause significant spinal distortion, for instance. **Osteoporosis** is a major contributor to hyperkyphosis. Scheuermann disease is a type of hyperkyphosis seen most often in young men.

Postural deviations can also cause complications. Scoliosis can lead to **peripheral neuropathy, spondylosis,** and serious heart and lung problems arising from a severely restricted rib cage. Hyperlordosis can be a factor in many low back pain scenarios, including ligament irritation and **disc disease.**

Signs and Symptoms

• Range from subtle to very obvious
• Postural distortion in some combination of directions
• Associated back, shoulder, neck pain
• Loss of range of motion
• Possible complications (described above)

Treatment Options

Mild scoliosis, which is any curve less than 30 to 40 degrees is treated, if at all, with any combination of exercise, chiropractic, a corrective brace, and electromuscular stimulation to strengthen the muscles of the stretched side of the spine. If the scoliosis appears at over 40° in childhood, the chances that it will worsen are very great. It typically progresses at 1° every year. Surgery for scoliosis involves inserting rods that straighten and fuse the affected vertebrae. This limits spinal mobility, but it can definitely improve the quality of life for people with advanced scoliosis.

Hyperkyphosis and hyperlordosis, when they are treated at all, may be addressed with physical therapy, exercise, and braces. Massage can certainly play a role here as well.

Medications

Postural deviations are not treated with medication, except for analgesics for pain relief.

🖐 Massage Considerations

Risks

- Massage has few risks for clients with postural deviations, as long as any underlying weakness (osteoporosis, central nervous system problems) are recognized and accommodated.

Benefits

- Massage can contribute to muscular balance and ligament health for clients with postural deviations.
- If bony adaptation has not yet taken place, massage along with increased postural awareness and new movement patterns may contribute to a long-term solution for these problems.

pre-eclampsia: see pregnancy-induced hypertension

---

pregnancy

Pregnancy is the condition a woman is in when she is carrying a fetus. It is important to point out that this is not a disease; rather, it is a condition that changes the way a person functions, and it has some implications for massage.

Many complications of pregnancy can occur. A prematurely expelled fetus leads to spontaneous **abortion** or miscarriage; **pelvic inflammatory disease, endometriosis,** or other factors can cause scarring around the uterine tubes, increasing the risk of ectopic pregnancy; and a woman may develop gestational **diabetes. Pregnancy-induced hypertension** can lead to dangerous consequences for both the mother and the child. Finally, both pregnancy and postpartum states dramatically increase the risk of **thrombophlebitis** and **deep vein thrombosis.**

Signs and Symptoms

- Specifically related to massage
    - Loose ligaments, muscle spasm
    - Fatigue
    - Changing proprioception, clumsiness

🖐 Massage Considerations

Risks

- The risks of massage for pregnant women vary by the stage of pregnancy and any complications.

- Pregnancy contraindicates deep abdominal massage.
- Many experts suggest avoiding reflexology points on the hand and ankle that might stimulate uterine contractions.
- A client's needs for positioning change as the pregnancy progresses; it is important to be prepared to bolster appropriately.

Benefits
- Massage can ameliorate many of the negative experiences of pregnancy (muscle spasms, fatigue, clumsiness), but it must be administered by appropriately trained therapists.

Practitioner Advice
- Special education in massage for pregnant women is available and highly recommended. Although this population can derive wonderful benefits from bodywork, they have some specific needs that can be best addressed by therapists who are well educated.

pregnancy-induced hypertension

Pregnancy-induced hypertension (PIH), also called toxemia, is one of hundreds of possible complications that can occur during pregnancy, and it has especially serious implications for massage therapy.

PIH is a condition in which the blood pressure of a woman with no history of hypertension before she got pregnant increases to a dangerously high level (over 140/90 on at least two occasions that are separated by several hours). It has three stages: hypertension alone; preeclampsia, which is hypertension along with elevated proteins in the urine and possible systemic edema; and eclampsia, which is the same situation along with convulsions. HELLP (hemolytic anemia, elevated liver enzymes, and low platelet count) syndrome is related to PIH and involves severe problems with blood cells, bleeding risk, and liver damage.

Elevated maternal blood pressure reduces the delivery of nutrients to the fetus, leading to a risk of underdevelopment or even spontaneous **abortion**. Complications of PIH for mothers include **renal failure**, hemorrhagic **stroke**, liver damage, and blindness. Risks to the baby include impaired growth or stillbirth from poor circulation and placenta abruptio, a condition in which the placenta prematurely separates from the uterus.

Signs and Symptoms
- Range from subtle to extreme
- Hypertension alone
- Sudden weight gain
- Any combination of dizziness, headache, nausea, pitting edema
- Vision changers
- Reduced urination, protein in the urine
- Possible seizures

Treatment Options
Treatment options for PIH are somewhat limited because many antihypertensive drugs are not well tolerated by fetuses. Bed rest and frequent monitoring of maternal and fetal health are usually recommended. It is not unusual for the babies of mothers with PIH to be delivered by cesarean section at 37 weeks (normal gestation is 40 weeks).

Medications
Steroids to speed the development of the baby's lungs may be administered in preparation for an early delivery.

Massage Considerations

Risks

- PIH contraindicates rigorous circulatory massage.

Benefits

- If the client is positioned comfortably (this varies with the stage of pregnancy), reflexive or energetic techniques may help lower the blood pressure and increase parasympathetic effect without challenging the cardiovascular system.

---

premenstrual syndrome

Premenstrual syndrome (PMS) is a collection of signs and symptoms that combine to interfere with a woman's ability to function normally during the luteal phase of the menstrual cycle (the time between ovulation and menstruation).

Some of the theories for the causes or triggers of PMS include hormonal imbalances; nutritional deficiencies; neurotransmitter imbalances; and other factors, including stress and genetic predisposition.

Several other conditions create overlapping symptoms with PMS, including **diabetes, hypothyroidism, eating disorders, depression, chronic fatigue syndrome, irritable bowel syndrome,** or any combination of these disorders. Only PMS will show a cessation of symptoms during and after menstruation, however, so patients are often counseled to keep a "PMS diary" to track any cyclical changes in their symptoms.

Signs and Symptoms

- Physical symptoms
    - Bloating
    - Breast tenderness
    - Acne
    - Craving for salt, sugar
    - Headache
    - Backache
    - Insomnia
    - Digestive upset (diarrhea, constipation)
    - Dizziness
    - Asthma
    - Possible seizures
- Emotional symptoms
    - Confusion
    - Depression
    - Anxiety, panic attacks
    - Mood swings, irritability

Treatment Options

Women with PMS are strongly recommended to make sure they get the best quality sleep they can muster during their difficult time and to exercise regularly. Some health professionals may recommend that patients follow a low-fat vegetarian diet to avoid excessive estrogen exposure and that they avoid salt, sugar, caffeine (specifically in soda, coffee, tea, and chocolate), and alcohol. Many alternative remedies have been reported to help women with PMS; some of the more common herbal recommendations include borage or evening primrose, black cohash, and dong quai.

Medications

Women who consult conventional physicians for this disorder may be prescribed low-dose birth control pills to control estrogen and progesterone levels, diuretics to control water retention, or antidepressants to address serotonin levels.

✋ Massage Considerations

Risks
- PMS holds no specific risks for massage or other types of bodywork.

Benefits
- PMS indicates massage, which has been shown to reduce depression and anxiety, and to help ameliorate some of the fluid retention that makes PMS so physically uncomfortable.

pressure sores: see decubitus ulcers

prickly heat: see miliaria rubra

prostate cancer

The prostate is a donut-shaped gland that lies inferior to the bladder and encircles the male urethra. It produces the fluid that allows for the motility and viability of sperm, and it controls release of the urine from the bladder. Most men experience some enlargement of the prostate as they age (i.e., **benign prostatic hypertrophy**), but sometimes the enlargement is caused by cancer.

The precise causes of prostate cancer are unknown. It has been observed that tumors must have access to testosterone from fully functional testes; this disease is unknown in men who have been castrated, and castration has also been shown to shrink cancerous tumors. Genetic predisposition, a high-fat diet, age, and race are other risk factors.

Prostate cancer has some complications that are occasionally the first clue to the presence of the disease. These include **urinary tract infections**, **pyelonephritis**, and **erectile dysfunction**.

Signs and Symptoms
- Problems with urination: pain, frequency, incomplete emptying, nocturia (the need to urinate during the night)
- Blood in the urine
- Difficulty maintaining an erection
- Low back pain
- Pain in the buttocks, legs with pressure on the pelvic nerves

Treatment Options

Treatment options for prostate cancer include radiation from internal or external sources, surgery to remove part or all of the prostate or the testes, and hormone therapy. Most treatment options for prostate cancer involve serious complications, including incontinence, impotence, and the development of feminine characteristics. Elderly men with slow-growing tumors may simply opt not to treat their disease because their quality of life would be so seriously impacted.

Medications

Prostate cancer is often treated with hormones that counteract tumor activity. Chemotherapy is generally reserved for patients with very advanced cases.

Massage Considerations

Risks

- Chemotherapy, surgery, and radiation carry cautions for massage, specifically in relation to infection risk, side effects, and general fragility.
- Clients who opt not to have their prostate cancer treated should not receive deep abdominal massage.

Benefits

- If the cautions related to cancer treatments are respected, massage therapists working as part of a health care team can certainly improve the quality of the lives of prostate cancer patients by providing supportive, informed touch during a time of great stress and challenge.

prostate enlargement, hypertrophy: see benign prostatic hypertrophy

prostatitis

Prostatitis is general term for a group of disorders in which the prostate becomes enlarged and possibly inflamed. It usually involves significant pain throughout the pelvis and groin.

Four types of prostatitis have been identified:

- Type 1: Acute bacterial prostatitis is an acute infection of the prostate, often related to a sexually transmitted infection or the use of a contaminated catheter to drain the bladder.
- Type 2: Chronic bacterial prostatitis is a recurrent, low-grade infection of the prostate.
- Type 3: Chronic nonbacterial prostatitis or chronic pelvic pain syndrome (CPPS) is prostate enlargement with no demonstrable infection. It can occur with or without signs of inflammation in prostate secretions. It is the most common form of prostatitis.
- Type 4: Asymptomatic inflammatory prostatitis (AIP) is silent, but white blood cells are found in prostate secretions or in prostate tissue during an evaluation for other disorders.

When a man has any difficulty with urination, an enlarged prostate is a logical assumption. Prostatitis, **benign prostatic hyperplasia**, and **prostate cancer** are all possibilities, and each requires a different treatment option, so it is important to obtain an accurate diagnosis.

Acute prostatitis is often related to a sexually transmitted infection such as **chlamydia** or **gonorrhea**; it is important to treat these thoroughly and to treat any sex partners as well.

A complication for any type of prostatitis is the risk of urethral obstruction. If enough pressure is exerted deeply on the urethra, acute urinary retention may develop. This is a medical emergency that requires immediate intervention.

Signs and Symptoms

- Pain, burning with urination
- Urinary frequency and urgency
- Pain in the low back, pelvis, perineum, testicles, penis
- Penile discharge, fever (with infection)
- Prostate is intensely painful on palpation
- Prostate is hot on palpation (with infection)

Treatment Options

Treatment for prostatitis depends on what type is present. Infections are treated with antibiotics. CPPS is treated symptomatically with some medications and with hydrotherapy and biofeedback to increase awareness of tightness in the perineal muscle, which can refer pain into the pelvis.

Medications

Acute bacterial infections respond well to antibiotics, but chronic infections may require a longer course. CPPS may be treated with smooth muscle relaxants and anti-inflammatory drugs.

Massage Considerations

Risks

- Acute infection contraindicates massage.

Benefits

- Clients with chronic low-grade infections may benefit from gentle massage that supports immune system function.
- Clients with chronic pelvic pain syndrome without infection may appreciate any general pain relief that massage can offer.
- Clients who have had prostatitis can enjoy the same benefits from massage as the rest of the population.

pseudomembranous colitis: see Clostridium difficile *infection*

---

psoriasis

Psoriasis is a chronic skin disease with occasional acute episodes in which epithelial cells in isolated patches replicate too rapidly. The result is a pile-up of excess cells that are itchy, red or pink, and scaly. This condition comes and goes but has no permanent cure.

Plaque psoriasis is the most common form of this condition. Other types are less common but can be more serious. They include guttate psoriasis, pustular psoriasis, inverse psoriasis, and erythrodermic psoriasis.

Psoriasis is seldom a life-threatening condition, although in severe cases, profound drying and cracking of the skin can lead to infection, fluid loss, and shock. **Psoriatic arthritis** is a joint inflammation that affects about 10% of all psoriasis patients.

Signs and Symptoms

- Plaque psoriasis: raised, itchy red or pink patches; may develop a silvery scale on the top
- Usually found on the knees, elbows; more rarely on the trunk, scalp, palms, soles of the feet
- Cycles of flare-ups and remissions
- Discolored skin between flare-ups

Treatment Options

Topical applications for psoriasis include coal tar, vitamin D ointments, salicylic acid, oatmeal, Epsom salt baths, and various strengths of steroid creams.

Phototherapy involves limited exposure to sunshine or carefully regulated doses of exposure to ultraviolet A or ultraviolet B lights.

Medications

Medications for psoriasis include oral or topical steroidal anti-inflammatory drugs, retinoids to limit sebaceous secretions, and cytotoxic drugs to limit the activity of those skin cells that have become overactive.

Topical and systemic therapies are often combined with phototherapy. PUVA treatment is a common example. It is a combination of a systemic medication (psoralen) and ultraviolet light exposure.

 Massage Considerations

Risks

- Psoriasis locally contraindicates any type of bodywork that might exacerbate itchiness.

Benefits

- Psoriasis is not contagious, and outbreaks are sometimes triggered by stress. It indicates any massage that promotes relaxation without increasing itchiness.

---

psoriatic arthritis

Psoriatic arthritis is a condition in which a person who has psoriasis develops painful inflammation in some joints and elsewhere in the body; the heart, eyes, lungs, cartilage, and tendons may all be involved.

Several subtypes of psoriatic arthritis have been identified. They range from mild to completely debilitating.

The cause and symptom profile of psoriatic arthritis are similar to those of several other disorders, including **rheumatoid arthritis**, **ankylosing spondylitis**, and the arthritides that may accompany inflammatory bowel disease (**Crohn disease** and **ulcerative colitis**).

In addition to causing significant inflammation in several joints, psoriatic arthritis can also cause inflammation in other places in the body. **Iritis** and **conjunctivitis** occur with inflammation of the eyes, **costochondritis** can occur if the rib cartilage is affected, **pleurisy** develops with inflammation of the pleural membranes, and inflammation of the aortic valves of the heart can lead to **heart failure**.

Signs and Symptoms

- Ridges or pitting in the fingernails and toenails
- Hot, swollen joints during flare in the knees, ankles, feet, fingers
- SAPHO: synovitis, acne, pustules, hyperostosis (bone enlargement), osteitis (bone inflammation)

Treatment Options

Psoriatic arthritis has no cure; this condition is managed mainly with medication.

Medications

Treatment for psoriatic arthritis usually begins with nonsteroidal anti-inflammatory drugs along with gentle exercise. Steroids and other medications may be recommended if these interventions are not successful. A class of medications called DMARDs (disease-modifying antirheumatic drugs) includes antimalarials, gold salts, and other drugs that can slow the progress of several types of arthritis. DMARDs can be effective, but they are slow acting, so pain relievers may be prescribed along with them.

🖐 Massage Considerations

Risks

- Acute joint pain and inflammation contraindicate massage.
- Psoriatic arthritis may involve inflammation away from the joints; information about this risk can inform decisions about massage.

Benefits

- Massage for affected joints when they aren't inflamed can help preserve mobility, reduce local muscle tension, and relieve pain.
- Clients with psoriatic arthritis can enjoy general benefits of massage in areas that are not affected by this condition.

pulmonary embolism: see embolism, thrombus

pyelonephritis

Pyelonephritis is an infection of the nephrons in the kidney, although the renal pelvis may also be involved. Infections may be acute and severe or chronic with few or no symptoms.

Pyelonephritis is often a complication of a **urinary tract infection** with *Escherichia coli* bacteria. Other kidney infections can develop from more obscure pathogens, they can be related to **diabetes** or **pregnancy**, they can arise from a neurogenic bladder, or they can develop because of surgical or medical instrumentation such as catheters or cystoscopes. Some kidney infections can be complications of a **kidney stone** or tumor that blocks the ureters.

Complications of untreated pyelonephritis include **hypertension**, **renal failure**, and **septicemia**.

Signs and Symptoms

- Acute pyelonephritis
    Sudden onset of fever, headache, malaise, nausea, vomiting
    Burning, frequency of urination
    Back pain, flank pain
- Chronic pyelonephritis
    May be subtle or silent while kidney damage accrues

Treatment Options

Pyelonephritis is treated with medication.

Medications

Most kidney infections clear up satisfactorily with antibiotic therapy.

🖐 Massage Considerations

Risks

- Acute infection contraindicates massage, especially because the kidneys are responsible for fluid management.
- Chronic infections require modality adjustments to avoid overwhelming a compromised system.

Benefits
- Clients with chronic kidney infections may benefit from immune support and pain relief offered by energetic and reflexive techniques.
- Clients who have fully recovered from pyelonephritis can enjoy the same benefits from massage as the rest of the population.

Ramsay-Hunt syndrome

Ramsay-Hunt syndrome is a complication of **herpes zoster**, also called shingles. It occurs when inflammation compresses the facial nerve, leading to pain and weakness on the affected side of the face, neck, and scalp.

Ramsay-Hunt syndrome occurs only with an outbreak of herpes zoster, but it closely resembles **Bell palsy**, which is compression of the facial nerve usually caused by **herpes simplex** infection. The distinguishing feature is that Bell palsy does not involve painful blisters.

Many other conditions can cause pain and weakness or paralysis of the face; these must be ruled out before assuming symptoms are related to herpes zoster or herpes simplex. Some causes of facial paralysis include **Lyme disease**, **stroke**, tumors, and **traumatic brain injury**.

Signs and Symptoms
- Extreme, intense facial pain
- May occur with diarrhea, nausea, and fever
- Blisters on a red base (sign of herpes zoster) in the ear canal, in the mouth, behind the ear
- Facial weakness or paralysis after blisters subside; may persist for 6 to 12 months
- Dry eye on the affected side
- Other sensory dysfunction: distorted taste, tinnitus

Treatment Options
Ramsay-Hunt syndrome is related to a viral infection that typically has to run its course. Interventions to limit pain and to keep the eye on the affected side free from damage are the mainstays of treatment.

Medications
The antiviral agent acyclovir is often recommended, but it is not clear that it shortens the duration or reduces the severity of this disorder. Steroidal anti-inflammatory drugs may also be prescribed along with analgesics to help manage pain.

Massage Considerations

Risks
- Acute shingles contraindicates massage because of the pain and the risk of communicability.
- Ramsay-Hunt syndrome may involve numbness; this is a caution for any massage that deeply or intrusively manipulates tissue.

Benefits
- If sensation is intact and the face is not painful, then massage can be a useful part of a treatment protocol for Ramsay-Hunt syndrome. Muscles degenerate quickly without nerve impulses; massage can support circulation and mobility while the motor neurons heal.
- Clients who have recovered from shingles or Ramsay-Hunt syndrome can enjoy the same benefits from massage as the rest of the population.

Raynaud syndrome

Raynaud syndrome is a condition involving constriction of the arterioles in the hands and feet, although it can also affect the nose, ears, and lips. During an episode, arterioles in the extremities experience sudden and extreme vasospasm, leading to pain, tingling, and discoloration in the affected areas. It occurs in temporary episodes at first, but the vasoconstriction can become a permanent situation.

Raynaud disease is a primary problem, meaning that it is unconnected to the underlying pathology. It can be related to stress, repeated percussive force, exposure to cold, or other factors. It generally has a slow onset and usually affects the hands or feet.

Raynaud phenomenon is extreme vasoconstriction that arises as a complication of another disorder such as **diabetes**, **scleroderma**, or **lupus**. Vasoconstriction in the extremities can also occur as a drug reaction or in response to neurologic entrapment, as seen with **carpal tunnel syndrome**.

Signs and Symptoms
- Cycle of color change in the fingers or toes: white to blue to red
- Episodes last minutes to hours
- Raynaud phenomenon can be severe with skin damage and a risk of gangrene

Treatment Options

Generally, a noninvasive approach is taken for Raynaud syndrome. Quitting smoking, immersing in warm water, dressing appropriately for the weather, protecting the hands when working with cold or frozen foods, making sure that shoes aren't too tight, and even moving to a warmer climate are all suggested before other interventions are suggested.

Medications

Vasodilators may be prescribed if other interventions are unsuccessful. Other drugs work to counteract norepinephrine, the stress-related hormone that initiates vasoconstriction.

✋ Massage Considerations

Risks
- If symptoms are related to an underlying pathology, it must be addressed in decisions about massage.
- Any skin damage in areas with poor circulation has a high risk of infection.

Benefits
- Massage can mechanically and reflexively improve blood flow for clients with primary Raynaud disease, and it can work to restore parasympathetic balance that may add to long-term improvement in function.

reactive arthritis

Reactive arthritis is a situation in which a trigger leads to inflammation of one or more joints and other tissues. As its name implies, this is a reactive process rather than an attack on joint structures. The majority of people with this disorder are male and have a genetic marker that is known to be a predisposing factor for other inflammatory conditions, including **ankylosing spondylitis** and **psoriatic arthritis**. Reactive arthritis is sometimes called Reiter syndrome; it was named after the doctor who first documented this pattern in 1915.

Reactive arthritis is often triggered by a bacterial infection of the genitourinary tract (**chlamydia**) or the digestive tract (**gastroenteritis**). It mimics several other types of joint inflammations. Ankylosing spondylitis and psoriatic arthritis can have similar symptoms, and they affect men more often than women; these can be confusing factors. **Rheumatoid arthritis, lupus, rheumatic fever**, and **septic arthritis** should also be considered.

Inflammation of the knee can cause the enlargement or even rupture of the joint capsule; this is a form of **Baker cyst**, but it can mimic **deep vein thrombosis**. Reactive arthritis can be an early indicator for **HIV** infection.

Signs and Symptoms

- Inflammation of a joint (low back or extremity)
- Painful swelling of a finger or toe ("sausage digit")
- Inflammation of the eye
- Inflammation of the genitourinary tract
- Possible inflammation of tendons, ligaments
- Inflammation persists for several months and may recur

Treatment Options

Careful exercise for strength and the maintenance of range of motion is another important part of the recovery from reactive arthritis. Many patients report that their symptoms are worse with immobility, so exercise may also provide some symptomatic relief.

Medications

Early and aggressive treatment with nonsteroidal anti-inflammatory drugs has been shown to limit overall joint damage, so it is important to begin it as soon as possible. Reactive arthritis caused by chlamydia infection typically responds well to antibiotic therapy. Injections of steroidal anti-inflammatory drugs into affected joint space are sometimes recommended.

 Massage Considerations

Risks

- Acute reactive arthritis locally contraindicates massage, which may exacerbate pain.
- Clients with this condition may use large doses of anti-inflammatory drugs that can obscure tissue response and increase the risk of overtreatment. In these situations, massage must be especially conservative to avoid doing inadvertent damage.

Benefits

- Clients recovering from reactive arthritis can use massage along with exercise and stretching to maintain the health and integrity of the affected joints.
- Clients who have fully recovered from reactive arthritis can enjoy the same benefits from massage as the rest of the population.

reflex sympathetic dystrophy syndrome: see complex regional pain syndrome

reflux esophagitis: see gastroesophageal reflux disorder

Reiter syndrome: see reactive arthritis

renal calculi: see kidney stones

---

renal cancer

Renal cancer is the development of malignant cells in the kidney. The most common form starts in the nephrons. It is called renal cell cancer, adenocarcinoma, or hypernephroma, and it accounts for about 90% of all renal cancer diagnoses. Other forms of renal cancer include transitional cell carcinoma, which starts in the renal pelvis and shares symptoms and treatment options with bladder cancer, and Wilms tumor, a type of malignancy found mostly in children.

Polycystic kidneys or **pyelonephritis** can show the same signs as kidney cancer, so it is important to rule these out in the diagnostic process.

Renal cancer is associated with a risk of metastasis through the lymph system to the bones, liver, and lungs.

Risk factors for renal cancer include age, gender, smoking, uncontrolled high blood pressure, and obesity. Long-term dialysis increases the risk of this disease, as does working with coal ovens, asbestos, or cadmium. Some genetic anomalies are also associated with an increased risk of renal cancer.

Signs and Symptoms

- Silent in the early stages
- Painless blood in the urine
- Palpable mass or lump in the abdomen
- Back pain on the affected side
- Low-grade fever with malaise
- Signs of kidney dysfunction: high blood pressure, protein in the urine, anemia

Treatment Options

Surgery for renal cancer can range from a partial nephrectomy (removal of the tumor and a small margin of surrounding tissue) to a radical nephrectomy (removal of the whole kidney along with the attached adrenal gland and nearby lymph nodes). Embolization is a procedure in which a substance is injected into the renal artery to clog it, thereby starving the tumor. This can be a treatment in itself or can be a strategy to shrink a growth in preparation for surgery.

Medications

Renal cancer may be treated with biologic response modifiers. These are immune system chemicals (interferon and interleukin-2) that enhance the immune response against tumor cells. Hormone therapy, radiation, and chemotherapy may all also be used to control kidney cancer.

Massage Considerations

Risks

- The risks for clients with renal cancer are the same as those for other cancer patients; the challenges of cancer treatments and complications must be considered in designing a session.

Benefits

- Carefully administered massage can boost immune system function, promote good-quality sleep, improve appetite, and be generally supportive for the healing process.

renal failure

Renal failure means that for various reasons, the kidneys are not functioning adequately.

If the kidneys lose significant function in a short time, it is referred to as acute renal failure. Cumulative damage that accrues over many years is called chronic renal failure. In either case, the kidneys are still working, but they are simply unable to keep up with the body's demands. In these situations, the kidneys can no longer adequately control blood volume, blood pressure, water balance, toxicity of the blood, and other factors.

Acute renal failure is typically a result of trauma and circulatory shock, an aggressive *Escherichia coli* infection, or an arterial **embolism**. Chronic renal failure is most likely to be linked to long-term **hypertension** or **diabetes** mellitus. In either case, hypertension, **edema**, **anemia**, rashes, muscle **cramps**, and other problems may be the result of the loss of kidney function.

Signs and Symptoms

- Decreased urine output
- Systemic edema
- Arrhythmia
- Anemia
- Osteomalacia (bone thinning)
- Rashes, skin discoloration
- Lethargy, fatigue, headache, malaise
- Loss of sensation in the hands and feet
- Muscle cramps
- Tremors, seizures
- Easy bruising, bleeding
- Changes in mental or emotional state

Treatment Options

Treatment goals for renal failure are to control symptoms, prevent further complications, and slow the progress of the disease. Fluid and salt intake may be restricted until kidney function can keep up with the body's demands.

If a patient's kidneys are simply incompetent regardless of these interventions, dialysis may become necessary. Many dialysis patients are waiting for a healthy kidney to become available for transplant.

Medications

Medication to control potassium levels in the blood is important to avoid heart problems. Diuretics are sometimes prescribed to help the kidneys process fluids.

Massage Considerations

Risks
- Renal failure contraindicates rigorous circulatory massage that puts stress on kidneys that are already challenged.

Benefits
- Reflexive or energetic work that promotes relaxation without mechanically impacting the circulation may be welcomed by a client in renal failure.

Practitioner Advice
- Clients who have received kidney transplants need to take immunosuppressant drugs for the rest of their lives; massage therapists and other bodyworkers need to be especially cautious about hygiene and the risk of carrying infection to these immunocompromised clients.

respiratory syncytial virus

Respiratory syncytial virus (RSV) is a viral attack on the respiratory system that is especially common among infants younger than 6 months old. It is spread through respiratory secretions in the air or on surfaces that contact the eyes, nose, or mouth of infants.

In babies who are premature or who have weak lungs, hearts, or immune systems, RSV can quickly become life-threatening **acute bronchitis** or **pneumonia**.

The vast majority of children have been exposed to RSV by age 2 years. It is possible to have subsequent infections, but they tend to be mild and indistinguishable from the **common cold**.

Signs and Symptoms
- Fever, runny nose, cough, wheezing, headache
- In infants, a high risk of complications in the lower respiratory tract
- In toddlers and older people, symptoms resemble those of the common cold

Treatment Options
Mild cases of RSV are treated with rest, humidifiers, and lots of liquids. Most hospitalizations occur when the infection is in a child younger than 6 months old. These patients may need to supplement oxygen or use a mechanical ventilator until the infection resolves.

Medications
Antibiotics are ineffective against this viral infection, and because several strains of the virus exist, no vaccine for RSV has yet been developed. Patients may be treated with fever reducers and bronchodilators.

 Massage Considerations

Risks
- Any acute respiratory infection contraindicates rigorous circulatory massage until the symptoms have subsided.

Benefits
- Circulatory massage modalities have no specific benefits for clients with acute RSV, but energetic or reflexive techniques may be soothing and supportive while the child goes through the crisis.

Practitioner Advice
- RSV in adults is essentially indistinguishable from a common cold. For this reason, massage therapists who have what feels like a cold should do everything in their power to recover quickly and to inform their clients that although they take the best possible precautions to prevent the spread of infection, a risk may be present. In this way, if a client or a therapist spends time with a new baby, he or she can make the best possible decisions about exposure.

restless leg syndrome

Restless leg syndrome (RLS) is a condition in which a variety of unpleasant sensations in the legs causes an uncontrollable urge to move. The condition is typically worse at night, leading to severe sleep deprivation.

Most people with RLS also have another type of sleep disorder: periodic limb movement disorder. This is involuntary jerking or twitching of the legs, which may be severe enough to interrupt sleep. RLS and **fibromyalgia** frequently overlap; both conditions are linked to poor-quality sleep.

RLS has been traced to an iron deficiency in the brain. A number of other conditions can cause iron deficiency, leading to secondary RLS. These conditions include **pregnancy**, end-stage **renal failure**, and **gastric bypass surgery**.

Signs and Symptoms
- Pulling, drawing, itching sensation in the legs ("creepy-crawlies")
- Irresistible urge to move the legs
- Symptoms are worse at night
- Symptoms are worse at rest than during activity
- Symptoms are relieved by movement, warm baths, massage

Treatment Options
The first step for a person with RLS is to evaluate his or her sleep habits. Eliminating caffeine is sufficient to control symptoms for some people. If massage and warm baths are inadequate for relief, patients may use medication.

Medications
RLS often responds well to dopamine agonists. Other medications used for RLS include antiseizure drugs.

🖐 Massage Considerations
Risks
- Massage has no specific risks for clients with RLS unless an underlying condition such as end-stage renal failure or pregnancy is also present.

Benefits
- Massage is frequently recommended to treat RLS during episodes. No evidence has yet shown that daytime massage reduces nighttime RLS symptoms, but it is unlikely to make the symptoms worse.

rhabdomyolysis

Rhabdomyolysis is a medical emergency in which muscle cells are destroyed and the release of their cellular byproducts results in shock and kidney damage.

Many factors can cause muscle damage. Rhabdomyolysis was first recognized in crushing injuries of victims of the London bombing raids during World War II, but it has also been seen with extreme exertion, malignant **hyperthermia**, **frostbite**, thyroid storm (**hyperthyroidism**), **alcoholism** with tremors, **burns**, **seizure disorders**, electrical injury, Duchenne **muscular dystrophy**, arterial **embolism**, bacterial infections, acute compartment syndrome (**shin splints**), and other conditions. Rarely, reactions to cholesterol-lowering medications can also cause rhabdomyolysis.

When muscle tissue is injured in this way, myoglobin (an oxygen-binding protein pigment in muscle cells) accumulates in the kidneys, leading to a risk of **renal failure**. Cellular phosphates, sulfate, and potassium also flow into the bloodstream, dangerously altering pH balance. Finally, interstitial fluid flows into the muscle cells to the extent that blood volume decreases and circulatory shock is a potential risk.

Signs and Symptoms
- Dark red or brown urine
- The affected muscle is tender, weak, often not acutely painful

Treatment Options

This condition is treated by quickly and aggressively flushing toxins out of the kidneys while also restoring blood volume. Drugs that speed this process may be administered, as well as chemicals to restore the correct pH balance to the blood.

Medications

Drugs for rhabdomyolysis include diuretics and potassium transporters to restore kidney function and correct the pH balance as quickly as possible.

Massage Considerations

Risks
- This condition is a medical emergency and contraindicates any circulatory massage.

Benefits
- Massage has no specific benefits for clients with acute rhabdomyolysis.
- Clients who have fully recovered from rhabdomyolysis with no long-term repercussions can enjoy the same benefits from massage as the rest of the population.

rheumatic fever

Rheumatic fever is a complication related to an untreated infection with a particular strain of group A *Streptococcus* (GAS) bacteria. This infection usually takes the form of strep throat, but scarlet fever may also be a trigger. Some strains of GAS bacteria can express enzymes that initiate a very extreme immune reaction, often against tissues that simply resemble the antigens rather than the antigens themselves.

Tissues that typically come under attack with this condition include the heart (all three layers but especially the endocardium that forms the valves); large joints (knees, ankles, elbows, wrists); and in some cases, the kidneys.

This condition sometimes also involves **glomerulonephritis**, which is inflammation in the glomeruli that may interfere with kidney function. Extensive damage to the heart valves increases the risk of life-threatening **heart failure**.

Signs and Symptoms

- Typically develops after strep throat infection
- Fever, fatigue
- Painful swollen joints
- Joint pain may move around the body (migratory arthritis)
- Chest pain, shortness of breath
- St. Vitus' dance: involuntary twitching that is more extreme on one side than the other
- Symptoms persist for several weeks and then subside

Treatment Options

Rheumatic fever is treated primarily with medication, rest, and good nutrition. If a bout of rheumatic fever causes significant weakness and scarring of the heart valves, corrective surgery may be suggested.

Medications

Strep throat infections are treated aggressively with antibiotics to not only shorten the duration of the throat infection but also to reduce the risk of rheumatic fever as a complication.

After rheumatic fever develops, it is treated symptomatically with nonsteroidal anti-inflammatory drugs for joint pain, steroidal anti-inflammatory drugs for heart inflammation, and a long course of antibiotics to eradicate any lingering streptococcus bacteria.

 ## Massage Considerations

Risks

- Acute rheumatic fever contraindicates rigorous circulatory massage.
- Clients who have a history of this infection may have heart damage that influences their ability to adapt to the changes that some types of massage may bring about.

Benefits

- Energetic or reflexive massage may be supportive and soothing for clients with acute rheumatic fever.
- Clients who have recovered from rheumatic fever without any evidence of heart damage or other repercussions can enjoy the same benefits from massage as the rest of the population.

rheumatoid arthritis

Rheumatoid arthritis (RA) is an autoimmune condition in which immune system cells mistakenly attack the synovial membranes of various joints. This leads to all the cardinal signs of inflammation, including heat, pain, redness, swelling, and loss of function at the affected joints. Inflammation inside the joint capsule destroys the articular cartilage and stretches the joint capsules, which is why joints with RA look so extremely disfigured.

In later stages, the overactive antibodies may also attack the pericardium, blood vessels, lungs, and fascia. When RA flares involve tissues outside the joint capsules, several problems can develop. Pathologically dry tear and salivary ducts (**Sjögren syndrome**), **pleurisy**, **pericarditis**, **vasculitis**, **Raynaud phenomenon**, skin ulcers, and gastrointestinal **ulcers** are all possible complications of RA.

Furthermore, deformed and bone-damaged joints may dislocate or even collapse. The tendons that cross over distorted joints sometimes become so stretched that they snap. If the disease is at the C_1–C_2 joint and the joint collapses, the resultant injury to the spinal column may result in **paralysis**.

Signs and Symptoms

- Runs in cycles of flare and remission
- During flare
    Malaise, low fever, muscle pain
    Becomes sharp, specific joint pain
    Joints are hot, painful, stiff
    Knuckles in the hands and feet are commonly affected areas
- During remission
    Permanent rheumatic nodules on the fingers, elbows, other areas

Treatment Options

The goals of RA treatment are to reduce pain, limit inflammation, halt joint damage, and improve function. Medications and physical therapy are used to limit the progression of the disease.

Surgery can be a successful option for RA patients if their disease has affected joints that can be easily treated. Joint replacement surgery is sometimes an option along with surgery to rebuild damaged or ruptured tendons and to remove portions of affected synovial membranes. The synovial membranes grow back, however, so this surgery is a temporary measure.

Medications

Treatment usually begins with nonsteroidal anti-inflammatory drugs to limit inflammation and pain. If these are inadequate, other medications can also interfere with the disease process. These include steroidal anti-inflammatory drugs and immunosuppressant drugs. They often give significant relief, but they are also associated with a long list of serious side effects and cannot be used for long-term care.

Massage Considerations

Risks

- RA in its acute stage or flare-up contraindicates rigorous massage that may exacerbate symptoms.

Benefits

- During a flare, reflexive or energetic modalities may be soothing and supportive.
- During remission, massage may improve mobility and the health of the soft tissues surrounding the joints.

- Massage as a health maintenance and stress management strategy may help reduce the risk of flare of RA.

rickets: see osteomalacia

ringworm: see fungal infections

Rocky Mountain spotted fever

Rocky Mountain spotted fever (RMSF) is a tick-borne bacterial infection that can rapidly become life threatening. It is caused by the tick *Rickettsia rickettsii* and is spread through the bites of hard-bodied (*Ioxid*) ticks, notably American dog ticks and wood ticks.

When these ticks bite a human, the bacteria flow from their saliva into the host's bloodstream. These bacteria invade the cells that line small- and medium-sized blood vessels. Eventually, plasma leaks from these damaged vessels into the tissues, or tiny hemorrhages may develop into the skin or internal organs. The cumulative loss of blood pressure can lead to acute renal failure, shock, and death.

RMSF got its name because it was first documented in the Snake River Valley of Idaho (where it was initially called "black measles"), but it is uncommon in the Mountain West. It occurs in highest incidence in South Carolina and Oklahoma. It has not been reported in Alaska, Hawaii, Maine, or Vermont, but every other US state has at least one case on record.

RMSF can lead to several serious complications, including **jaundice**, **encephalitis**, and **renal failure**. Long-term complications of this infection include **gangrene** requiring amputation, partial **paralysis** of the extremities, hearing loss, and loss of bowel or bladder control.

Signs and Symptoms

- High fever, chills, malaise, nausea
- Later: dark, nonitchy patches on the extremities (palms, soles)
- Patches appear over the whole limb toward the trunk
- Internal organ damage, especially of the liver, gastrointestinal tract
- Can affect the central nervous system
- Can lead to death from renal failure, circulatory shock

Treatment Options

RMSF is treated with medication.

Medications

RMSF responds well to antibiotics, but an early diagnosis is important to avoid serious long-term damage.

Massage Considerations

Risks

- Acute RMSF, which can involve a hemorrhagic rash, contraindicates any massage until the infection has been completely resolved.

- Clients who have had RMSF may have permanent kidney damage; this influences decisions about bodywork.

Benefits
- Massage has no specific benefits for clients with RSMF until the infection has been identified and treated.
- Clients who have fully recovered from RMSF with no long-term repercussions can enjoy the same benefits from massage as the rest of the population.

Practitioner Advice
- Massage therapists are in a unique position to see ticks where our clients might miss them. Ticks are most likely to latch onto the skin at the popliteal fossa, the axilla, in or around the ear, and anywhere on the scalp or hairline.
- If a massage therapist finds a tick on a client's body, the client should be informed. If both the therapist and client consent, the tick should be removed with tweezers squeezed as close to the skin as possible; the tick should be pulled directly upward, not twisted out. The area should be disinfected, and the tick should be put into a plastic bag and frozen to take to the doctor in case symptoms develop. If any mouthparts are left in the host, a doctor should be consulted immediately, regardless of whether symptoms develop.
- The Centers for Disease Control and Prevention (CDC) warns that any liquid expressed from a tick could carry bacteria; the person removing a tick should avoid coming into direct contact with it. The CDC further advises that exposing the tick to toxins or a hot match may cause the animal to regurgitate into the host, increasing the risk of infection.

rosacea: see acne rosacea

rubella

Rubella, also known as German measles or 3-day measles, is a viral infection leading to a mildly itchy rash of small pink spots all over the body. It is not a serious disease for children or adults, but it is significantly dangerous to fetuses in utero. Many fetuses of infected mothers are miscarried or stillborn. Babies born to women who have rubella while they are pregnant can have any combination of blindness, hearing loss, mental disability, or heart damage. This group of problems is called congenital rubella syndrome.

Signs and Symptoms
- Rash of small pink spots
- Appear on face and then spread all over the body
- Fever, headache, swollen lymph nodes, fatigue, joint pain
- Symptoms persist for about 3 days

Treatment Options

Rubella is a mild viral infection; it has no treatment but rest and time. It is preventable through vaccination. This vaccination, which is given in childhood, protects pregnant women that a child may encounter and protects women throughout their pregnancies.

Medications

Rubella is not treated with medication.

Massage Considerations

Risks

- Acute rubella is a systemic viral infection, and it systemically contraindicates massage.
- Clients with congenital rubella syndrome may have heart problems that influence decisions about massage.
- Clients who are mentally disabled because of a prenatal exposure to rubella are best receiving massage in a setting where a caregiver is readily accessible in case the client feels uneasy.

Benefits

- Massage has no specific benefits for clients with a current case of rubella.
- Clients who have fully recovered from rubella can enjoy the same benefits from massage as the rest of the population.

Practitioner Advice

- Rubella is contagious. Massage therapists who have not been vaccinated must consider communicability issues before working with clients who may be able to spread the infection.

S

sarcoidosis

The term sarcoidosis comes from the Greek for "flesh" and "condition," referring to multiple bumps or fleshy tumors that accumulate in the skin and other tissues with this disease. Sarcoidosis is an idiopathic condition involving an ineffective immune response in various organs throughout the body. This response leads to the formulation of granulomas, which are small masses of inflamed cells that collect in the lungs, eyes, skin, or other locations.

The signs and symptoms of sarcoidosis resemble those of many other conditions; these must be ruled out to get an accurate picture of the problem. The differential diagnosis must include tests for **tuberculosis; lymphoma; rheumatoid arthritis; rheumatic fever; aspergillosis**; and some other more obscure problems.

If sarcoidosis affects the central nervous system, flaccid facial paralysis may develop. This must be differentiated from **Bell palsy**, which has a different trigger.

Signs and Symptoms

- Lungs: dry cough, chest pain, shortness of breath; scar tissue may permanently decrease lung capacity and function
- Lymph nodes: enlarged nodes at the submandibular, cervical, axillary, or inguinal groups; enlarged spleen
- Skin: painful, inflamed red bumps on the face, arms, shins; discoloration of the nose, cheeks, lips, ears
- Eyes: dryness and photophobia, uveitis, glaucoma, cataracts, possible blindness
- Musculoskeletal system: painful joints and stiff muscles
- Other: weight loss, fever, fatigue, night sweats, malaise

Treatment Options

Sarcoidosis is treated by its symptoms, with the goal of reducing inflammation and promoting good function. People with mild cases may not undergo any treatment.

Medications

Long-term, low doses of corticosteroids are the most commonly prescribed intervention along with creams for skin lesions, drops for uncomfortable eyes, or inhalants to improve lung function.

Massage Considerations

Risks

- Symptoms of sarcoidosis can range from mild to severe. The safety of bodywork depends on the degree of dysfunction this disease brings about.
- If the lungs have been damaged, the client may be uncomfortable lying flat on a table.
- Tender bumps in the skin can be painful and inflamed; these locally contraindicate massage.
- Clients with central nervous system involvement may have paralysis or numbness; these conditions require adjustments in massage strategies.
- Clients with sarcoidosis may use medication that alters their inflammatory response or immune system efficiency. These factors must be addressed in designing a massage session.

Benefits

- Massage has no specific benefit for clients with sarcoidosis.
- If the client is comfortable on a table, gentle massage may be a supportive, soothing intervention.

scabies: see mites

Scheuermann disease: see postural deviations

schistosomiasis

Schistosomiasis, also called bilharzia, is an infestation with any of five different species of parasitic worms. Symptoms are initiated not by the worms themselves but also by an immune system reaction against their eggs.

The five species of Schistosoma worms go through several stages of growth. In the infectious stage, the organisms, called cercaria, swim freely in fresh water. They can penetrate the skin of waders, swimmers, or people washing in the contaminated water. After they are inside a human host, the worms mature in the liver or the lungs. In the next life phase, they migrate to their preferred tissues; this is determined by which species of worm is present. The most commonly invaded tissues are the bladder, rectum, intestines, liver, portal system, spleen, and lungs. In rare cases, the central nervous system may be colonized.

The eggs they lay may stay local or wind up in the urinary tract and the intestines to be shed with urine or feces. If the host urinates or defecates where the waste can contaminate fresh water, the eggs are released there. They mature to the next stage in the bodies of freshwater snails. Then the infectious organisms leave the snails to swim freely in water and begin the cycle again.

Signs and Symptoms
- Symptoms don't always develop
- Early symptoms
  Itchy rash ("swimmer's itch")
  Fever, chills, coughing, muscle ache
- Late symptoms (determined by where the worms colonize)
  Liver damage
  Urinary tract obstruction
  Chronic renal failure
  Increased risk of bladder cancer
  Pulmonary hypertension, right-sided heart failure
  Seizures, encephalitis, meningitis

Treatment Options
This condition is easily treated with medication.

Medications
The medications used to eradicate parasitic worms are called antihelminthics. They are typically very effective and relatively inexpensive, making schistosomiasis a highly treatable condition. Reinfection is common if the contaminated water that is the source of the parasites isn't treated.

Massage Considerations

Risks
- Clients with a history of schistosomiasis may have kidney, liver, and lung health issues; this information is important for making decisions about massage.

Benefits
- Massage has no specific benefits for clients with schistosomiasis.
- If clients with a history of this condition have no long-term damage to the heart, lungs, kidneys, or urinary tract, they may enjoy the same benefits from massage as the rest of the population.

schizophrenia

Schizophrenia is a mental illness involving delusions (deeply held beliefs) and hallucinations (perceptions of sights, smells, sounds, or tastes that aren't there) along with disrupted emotional responsiveness, withdrawal, and a progressive loss of function in private and work-related settings. It is considered a type of psychosis (a condition in which the interpretation of reality is abnormal and disorganized).

Diagnosis of schizophrenia is difficult because although its hallmarks are hallucinations and paranoid delusions, other central nervous system problems may also cause these symptoms. Other factors, such as **depression**, **hypothyroidism**, **chemical dependency**, side effects of other medications, and brain tumors, must be ruled out before it is possible to diagnose schizophrenia.

Signs and Symptoms

- Negative symptoms (lost function)
    Dulled emotional responses
    Speaking in a monotone
    Withdrawal from social situations
    Loss of connection with the world
    Loss of hygiene habits
    Catatonia
- Positive symptoms (new behaviors)
    Auditory, visual hallucinations
    Delusions involving paranoia
    Disorganized thinking, behavior

Treatment Options

Many people find that treatment for schizophrenia is most successful when medication is enhanced by individual and family therapy, as well as participation in other support groups.

For most patients, schizophrenia may be a lifelong condition; only a small number ever find that they "get over" this disease.

Medications

Schizophrenia is treatable with medications, but the nature of this disease is that the person who has it doesn't believe he or she is sick. Furthermore, some drugs have serious side effects. Consequently, although a number of antipsychotic drugs work well, compliance may be poor, and most people find that medication is only one part of a multifaceted treatment program.

Massage Considerations

Risks

- The appropriateness of massage for clients with schizophrenia is determined by the client's perception of safety. If the client doesn't feel safe, the session must be adjusted or terminated.

Benefits

- If the client feels at ease, massage is probably a helpful coping strategy for a client who has schizophrenia. The experience of receiving safe and educated touch may contribute to a clearer, more accurate perception of the world as a good place to be.

sciatica

Sciatica, also called lumbar radiculopathy, is a term used to describe the consequences of compression or irritation to some part of the sciatic nerve. The source of irritation can be inside the spinal canal, usually at the L5 or S1 nerve roots. Factors can include **disc disease**, lumbar stenosis, **spondylosis, spondylolisthesis**, or spinal tumors. Sciatic pain can also originate outside the spine, with **piriformis syndrome** or **osteoarthritis** at the sacroiliac joint.

When low back pain is accompanied by bilateral numbness in the groin or loss of bladder or bowel control, it is an indicator of cauda equina syndrome (pressure directly on the nerve roots in the spinal canal), which is a medical emergency.

Signs and Symptoms

- Low back, buttock pain on the affected side
- The leg may feel weak, cold, heavy
- Sharp, shooting, electrical pain in a radicular pattern
- Paresthesia ("pins and needles") on the affected side
- Symptoms elicited by sitting, sneezing, coughing

Treatment Options

Treatment for sciatica is determined by the source of the irritation. Disc disease is responsible for most cases, and many people find that the situation resolves without surgical intervention within about 6 weeks. Using hot or cold applications to the painful areas helps some people manage the pain.

If other interventions are not successful and pain is still disabling 3 months after onset, surgery to remove the bulging disc may be performed.

Medications

Nonsteroidal anti-inflammatory drugs, muscle relaxants, or other analgesics may also be prescribed. Some orthopedists suggest an epidural steroid injection at the inflamed nerve root.

Massage Considerations

Risks

- The safety of massage for clients with sciatica is determined by what is causing the compression to the sciatic nerve.
- Avoid positions or pressure that could elicit symptoms.

Benefits

- Depending on the source of the irritation, massage may offer some temporary or even long-term relief for clients with sciatic pain.
    Massage can help decrease spasms of the piriformis.
    Massage may help decrease inflammation and irritation at the sacroiliac joint.
    Massage can work to decompress the lumbar curve.

scleroderma

Scleroderma is a chronic autoimmune dysfunction in which faulty antibodies attack and damage arterioles. Damage to these small blood vessels causes local edema and the stimulation of nearby fibroblasts to spin out huge amounts of collagen (the basis for scar tissue). Eventually, the edema subsides, but the scar tissue deposits remain hard and unyielding for years at a time. "Sclero" comes from the Greek for "scar," and "derma" refers to the skin.

Scleroderma takes two forms: localized or systemic. Localized scleroderma is usually limited to the skin of the hands and face. The initial edema may last for several weeks or months, and the thickening of the skin may accumulate over a course of about 3 years. Then the symptoms gradually stabilize or even reverse.

Systemic scleroderma can affect the internal organs and other tissues as well as the skin. The tissues most at risk are in the digestive tract, the heart and circulatory systems, the kidneys and lungs, and various parts of the musculoskeletal system (especially the synovial membranes in the joints and around the tendons). When systemic scleroderma attacks the lungs, kidneys, or heart, the prognosis becomes much more serious. This disease can be fatal.

Complications of scleroderma include **gastroesophageal reflux disorder, Raynaud syndrome, tenosynovitis, angina,** arrhythmia, **heart failure, renal failure, trigeminal neuralgia,** and **Sjögren syndrome.**

Signs and Symptoms

- CREST syndrome
  Calcinosis: accumulation of calcium deposits in the skin
  Raynaud syndrome
  Esophageal dysmobility: sluggishness of the digestive tract and chronic gastric reflux
  Sclerodactyly ("hardening of the fingers")
  Telangiectasia ("spider veins")
- Skin ulcers, changes in pigmentation, hair loss
- Weak muscles, swollen tendons, tenosynovitis
- Trigeminal neuralgia
- Sjögren syndrome
- Pulmonary edema
- Angina, arrhythmia, risk of heart failure
- Kidney damage, risk of renal failure

Treatment Options

Scleroderma is typically treated by its symptoms. Medications can address some issues. Physical or occupational therapies are often used to maintain flexibility in the hands. Patients are usually advised to avoid smoking, cold conditions, and spicy foods to minimize their symptoms.

Medications

Calcium channel blockers may be recommended for Raynaud syndrome. Diuretics are prescribed to improve kidney function. Antacids can relieve gastric reflux. Nonsteroidal anti-inflammatory drugs are used for muscle and joint pain.

Massage Considerations

Risks

- Scleroderma can compromise the circulatory and urinary systems; this contraindicates rigorous circulatory massage.

Benefits

- Scleroderma patients who use physical therapy to maintain health can probably also adapt to the changes that massage brings about.
- Reflexive or energetic techniques can offer important stress-relieving, immune system–boosting benefits for clients who struggle with this difficult disorder.

scoliosis: see postural deviations

seasonal affective disorder: see depression

sebaceous cysts

Sebaceous cysts are connective tissue wrappings around a deep and usually long-term **acne** infection. Building a connective tissue wall around an old infection site is a strategy for "removing" this foreign material from the rest of the body.

Signs and Symptoms

- Small, painless bumps under the skin
- Can move with the mobility of the surrounding fascia
- Most common on the scalp, neck, shoulders

Treatment Options

Most cysts require no treatment unless they cause pain, but they can be removed for cosmetic reasons. If the connective tissue wrapping has adequately isolated the cyst, it can generally be removed with a simple surgery.

Medications

Sebaceous cysts are not treated with medication.

Massage Considerations

Risks

- Sebaceous cysts locally contraindicate intrusive massage, which can be irritating.

Benefits

- Massage has no specific benefits for sebaceous cysts, but any work in the area that does not cause pain is safe and appropriate.

Practitioner Advice

- If a client has a questionable or new cyst that hasn't been diagnosed, it is good practice to recommend that he or she have it diagnosed before the next appointment. Most painless bumps under the skin are not dangerous, but diagnosis is not within the scope of practice of massage therapists.

seborrheic eczema: see eczema/dermatitis

seizure disorders

A seizure disorder is any kind of problem that causes seizures as one of its symptoms.

When interconnecting neurons in the brain are stimulated in a certain way, a tremendous burst of excess electricity may stimulate the neighboring neurons. The reaction is repeated, and soon millions of neurons in the brain are giving off electrical discharge. This is the central nervous system "lightning storm" of a seizure, and it affects the rest of the body in a number of different ways.

In some cases, the cause of seizures can be definitively linked to a mechanical or chemical problem in the brain. Birth trauma, **stroke, traumatic brain injury,** shaken baby syndrome, brain tumors, and penetrating wounds can all cause seizures, as can some types of metabolic disturbances, infections, exposure to some toxins, and extreme hypotension or hemorrhage. Rarely, seizures can be traced to a hereditary problem.

Epilepsy is one type of seizure disorder. It is identified as a specific disorder when a person has two or more seizures that are not related to any identifiable cause such as head injury, stroke, infection, or fever. This rules out about 75% of all people who have a history of seizure.

Seizure triggers for people with epilepsy vary. For some people, sudden changes in light level trigger a seizure. For others, flashing or strobing lights or the strobing effect created by ceiling fans are triggers. For still others, certain sounds or even particular notes of music cause seizures. Anxiety or other sicknesses such as **cold** or **flu** may also lead to seizures.

Signs and Symptoms

- Generalized seizures (affect the whole brain)
    - Absence seizures: very short (5 to 10 seconds) episodes of loss of consciousness
    - Myoclonic seizures: bilateral muscular jerking; may be subtle or obvious
    - Tonic-clonic seizures ("grand mal" seizures): uncontrolled movement of the face, arms, and legs followed by loss of consciousness
    - Status epilepticus: life-threatening variation of tonic-clonic seizures; a medical emergency that persists for more than 20 minutes
- Partial seizures (abnormal activity in isolated areas of the brain)
    - Simple partial: no change in consciousness; weakness, numbness, sensory hallucinations, vertigo, muscle tics, or twitching
    - Complex partial: repetitive behaviors, including pacing in a circle, rocking, or smacking the lips

Treatment Options

Some epilepsy patients find that their seizures are less frequent and less extreme when they follow a strict high-fat, low-fiber ketogenic diet.

Surgical intervention for seizure disorders is reserved for when an isolated and expendable mass (i.e., a tumor or clump of scar tissue) can be determined to be the cause of the seizures. Tonic-clonic seizures can be successfully controlled in some patients by severing the corpus callosum.

Medications

Seizures are generally treated with anticonvulsant medication, which makes neurons in the brain harder to stimulate.

☝ Massage Considerations

Risks
- A client who is undergoing a seizure cannot receive massage.
- Massage has no other risks specifically related to seizure disorders.

Benefits
- Massage has no specific benefits for clients with seizure disorders.
- Massage is safe for clients with a history of seizures, but if their seizures tend to come on fast with no warning, the therapist should be alert to the possibility that it may happen during a session.

Practitioner Advice
- In the event of a tonic-clonic seizure, the practitioner's job is to make sure the client is safe. The practitioner should call 911 or the local emergency number and wait until the seizure has subsided.

septic arthritis

Septic arthritis is a form of arthritis brought about by a bacterial infection. *Neisseria gonorrhea* and *Staphylococcus aureus* are the most common infectious agents.

The most common ways for infections to be introduced into a joint capsule are through puncture wounds; contaminated needles; or as a complication of an underlying illness, especially **gonorrhea, rheumatoid arthritis,** or **diabetes**. When it occurs in the spine, it may resemble **ankylosing spondylitis**. It is important to obtain an accurate diagnosis because treatment protocols are very different.

Signs and Symptoms
- Redness, pain, heat, swelling at the joint
- Mild to high fever
- Most common at the knees and hips
- When related to gonorrhea, it may start at sacroiliac joints and move superiorly up the spine

Treatment Options

Infected joints are repeatedly aspirated with either needles or open shunts. Arthroscopic surgery may be performed to débride or scrape the insides of the synovial capsule to make sure all bacteria are removed. After the infection has subsided, the patient is recommended for physical therapy to prevent or limit permanent loss of function.

Medications

Antibiotic drugs are administered orally, as an injection into the joint, or both.

Massage Considerations

Risks
- Septic arthritis contraindicates any bodywork that physically manipulates the joints or soft tissues while the infection is active.

Benefits
- After the infection has past, massage may help restore normal range of motion and restore suppleness to the affected joint and surrounding structures.
- Clients with a history of septic arthritis and no permanent dysfunction can enjoy the same benefits from massage as the rest of the population.

septicemia

Septicemia is an umbrella term that refers to a system-wide infection occurring in a continuum of severity. Another term for septicemia is blood poisoning. Viruses or fungi can cause septicemia, but the most common cause is bacteria.

Septicemia typically begins with an infection that enters the bloodstream. The infectious agents are often endogenous (usually harmless colonies of bacteria in the lungs, digestive tract, skin, or throat). But age, underlying illness, or a weak immune system may allow these bacteria to become more dangerous. Septicemia can also arise from the use of catheters or other invasive equipment.

Several factors have contributed to an increasing incidence of septicemia. Aggressive use of immunosuppressant therapies (chemotherapy, radiation, steroids) reduces bacterial resistance; people with chronic diseases are living longer, which increases their risk for serious infections; more invasive devices (catheters, insulin pumps, ostomy bags) are being used, and they may become contaminated; and the long-term indiscriminate use of antibiotics has led to the development of new drug-resistant strains of bacteria, such as **methicillin-resistant *Staphylococcus aureus* and *Clostridium difficile*.**

The prognosis for survival from septicemia depends largely on the invading pathogens, the underlying health of the patient, and the stage at which treatment is given. This is can be a fatal condition if intervention is delayed.

Signs and Symptoms
- Fever, chills, malaise
- Rapid heart rate
- Confusion
- Shock
- Subdermal hemorrhaging
- Possible organ failure

Treatment Options
The three top priorities in treating septicemia are to stabilize the patient, clear microorganisms from the blood, and identify and treat the original site of infection. These are hospital-based interventions that are outside the scope of home care.

Medications
Septicemia is aggressively treated with antibiotics when the infectious agents have been identified.

Massage Considerations

Risks
- Septicemia systemically contraindicates any massage that has mechanical impact.

Benefits
- Energetic or reflexive modalities can support the rallying of the immune system against this life-threatening infection, but no other type of bodywork has any significant benefit for clients with septicemia.
- Clients who have fully recovered from septicemia with no long-term damage can enjoy the same benefits from massage as the rest of the population.

Shigella infection: see gastroenteritis

shingles: see herpes zoster

shin splints

"Shin splints" is a term used to describe a variety of lower leg problems that are often related to overtraining, not allowing adequate warm-up or cool-down time, or using worn-out shoes.

Technical terms for the injuries that often appear under this heading include medial tibial stress syndrome, periostitis, stress fractures, and chronic or acute exertional compartment syndrome. Of these, acute exertional compartment syndrome is the most serious. Because the fascia on the lower leg is such a tough container, acute swelling there can cause tissue death if it is not resolved naturally or with surgical intervention. This is an emergency situation and should be treated as quickly as possible.

Acute exertional compartment syndrome can mimic or occur simultaneously with **rhabdomyolysis**. This is another medical emergency that involves muscle injury, but it carries a high risk of kidney damage.

Signs and Symptoms

- Pain (mild to severe)
- The location varies according to site of injury
- Exacerbated by dorsiflexion, inversion, plantarflexion of the foot

Treatment Options

Shin splint treatment depends on the source of the injury. Most situations can be avoided or prevented with adjustments in training schedules and footwear. Muscle and fascia injuries may be treated with careful exercise and stretching. Acute compartment syndrome may be treated surgically or with injections of cortisone. Stress fractures only heal with appropriate rest.

Medications

People with shin splints may take nonsteroidal anti-inflammatory drugs to help with pain and inflammation.

Massage Considerations

Risks

- Acute inflammation locally contraindicates massage. Otherwise, massage has no specific risks for shin splints.

Benefits

- Shin splints that are not acutely inflamed indicate massage, which can improve fluid turnover and can help stretch lower leg muscles that are otherwise difficult to access.

Shy-Drager syndrome: see multiple system atrophy

sick building syndrome

Sick building syndrome (SBS) is a situation in which people experience serious compromises to comfort and health, and these symptoms develop in relation to how much time they spend in a particular building or area within a building. By definition, SBS is not related to a specific identified cause but is probably caused by a combination of several factors.

Contributors to SBS include any combination of indoor chemical contaminants (formaldehyde, tobacco smoke, carbon monoxide), outdoor chemical contaminants (motor vehicle and other exhaust that can be drawn into a ventilation system), and biological contaminants (molds, fungi, viruses, bacteria).

Signs and symptoms of SBS mimic several other low-grade chronic hypersensitivity conditions, especially **multiple chemical sensitivity syndrome**. The difference is that several people in the same environment all develop symptoms in relation to exposure to the building or room in question.

Signs and Symptoms

- Vary widely according to irritants and occupants
- Headache
- Eye irritation
- Nose, throat irritation; dry cough
- Dizziness, nausea
- Fatigue, poor concentration
- Hypersensitivity to odors

Treatment Options

Treatment for SBS focuses on the building, not on the people. Improving ventilation is usually the first step, along with removing or modifying any pollution source and using air filters if necessary.

Recovery from SBS can take several weeks or months, but after the irritating triggers are removed, people without other underlying disorders should return to normal.

Medications

Some medications may treat the symptoms of SBS (e.g., analgesics for headache), but this condition is best treated by addressing the contaminants that are the cause of the symptoms.

Massage Considerations

Risks

- As long as the client can be made comfortable, massage has no particular risks for clients with SBS.

Benefits

- Massage has no specific benefits for clients with SBS except for those enjoyed by the rest of population.
- Massage may improve headache and the ability to focus and concentrate and may provide a general sense of well-being, but these effects only persist while the client is removed from the site of contamination.

sickle cell disease

Sickle cell disease is a type of hemolytic **anemia**, a condition in which red blood cells (RBCs) are prematurely destroyed. It is an inherited disorder, requiring two sickle cell genes, one from each parent.

The presence of two sickle cell genes alters the formation of hemoglobin, the oxygen-carrying molecule that makes up the bulk of RBCs. The most common form of sickle cell disease involves the formation of hemoglobin-S (the S is for sickle), which forms long rods after it gives up its oxygen. This distorts the RBC into a sharp, collapsed disc, or sickle shape.

The lifespan of a sickled RBC is 10 to 20 days, as opposed to the 120-day life span of normal RBCs. Pulling dead RBCs out of the bloodstream puts a heavy load on the spleen, which is typically destroyed by age 4 years in these patients. Losing the spleen puts people with sickle cell disease at increased risk for infections. The liver can take over for spleen function, but the risk for **jaundice** and **gallstones** is high for this population. A tendency toward excessive blood clotting also increases the risk of ischemic **stroke**.

Signs and Symptoms

- Anemia, pallor, fatigue, poor stamina
- Shortness of breath
- Frequent infections
- Jaundice
- High risk of ischemic stroke
- Sickle cell crisis: sickled RBCs completely block an arteriole

Treatment Options

Sickle cell disease is typically treated with medication. Folic acid supplementation can support the formation of new RBCs to replace the damaged ones. Transfusions can offer temporary relief but are not a long-term solution.

Medications

Young children with sickle cell disease are often put on prophylactic doses of antibiotics to forestall the possibility of bacterial infections. Vaccinations against bacterial infections are highly recommended.

Some drugs may slow or even prevent RBC degeneration.

Other than these interventions, the only other treatment option for this disease is pain management for acute sickle cell crises.

Massage Considerations

Risks

- Sickle cell disease contraindicates any massage that forcefully pushes fluid through a compromised system.

Benefits

- Gentle massage and reflexive or energetic techniques can address the chronic pain that many sickle cell disease patients live with.

Silk Road disease: see Behçet disease

sinusitis

Sinusitis, or inflammation of the sinuses, occurs in two forms: noninfectious and infectious. Noninfectious sinusitis may also be called allergic rhinitis or hay fever. Infectious sinusitis involves a pathogenic invasion followed by an inflammatory response that creates a vicious cycle. The body creates excessive mucus to help remove infectious agents, but the inflamed tissues make drainage of that mucus (which is an ideal growth medium for many types of bacteria) impossible. Infectious sinusitis may be linked to viruses, bacteria, fungi, nasal polyps, and other factors. It can be chronic or acute.

Sinusitis is often related to an **allergic reaction**, but it can also be a sign of **aspergillosis** or **nasal polyps**. Possible complications of sinus infections include **osteomyelitis** and **meningitis** as the infection invades deeper tissues.

Signs and Symptoms

- Severe headache
- Swelling, puffiness, tenderness of the face
- Fever, chills with infection
- Sore throat, cough, congestion, runny nose
- Fatigue
- With allergies: thin, clear, runny mucus
- With infection: streaked, opaque, thick, sticky mucus

Treatment Options

Treatment for sinusitis begins with self-help measures, including staying in humid air, increasing daily water intake, and using air filters to remove irritating particles from the air. In very extreme cases, surgery is recommended to correct any structural anomaly. (Antihistamines are most appropriate for allergies, not infectious sinusitis.)

Medications

Drugs prescribed for sinusitis begin with antibiotics if the infection is bacterial, but the prescription may be long term for this tenacious infection.

Decongestants are sometimes recommended to shrink the mucous membranes, but they are only appropriate for short-term use because they can create a "rebound effect" when usage is stopped. Corticosteroids in nasal spray form can reduce swelling, but they are also best used in short-term doses.

🖐 Massage Considerations

Risks

- Acute infection with fever contraindicates rigorous circulatory massage.
- Clients with severe nasal congestion may need some accommodations in positioning.

Benefits

- Careful massage of the face may improve sinus drainage for clients with allergic sinusitis.
- Massage has no specific benefits to address chronic sinus infections, but clients may enjoy this supportive intervention in their efforts to overcome a stubborn illness.
- Clients who have had either kind of sinusitis but who have no current symptoms can enjoy the same benefits from massage as the rest of the population.

Sjögren syndrome

Sjögren syndrome is an autoimmune condition in which antibodies attack tear ducts and mucous membranes. It can occur as a free-standing primary disease or as a complication or symptom of some other autoimmune disease. It often accompanies **rheumatoid arthritis**, **scleroderma**, and **lupus**. It is also associated with Hashimoto thyroiditis (**hyperthyroidism**),

gastroesophageal reflux disease, and **Raynaud syndrome**. Some studies show that Sjögren syndrome is associated with an increased risk of **lymphoma**. People with this condition should be vigilant about other signs and symptoms.

Signs and Symptoms

- Pathologically dry eyes, poorly functioning tear ducts
- Dry salivary ducts
- Dry nasal passages
- Impaired vaginal secretion

Treatment Options

Sjögren syndrome is treated according to the symptoms. Eye drops, careful oral hygiene, and humidifiers can help make people with this disorder more comfortable.

Medications

If symptoms extend beyond the mucous membranes to affect the blood vessels or other tissues, immunosuppressant drugs may be used to interfere with this autoimmune disorder.

✋ Massage Considerations

Risks

- The risks of massage for a person with Sjögren syndrome are determined by what (if any) autoimmune disorders are also present; each of these disorders has impact on decisions about massage.
- Clients with very dry eyes may not be comfortable in a face cradle.

Benefits

- Massage has no specific benefits for clients with Sjögren syndrome.
- Clients with this condition who have no current symptoms can enjoy the same benefits from massage as the rest of the population.

---

skin cancer

Skin cancer is an umbrella term for four conditions that involve uncontrolled replication of cells in various layers of the skin.

Actinic Keratosis

Also called solar keratosis, actinic keratosis (AK) is a relatively benign condition, but it has the potential to become squamous cell carcinoma, which can be dangerous. It usually occurs on the head and face or on the hand, arms, and legs where exposure to sunlight has taken place.

Basal Cell Carcinoma

Basal cell carcinoma (BCC) is the most common type of skin cancer, accounting for about 75% to 90% of all skin cancer cases. It is a slow-growing, nonmetastasizing tumor of epithelial cells in the stratum basale of the epidermis. It is not usually dangerous, although if the tumor is left untreated, it can erode into vital tissues.

Squamous Cell Carcinoma

Squamous cell carcinoma (SCC) is a malignancy of keratinocytes in the epidermis. It sometimes begins as AK, but it can develop independently as well. SCC can metastasize and become life threatening.

Malignant Melanoma

Malignant melanoma (MM) is cancer of the melanocytes, the pigment-producing cells of the dermis. It is the most dangerous and least common of all types of skin cancer. It metastasizes readily, so it is treated aggressively when found early.

Signs and Symptoms

- Nonmelanoma skin cancer: a sore that doesn't heal or that comes and goes in the same location
- May resemble a wart, blister, scab, pimple
- Common patterns
    AK: pink or red scaly spots in areas with sun exposure
    BCC: "rodent ulcer" with a pink, pearly border or a large tumor on the face
    SCC: can look aggressive and painful; may occur inside the mouth
- Malignant melanoma: "ABCDE" pattern
    Asymmetrical
    Indistinct borders
    Colors are mixed
    Diameter is large
    Elevated or evolving

Treatment Options

Nonmelanoma lesions are usually removed with liquid nitrogen or other methods if they are found early. Because SCC is potentially metastatic, removal of the lesion(s) may be followed by radiation or chemotherapy.

Malignant melanoma is an aggressive form of cancer and is treated accordingly. Surgical excision, radiation, and chemotherapy may be incorporated into a treatment plan. Skin grafts may be necessary to replace damaged tissue.

Medications

Analgesics are given after removal of nonmalignant growths. Chemotherapy can be used treat aggressive SCC or MM.

Massage Considerations

Risks

- Clients who are being treated for SCC or MM may be undergoing any combination of surgery, radiation, or chemotherapy. These interventions all have implications that may make rigorous circulatory massage too intense for some clients to tolerate.
- Clients who have recently been treated for AK or BCC may have sores or incisions where growths were removed; these locally contraindicate massage.
- Undiagnosed skin lesions at least locally contraindicate massage until more information has been gathered about the condition.

Benefits

- Massage has no specific benefits for clients with any form of skin cancer.
- Clients with AK or BCC that has been identified and treated can enjoy the same benefits of massage as the rest of the population.
- Clients who are being treated for more aggressive forms of cancer may enjoy the pain relief, improved sleep, increased appetite, and other benefits that reflexive or energetic techniques may offer.

Practitioner Advice

- Massage therapists see more of their clients' skin than clients themselves may see. Therefore, practitioners are in a position to recommend that a client with a suspicious lesion consult a dermatologist sooner rather than later for best results.

sleep apnea: see sleep disorders

---

sleep disorders

Sleep disorders are any conditions that interfere with the ability to fall asleep, to stay asleep for an adequate period of time, or to wake up feeling refreshed.

Sleep is such a vital process that without the proper balance of stages, people can develop disorders that range from slowed reflexes and lower cognitive skills to poor immune system efficiency, **fibromyalgia**, chronic pain, **depression**, hallucinations, and psychosis. Patients with sleep disorders also have an increased risk of on-the-job injuries, infertility, **stroke**, **hypertension**, and **diabetes**.

More than 70 different sleep disorders have been defined; this discussion will cover four of them: insomnia, sleep apnea, narcolepsy, and circadian rhythm disruption.

Insomnia

Insomnia can involve difficulty falling asleep, difficulty staying asleep, or difficulty sleeping long enough for the body to get the rest it needs. Insomnia can be described as transient when it occurs for less than 4 weeks at a time or chronic when a person can't sleep most nights for a period of more than 1 month at a time.

Sleep Apnea

"Apnea" means absence of breath. Sleep apnea is a disorder in which the air passage of a sleeping person temporarily shuts down, depriving him or her of oxygen for several seconds. Repeated episodes may occur dozens or even hundreds of time each night, reducing the quality of sleep, but more importantly, putting the person at risk for damage from oxygen deprivation.

- Obstructive sleep apnea is a mechanical problem in which the air passage collapses when muscles relax during sleep so that oxygen cannot enter during inhalation. When O_2 levels decrease, the muscles tighten slightly, and air re-enters the passageway with a loud snort or gasp.
- Central sleep apnea is a neurologic problem involving decreased respiratory drive. In some extreme cases, central sleep apnea has caused sudden death from respiratory arrest during sleep.

Narcolepsy

This chronic neurological dysfunction gets its name from the Greek *narco* for stupor and *lepsis* for seizure. It involves unpredictable "sleep attacks" at inappropriate times, often in response to intense emotional reactions, such as laughing or anger.

During an episode, a narcolepsy patient may experience cataplexy, which is a sudden loss in all muscle tone. These events can last anywhere from several seconds to 30 minutes. Narcolepsy patients often experience poor nighttime sleep, which adds to a general problem with drowsiness during the day.

Circadian Rhythm Disruption

Circadian rhythm disruption can occur in response to changing work shifts, losing a night's sleep, or changing time zones through travel. Short-term difficulties associated with this problem are excessive sleepiness along with degenerating reflexes and mental functioning that accompany exhaustion. Longer-term problems can include depression and other physical and psychological disorders brought about by sleep deprivation.

Signs and Symptoms

- Excessive daytime sleepiness
- Irritability, mood swings
- Decreased ability to concentrate, short-term memory loss

Treatment Options

Sleep disorders are generally treated with lifestyle changes that better support healthy sleep. These include changes in diet and exercise habits, quitting smoking, adjusting temperature or sound levels in the bedroom, and other simple interventions.

Sleep apnea can be treated in a variety of ways. Surgery to keep the airways open may be conducted or a device to provide continuous positive airway pressure (CPAP) may be used. It is especially important that sleep apnea patients not drink alcohol or use sleeping aids at night because these substances may interfere with their already challenged breathing mechanisms.

Medications

Prescription and nonprescription sleep aids can help the patient in bridging from wakefulness to sleeping, but they can be habit forming and don't necessarily provide sleep in organized and sufficient cycles.

Massage Considerations

Risks

- Massage has no specific risks for clients with any form of sleep disorder.

Benefits

- Massage has been seen to increase the amount of time clients spend in stages III and IV of sleep; this is a remarkable benefit people who rarely feel rested.

Practitioner Advice

- Massage therapists may be the first to notice the leading sign of sleep apnea, a lack of breathing followed by a sudden gasp for air. It is important to bring this habit to the client's attention because it may indicate a serious problem with air passages or central nervous system respiratory drive.

social anxiety disorder: see anxiety disorders

solar keratosis: see skin cancer

sore throat: see pharyngitis

spasmodic torticollis: see torticollis

spasms, cramps

A spasm is an involuntary contraction of a muscle. Clonic spasms are marked by alternating cycles of contraction and relaxation, and tonic spasms are sustained periods of hypertonicity. The difference between spasms and cramps is somewhat arbitrary; cramps are strong, painful, usually short-lived spasms. So, one could say that tight, painful paraspinals are in spasm and a gastrocnemius with a charley horse is a cramp.

Several things can trigger involuntary muscle contractions. Contributing factors include nutritional imbalance, the pain–spasm–ischemia cycle, exercise-induced cramping, and the splinting mechanism that stabilizes traumatized joints.

The electrolyte imbalances that can occur with **hyperthermia** and dehydration make painful cramps a common occurrence at very demanding athletic events.

Signs and Symptoms
- Involuntary, painful contraction of skeletal muscle

Treatment Options

Acute cramping in athletes suggests dehydration and electrolyte imbalance. Replacing fluids is the highest priority. Chronic, repeating cramps in nonathletes may point toward a nutritional deficiency.

Long-term spasms are often treated with heat, stretching, and massage. The goals are to improve circulation and address the proprioceptive patterns in posture and movement that may cause the unnecessary tightness to develop in the first place.

Medications

Acute muscle spasms, especially in relation to injury, are sometimes treated with muscle relaxants.

Massage Considerations

Risks
- Inappropriate massage can exacerbate muscle cramps.
- Muscles that tighten around an injured area are acting as a splint to stabilize a precarious situation. Massage that prematurely interferes with this process can put the client at risk for further joint damage.

Benefits
- Proprioceptive techniques are often effective for acute cramps.
- Massage to decrease tension in chronically tight muscles is usually successful, with the caution that it is usually preferable to aim for small, incremental improvements in function

so the client can incorporate these changes and make appropriate adaptations to a changing range of motion.

spina bifida

Spina bifida (literally, "cleft spine") is a neural tube defect in which the vertebral arch fails to close completely over the spinal cord. This defect can be so subtle that it is only found through incidental radiographs, or it can be so severe that it the spinal canal is open at birth or the baby may not survive the birth process. Three classes of spina bifida have been identified: spina bifida occulta (SBO), spina bifida meningocele, and spina bifida myelomeningocele.

In SBO, the vertebral arch doesn't completely fuse, but no signs or symptoms are obvious. Some people with SBO have a small dimple, birthmark, or tuft of hair on the spine at the location of the abnormality but no loss of function.

In spina bifida meningocele, the dura mater and arachnoid layers of the meninges press through at the site of the vertebral cleft, forming a cyst that is visible at birth. It is easily repairable with surgery and generally has little or no long-term consequences for the baby.

In spina bifida myelomeningocele, the spinal cord or extensions of the cauda equina protrude along with the meninges through several incompletely formed vertebral arches. Occasionally, the skin doesn't cover the protrusion, increasing the risk of serious central nervous system infection without immediate intervention.

Spina bifida is a complex disorder with several possible complications. Spinal cord damage leads to various levels of **paralysis**. Hydrocephalus is a common issue after a cyst has been reduced. This is usually dealt with by the insertion of a shunt that drains cerebrospinal fluid from the brain, down the neck, and into the abdominal cavity.

Although most children with spina bifida have normal intelligence, many of them experience mild to severe learning disabilities that may make it difficult to function in a mainstream classroom situation. Many spina bifida patients develop very severe **allergic reactions** to latex, which can lead to **anaphylaxis**. Other common complications include **decubitus ulcers**, digestive tract problems, **obesity**, and muscle imbalances that can lead to severe **postural deviations**.

Signs and Symptoms

- The symptoms of spina bifida are determined by how big the cleft is and whether material bulges through it. Specific descriptions are above.

Treatment Options

A baby born with cystic spina bifida needs to undergo surgery within a few days to reduce the cyst and preserve as much spinal cord function as possible. Afterwards, even tiny babies are supported with rigorous physical therapy and exercises to maintain function in the leg muscles as much as possible. As children mature and their functional levels become clear, they can learn to use crutches, braces, wheelchairs, or other equipment as necessary.

Many spina bifida patients undergo multiple surgeries, not only to reduce the protruding cyst but also to correct a "tethered cord" in which the spinal cord doesn't slide freely within the spinal canal, to deal with the complications of hydrocephalus, and to address whatever complications may be brought about by severe scoliosis or hyperkyphosis.

Medications

Medications for people with spina bifida are typically related to recovery from surgery or assistance with bladder and bowel control.

Massage Considerations

Risks

- Spina bifida has many serious possible complications that have implications for massage. Massage therapists must work with the rest of the health care team to achieve best results in the context of a high risk of infections along with muscle contractures and postural deviations.
- Massage where sensation is impaired or altogether missing must be conducted conservatively to avoid inadvertently damaging tissue.
- Massage for clients with shunts to drain cerebrospinal fluid must be conducted with care around the neck and head to preserve the equipment's function.

Benefits

- If a client with spina bifida is physically active, free of contraindicating complications, and has good sensation, massage can be a safe and useful adjunct to the other types of therapy he or she uses to achieve the best possible function.

spinal cord injury

Spinal cord injury (SCI) is damage to some percentage of nerve tissue in the spinal canal. Spinal cord injuries fall into three categories: concussions, in which tissue is jarred and irritated but not structurally damaged; incomplete injuries, in which only some of the neuron tracts in the spinal cord have been damaged; and complete injuries, in which all of the ascending and descending tracts have been interrupted at a specific level or levels.

When a SCI is new, the affected muscles may be hypotonic. As the inflammatory process subsides, the muscles supplied by damaged axons begin to tighten, and their reflexes become hyperreactive. Spasticity along with hyperreflexia is a hallmark of SCI. If the muscles stay flaccid and the reflexes are dull or nonexistent, the damage is probably to the nerve roots rather than to the spinal cord itself. Injuries to the low back often show this pattern because the spinal canal is occupied by the cauda equina nerve extensions from T12 down to the sacrum. Depending on the nature of the accident, it is possible to simultaneously sustain injury to both the spinal cord and the nerve roots.

SCI survivors are vulnerable to a number of serious complications, including **paralysis, decubitus ulcers**, heterotopic ossification (**myositis ossificans**), **deep vein thrombosis, pulmonary embolism, pneumonia, urinary tract infection, atherosclerosis** and other cardio-vascular diseases, autonomic hyperreflexia, spasticity, contractures, numbness, and pain.

Signs and Symptoms

- Motor and sensory impairment that indicates what level and part of the spinal cord has been damaged
    Anterior SCIs affect motor function.
    Posterior SCIs affect touch, proprioception, and vibration.
    Lateral SCIs affect pain and temperature sensation.

Treatment Options

When nerve tissue is directly compressed, emergency surgery to relieve the pressure is indicated.

Some later treatments for SCI include the implantation of electrodes in muscles that are controlled from an external computer or surgically extending the nearby tendons to do the work of muscles that are no longer innervated.

Long-term treatment for SCI survivors is designed to provide them with the skills they need to live as fully as possible. This includes work with physical and occupational therapists, as well as other specialists.

Medications

A critically important early intervention in SCI is the administration of powerful anti-inflammatory drugs that can help limit damage to the spinal cord.

Long-term SCI survivors may use prophylactic antibiotics to reduce the risk of pneumonia or urinary tract infections, anticoagulants to reduce the risk of deep vein thrombosis, and other medications to manage the complications of their condition.

Massage Considerations

Risks

- The complications related to SCI are serious, and most have implications for massage therapy; these must inform decisions about bodywork, but they don't necessarily rule it out.

Benefits

- Massage has many benefits to offer SCI survivors as long as other complications have been addressed.

    Massage can help keep functioning tissues elastic and mobile.

    Massage can help retrain the proprioceptors to help maintain or improve range of motion.

    Massage can improve the quality of life for clients who may often feel separated and isolated by the nature of their condition.

spondylolisthesis

Spondylolisthesis is a situation in which a vertebral body slips anteriorly. It happens most frequently at the L5–S1 connection. Spondylolysis, a related condition, is the development of stress fractures at the vertebral arch in lumbar vertebrae. This condition may be a precursor to spondylolisthesis. Arthritis at the spine, called **spondylosis**, is also part of the picture of bony distortion, poor alignment, and the risk of spinal cord or nerve root pressure.

Signs and Symptoms

- May be silent
- Low back pain
- Muscle spasms in the paraspinals, hip stabilizers
- Aggravated by spinal extension; relieved by spinal flexion

Treatment Options

Most cases of spondylolisthesis are treated with modified activity and physical therapy. If pressure is consistently exerted against the nerve roots or spinal cord, surgery to realign and fuse the spine may be recommended.

Medications

Nonsteroidal anti-inflammatory drugs are often used for their analgesic effects.

Massage Considerations

Risks
- Massage may exacerbate the pain associated with spondylolisthesis if the client is positioned in a way that emphasizes low back extension.

Benefits
- Massage doesn't correct the deep alignment problems that lead to spondylolisthesis, but it may address the secondary low back pain and holding patterns of other nearby muscles that influence function in the low back.

spondylosis

Spondylosis is **osteoarthritis** specifically in the spine, although it may also refer to stenosis or narrowing of the spinal canal. It usually develops in the lumbar and cervical regions, which are the most mobile areas. Bony remodeling of the vertebral bodies and joints leads to inflammation of surrounding tissues and restricted range of motion. Several factors may contribute to the process, including **disc disease** and chronic misalignment.

Spondylosis has some serious consequences. Hypermobility may develop in areas of the spine to compensate for the loss of movement in the affected area. Bone spurs may grow to put pressure on nerve tissue at the spinal canal or intervertebral foramina. Osteophytes may also put pressure on the vertebral arteries, which travel through the transverse foramina of the cervical vertebrae.

Signs and Symptoms
- May be completely silent
- Often a slow, painless loss of range of motion at the spine
- With nerve pressure from osteophytes: shooting electrical pain in a predictable pattern
- With lumbar involvement: low back and leg pain that is aggravated by standing and relieved by sitting or forward bending

Treatment Options

Treatment for spondylosis depends on which (if any) complications are present. Stretching and exercise can limit the progression after the damage has begun. If these interventions are insufficient, a variety of surgical procedures can create more space for nerve roots or the spinal cord.

Medications

Spondylosis is typically treated with nonsteroidal anti-inflammatory drugs for pain relief.

 Massage Considerations

Risks
- If inflammation is very acute, massage could exacerbate the symptoms of spondylosis.
- If bone spurs are present, the massage therapist must not position the client's head or neck in a way that puts pressure on nerves or blood vessels.
- Muscles in the neck may be hypertonic in an attempt to stabilize weakened joints. Massage that interferes with this process too rapidly may increase rather than decrease the risk of injury.

Benefits
- Massage that aims to carefully and incrementally loosen tight muscles in the neck or low back may help decrease pain and increase the range of motion for people with spondylosis.

sprains

Sprains are tears to ligaments, which are the connective tissue "strapping tape" that links bone to bone throughout the body. The severity of the injury depends on what percentage of the fibers is affected. First-degree sprains involve just a few fibers; second-degree injuries are much worse; and third-degree sprains are ruptures, meaning that the entire ligament has been ripped through and no longer attaches to the bone.

Sprains, **strains**, and **tendinopathies** are all tears of linearly arranged fibers. Sometimes it can be challenging to differentiate between these injuries, especially because several structures may be injured with any given trauma. Sprains tend to swell more than other tears, however, and are more painful on passive movement. Muscle and tendon injuries hurt more with active or resisted movement.

Sprains that don't heal well may develop masses of constrictive scar tissue, or the injured ligaments may elongate, which makes the joint unstable. This increases the risk of **osteoarthritis** because the affected joints have too much mobility.

Sprains of the anterior talofibular ligament (the most commonly sprained ligament in the body) can sometimes hide the signs of bone **fractures** in the foot. A sprained ankle that doesn't have significant improvement within a few days should be tested for bone damage.

Signs and Symptoms
- Acute stage: pain, heat, redness, pronounced swelling
- Exacerbation of pain with passive stretching
- Subacute stage: pain persists; swelling subsides

Treatment Options

RICE (rest, ice, compression, elevation) therapy is the best option for most sprains, with an emphasis on moving the joint and putting weight on it within pain tolerance as soon as possible. This reduces inflammation and supports the formation of the healthiest possible scar tissue.

Medications

A person with an acute sprain may use nonsteroidal anti-inflammatory drugs for pain relief.

🖐 Massage Considerations

Risks
- Acute sprains locally contraindicate massage that interferes with the process of producing and laying down new scar tissue.

Benefits
- Lymphatic techniques may help control the inflammation associated with an acute sprain.
- In the subacute or maturation phase of healing, massage can reduce adhesions and influence the direction of new collagen fibers. It can be an important intervention in the development of healthy, functional scar tissue.

- Clients who have fully recovered from a sprain with no lingering pain or dysfunction can enjoy the same benefits from massage as the rest of the population.

squamous cell carcinoma: see skin cancer

stomach cancer

Stomach cancer is the development of malignant tumors in the stomach. These tumors can block the passage of food through the digestive system, and they can spread to other organs, either through cells flaking off into the peritoneal space or through blood and lymph flow.

One of the risk factors for stomach cancer is the presence of *Helicobacter pylori* bacteria. These pathogens are also associated with **ulcers**.

Signs and Symptoms

- Feeling of fullness without significant food intake
- Vague abdominal pain, often above the navel
- Unintended weight loss
- Heartburn, ulcer symptoms
- Nausea, vomiting
- Ascites (excessive fluid in the peritoneal cavity)

Treatment Options

Stomach cancer is treated with chemotherapy, radiation, and surgery. Because it is not usually found in the early stages, many stomach cancer patients undergo combinations of therapies in an attempt to limit the spread of the cancer through the rest of the body.

Medications

Stomach cancer patients often use chemotherapy in their treatment process.

Massage Considerations

Risks

- As with many other types of cancer, the risk of massage for stomach cancer has more to do with cancer treatment than the cancer itself. Risks include the risk of postoperative infection, impaired immunity, and other side effects of chemotherapy and radiation.

Benefits

- Stomach cancer patients can enjoy the same benefits from gentle massage as other cancer patients, including a reinforced parasympathetic state, improved sleep, decreased pain perception, and immune system support during an especially challenging time.

strains

Strains involve injury to the muscle–tendon unit, with an emphasis on muscle tissue. Strains can be related to specific trauma, but they appear more often in the context of chronic, cumulative overuse patterns with no specific onset.

Strains are closely related to **tendinopathies** and **sprains**; the terms simply refer to which linear structure is injured.

Signs and Symptoms
- Mild or intense local pain; muscle stiffness
- Pain is worse with resisted movement or passive stretching of the muscle

Treatment Options
Muscle strains are most successfully treated by limiting inflammation followed by careful rehabilitation exercises. It is important to do just enough exercise to promote the formation of healthy scar tissue. Too much weight-bearing stress can reinjure a muscle; too little can allow scar tissue to stay dense and disorganized.

Medications
Nonsteroidal anti-inflammatory drugs are often used for pain relief.

Massage Considerations
Risks
- Acute injuries and inflammation locally contraindicate deep massage.
- Otherwise, massage has no specific risks for clients with muscle strains.

Benefits
- Lymphatic techniques can be used in the acute phase of a muscle strain to limit inflammation and promote the formation of healthy scar tissue.
- In the subacute or maturation phase, cross-fiber and linear friction and careful stretching can influence the way old scar tissue matures and new scar tissue lays down.

strep throat: see pharyngitis, rheumatic fever

stroke

Stroke, also called brain attack or cerebrovascular accident (CVA), is damage to the brain caused by oxygen deprivation. Strokes can be ischemic or hemorrhagic.

Two types of ischemic strokes are cerebral **thrombosis** (a clot develops in a cerebral artery and starves off nerve cells) and **embolism** (a clot travels from the heart or carotid arteries and lodges in the brain).

Ischemic strokes are closely related to another phenomenon, transient ischemic attacks (TIAs). In a TIA, a very tiny blood clot creates a temporary blockage in the brain, but it quickly disperses before any lasting damage occurs. Symptoms of TIAs are very similar to those of stroke except that they last only a few minutes or hours. They are, however, an important warning sign that a larger stroke may be imminent.

Ischemic strokes are closely linked to cardiovascular disease and the tendency to form blood clots that may break free and travel in the arteries. Arrhythmia, **atherosclerosis**, **hypertension**, and undertreated **diabetes** mellitus are all risk factors for ischemic stroke.

Two types of hemorrhagic stroke are cerebral hemorrhage (an **aneurysm** ruptures inside the brain) and subarachnoid hemorrhage (a vessel ruptures on the surface of the brain, filling the space between the brain and the cranium).

The amount of damage a stroke causes is determined primarily by the location and amount of tissue that is damaged by oxygen deprivation. Secondary responses to tissue damage, including inflammation, free radical activity, and other factors, can cause tissue damage that far exceeds the oxygen deprivation brought about by the stroke itself.

Signs and Symptoms

- During the initial event

   Sudden onset of unilateral weakness; any combination of numbness or paralysis of the face, arm, or leg

   Suddenly blurred or decreased vision in one or both eyes; asymmetrical dilation of the pupils

   Difficulty speaking or understanding simple sentences; confusion

   Sudden onset of dizziness, clumsiness, vertigo

   Sudden, very extreme headache

   Possible loss of consciousness
- Later signs and symptoms

   Partial or full paralysis of one side of the body (hemiplegia)

   Aphasia (loss of language)

   Memory loss

   Personality changes

   Sensory changes, including numbness, vision loss

Treatment Options

Ischemic strokes are treated with medication as quickly as possible. If the stroke is from a hemorrhage, however, thrombolytic treatment could be dangerous or even deadly. A brain aneurysm caught before it ruptures may be treated with surgery to take the pressure off or strengthen the affected artery.

After the initial trauma subsides, the stroke survivor must work to recover lost function. This needs to be started as quickly as possible to forestall atrophy and contractures of disused muscles. Physical, occupational, and speech therapy may all contribute to this process.

Medications

The immediate treatment of choice for ischemic stroke is anticoagulant medication to minimize the risk of more clotting. Severe brain damage may be averted if the anticoagulants and anti-inflammatory drugs are administered within a few hours of the stroke.

✋ Massage Considerations

Risks

- Stroke patients may have other cardiovascular weaknesses that influence decisions about massage.
- Massage around the carotid artery must be very conservative for clients with a risk of atherosclerosis in this area.
- Numbness contraindicates rigorous massage that may do damage without eliciting a pain response from the client.

Benefits

- Massage can be a useful tool for patients working to regain motor control of one side the body. Even muscles that have not been affected by nerve damage may degenerate if they are not stretched or exercised. Massage therapists can work with physical or other therapists to help clients regain the best possible use of their bodies.

sty: see folliculitis

superior vena cava syndrome

Superior vena cava syndrome (SVCS) is a situation in which the superior vena cava is compressed or even fully obstructed before it empties into the right atrium.

The vena cava is a thin-walled soft vessel with low blood pressure. This puts it at risk for compression from other nearby more rigid structures, such as the aorta or tumors. Obstruction of the superior vena cava can be entirely from outside the vessel (as with a tumor) or can be a combination of external pressure with thrombosis inside the vena cava itself.

When it was first documented in the 18th century, the most common causes for SVCS were **syphilis**-related aneurysms and **tuberculosis**. Now SVCS is usually related to pressure exerted by **lung cancer** tumors, lymph nodes enlarged with non-Hodgkin **lymphoma**, or an **aneurysm** in the aortic arch. Blood clots triggered by venous catheters or pacemaker wires account for a smaller number of SVCS cases.

Signs and Symptoms

- Dyspnea (shortness of breath), coughing, hoarseness
- Swelling of the face
- Distension of the neck veins
- Edema of the upper extremities and trunk
- Nausea, lightheadedness

Treatment Options

Treatment for SVCS depends on the underlying disease. Most cases occur in people with terminal lung cancer, and treating SVCS in these patients is a comfort issue. In some cases, surgery to create a bypass or to insert a stent may be conducted; this is usually done only when cancer is not the cause of the problem.

Medications

Medications for SVCS include diuretics to help with edema, chemotherapy to reduce compressing tumors, and thrombolytics to destroy any clots that might be blocking the vessel.

Massage Considerations

Risks

- SVCS indicates a serious problem or a medical emergency; massage is contraindicated until the problem has been addressed.

Benefits

- Massage has no specific benefits to for clients with SVCS.
- Clients with this disorder can enjoy the comfort and support that comes with gentle, nurturing, educated touch during a time of great stress and challenge.
- Clients who have fully recovered from SVCS and its underlying causes can enjoy the same benefits from massage as the rest of the population.

surgery: see bariatric surgery, joint replacement surgery, postoperative conditions

sycosis barbae: see folliculitis

syphilis

Syphilis is a sexually transmitted infection with a spirochetal bacterium called *Treponema pallidum*. It spreads through sexual contact and from mother to fetus. This bacterium is very fragile outside a host and does not last when exposed to air or sunlight.

Syphilis moves through the system in three specific stages. It is communicable only in the first two stages of infection. In the late stage, although it may cause very serious problems in the infected person, it is no longer contagious.

Similar to other bacterial sexually transmitted infections, syphilis significantly increases the transmission rate of **HIV**. Babies born with syphilis may not have symptoms immediately, but they may develop vision or central nervous system (CNS) problems along with syphilitic rhinitis; their respiratory secretions are highly contagious.

Signs and Symptoms

- Primary syphilis: chancre (open ulcer) appears 10 days to 3 months after exposure
- Secondary syphilis: open, brownish sores on the palms or soles appear several weeks after chancre heals; lesions come and go, and lesions can spread infection
- Tertiary syphilis: bacteria invade other systems, resulting in:
  Bones and joints: rheumatic pain
  Blood vessels: risk of aneurysm
  CNS: blindness, deafness, stroke, meningitis, psychosis

Treatment Options

Syphilis is treated with medication.

Medications

Syphilis is treatable with a single dose of penicillin. Treatment must be administered before organ damage takes place, however. Syphilitic damage to the CNS, blood vessels, and other structures is irreversible.

Massage Considerations

Risks

- Open syphilis lesions are contagious without sexual activity; these contraindicate and skin-to-skin contact.
- Tertiary syphilis is no longer contagious, but it can involve damaged blood vessels, joints, and nerve tissue; all of these also hold cautions for massage.

Benefits

- Massage has no specific benefits for clients with untreated syphilis.
- Clients who have completely recovered from a syphilis infection can enjoy the same benefits from massage as the rest of the population.

T

temporal arteritis: see vasculitis

temporomandibular joint disorders

Temporomandibular joint (TMJ) disorders are a collection of signs and symptoms indicating problems with function at the jaw.

The jaw is capable of exerting tremendous biting force. At the same time, its range of motion is extensive for a joint of its size. The mandible can elevate, depress, protract, retract, and move sideways. A fibrocartilage disc cushions the temporal bone and the condyle of the mandible, but this disc is sometimes pulled awry or injured, which can lead to problems in the joint. Also, the lateral pterygoid muscle that attaches directly to the fibrocartilage constantly pulls on the disc, acting as a high-tension spring. This makes the lateral pterygoid especially prone to **myofascial pain syndrome** trigger points, which can both mimic and precipitate TMJ problems.

In many cases, it is clear that TMJ disorders begin with a specific trauma such as a fall, a motor vehicle accident, or another episode. But in many cases, the factors that contribute to TMJ problems (especially bruxism, or grinding teeth) can also be the symptoms. Other contributors include misalignment of the bite and congenital malformations of the bones.

Several other problems, including **sprain** of a nearby ligament (Ernest syndrome), **trigeminal neuralgia**, occipital neuralgia, and **osteomyelitis**, have symptoms similar to the symptoms of TMJ disorders. TMJ disorders that result in damage to the cartilage and bone can be classified as a type of **osteoarthritis**, which is the culmination of wear-and-tear on the joint structures.

Signs and Symptoms

- Jaw, neck, shoulder pain
- Limited range of motion at the jaw
- Jaw popping and locking
- Bruxism (during waking and sleeping)
- Ear pain
- Headaches
- Subluxation of the cervical vertebrae

Treatment Options

Treatment for TMJ disorder is divided into nonsurgical and surgical options. Nonsurgical interventions include hydrotherapy, physical therapy, ultrasonography and massage for the jaw muscles, and jaw splints. If these noninvasive techniques are successful, the TMJ disorder may be averted before permanent bony distortion or cartilage damage inside the joint occurs.

Surgical options range from an outpatient procedure in which scar tissue and adhesions are dissolved by injections into the joint, to arthroscopic surgery to manipulate the cartilage, to full prosthetic joint replacement.

Medications

Medical interventions for TMJ disorders include anti-inflammatory drugs and injections of local anesthetics.

Massage Considerations

Risks

- Massage has no specific risks for TMJ disorders unless the therapist inadvertently aggravates the client's symptoms by working too aggressively.

Benefits

- TMJ disorders indicate massage that can address the jaw flexors.
- Massage can help increase the client's awareness of bruxism, resetting the proprioceptors in the jaw muscles.
- Massage can also help resolve trigger points and the referred pain patterns that can be a significant source of pain with this condition.

Practitioner Advice

- Some local massage ordinances may prohibit working with the intraoral muscles; this question should be answered before the therapist works with the lateral pterygoid muscles.

tendinitis: see tendinopathies

tendinopathies

Tendinopathy is a general term that refers to injury, inflammation, and poor healing in tendinous tissues.

Tendon tears happen most frequently at the tenoperiosteal junction or the musculotendinous junction, the points of transition between tissue types. Similar to other musculoskeletal injuries, tendon tears may be rated by severity: first degree for mild tears, second degree for moderate tears, and third degree for full ruptures.

Various forms of tendinopathies include tendinitis, tendinosis, and **tenosynovitis**. Tendinitis is a situation with an acutely inflamed tendon. Tendinosis refers to a tendon injury that healed poorly and is consequently weak; this appears to be the situation with many long-term, stubborn injuries. And tenosynovitis can involve weakened tendons with irritation at the tenosynovial sheath.

Tendinopathies can be difficult to differentiate from muscle **strains** or **sprains**. Furthermore, most injuries involve damage to multiple structures, so strains, sprains, and tendon damage may occur simultaneously. It is important to get the clearest picture possible about these injuries to design the best treatment protocols.

Signs and Symptoms

- Acute tendinitis: pain, heat, swelling
- Subacute or postacute tendinosis: pain on resisted movement or passive stretching; weakness

Treatment Options

New tendon injuries are typically treated with RICE (rest, ice, compression, elevation) therapy.

As the healing process progresses, friction, stretching, and carefully gauged exercise are excellent options for helping injured tendons heal with a minimum of adhesive scar tissue residue.

Medications

Nonsteroidal anti-inflammatory drugs may be recommended for short-term pain relief with a new tendon injury.

 Massage Considerations

Risks

- An acute, new tendon injury contraindicates rigorous massage that might increase swelling and disrupt the healing process.
- Massage has no specific risks for subacute or postacute tendinopathies.

Benefits

- New injuries may respond well to lymphatic techniques that limit inflammation and promote organized healing.
- Older injuries benefit from friction along with stretching and careful exercise to help speed healing, reduce scar tissue adhesions, and improve the quality of the repaired tissue.

---

tenosynovitis

Tenosynovitis is a situation in which the tendons that pass through a lubricating synovial sheath become irritated and possibly inflamed.

Repetitive stress, percussive movement, or constant twisting can cause the tendons inside tenosynovial sheaths to become irritated. The sheath may become inflamed and then shrink around the tendons in such a way that it inhibits freedom of movement.

Tenosynovitis is usually triggered by trauma, repetitive movement, or excessive exercise. It can happen anywhere synovial sheaths protect tendons, including the wrist, ankle, long head of the biceps, or near the thumb (where it is called de Quervain tenosynovitis).

Occasionally, tenosynovitis can be caused by a local infection that inflames the synovium or may be a complication of other inflammatory wrist problems, such as **rheumatoid arthritis** or **fractures**.

Signs and Symptoms

- Local pain, especially with movement
- Swelling and heat in extreme cases
- Flexion is easier than extension
- Crepitus: grinding sensation as the tendons move through the sheath

Treatment Options

If time and medications don't solve the problem of tenosynovitis, the synovium may be surgically split to make more room for the tendons to pass through.

Medications

Tenosynovitis caused by a bacterial infection is treated with antibiotics. Noninfectious tenosynovitis is typically treated with anti-inflammatory drugs and then steroid injections if necessary.

 Massage Considerations

Risks

- Tenosynovitis locally contraindicates massage when it is acutely painful.

Benefits
- When infection is not the cause, lymphatic techniques during acute inflammation may help limit swelling and promote a faster, more efficient healing process.
- When tenosynovial inflammation is not acute, massage can help create very specific movements of structures against each other to prevent the accumulation of scar tissue and adhesions.

testicular cancer

Testicular cancer is the growth of malignant cells in the testicles. These cells usually grow slowly, but they may metastasize through the lymph or blood systems.

Testicular cancer is typically divided into germ cell tumors and stromal cell tumors. Germ cell tumors are by far more common. They include seminomas, which grow slowly and are highly sensitive to radiation, and nonseminomas, which can be more aggressive and resistant to treatment.

Signs and Symptoms
- Painless lump on the testicle
- Sense of fullness or heaviness in the scrotum
- Dull ache in the lower abdomen or groin
- Possible enlargement or tenderness of breast tissue

Treatment Options

Treatment for testicular cancer begins with surgery to remove the affected testicle and any secondary tumors that might be found. If the cancer is identified as a seminoma, radiation therapy is done after surgery.

For mixed tumors and nonseminomas, chemotherapy may be given after surgery.

Follow-up care after testicular cancer treatment is critical to make sure no metastases have been missed. Furthermore, testicular cancer survivors have a small but significant risk of developing cancer in the other testicle.

Medications

Chemotherapy is used for mixed or nonseminoma testicular tumors.

✋ Massage Considerations

Risks
- The risks of massage for testicular cancer patients are tied to the treatments they are using. Surgery, chemotherapy, and radiation all carry cautions for massage, including the possibility of infection, bone thinning, skin damage, and other side effects.

Benefits
- With appropriate accommodations for client resilience, massage may improve the tolerance for cancer treatments by improving sleep and appetite, decreasing pain and anxiety, and generally supporting the healing process.
- Clients with a history of testicular cancer who are currently cancer free can enjoy the same benefits from massage as the rest of the population.

thalassemia

Thalassemia is a group of genetic disorders that lead to the production of inadequate or poorly functioning hemoglobin. Two parental genes must be present for a person to have this disorder; inheritance of only one gene results in thalassemia trait but not the disease.

When hemoglobin is not produced correctly or in adequate amounts, red blood cells (RBCs) cannot carry sufficient oxygen, and they tend to die earlier than normal RBCs. Both of these issues contribute to **anemia,** which is often the earliest sign of thalassemia. Without treatment, a person with thalassemia major experiences damage to the spleen, liver, and ultimately the heart. Children with untreated thalassemia major usually die of **heart failure** or infection before adolescence.

Several types of thalassemia have been named. Thalassemia alpha refers to problems with the production of alpha hemoglobin; thalassemia beta refers to production of beta hemoglobin. These disorders are also classified by severity as thalassemia major, intermediate, and minor.

Thalassemia has much in common with **sickle cell disease;** both are genetic disorders that must be inherited from both parents and both involve the formation of poor-quality hemoglobin and premature RBC destruction.

Signs and Symptoms

- Mild cases may be silent
- Intermediate and major versions present symptoms by age 2 years
    Anemia, pallor, fatigue
    Failure to grow
    Jaundice
- Later signs and complications
    Enlarged spleen
    Enlarged liver
    Enlarged heart, heart failure
    Thin, brittle bones, especially in the legs and hands

Treatment Options

Thalassemia is treated with repeated blood transfusions (every 3 to 4 weeks for some patients) that keep hemoglobin levels as close to normal as possible.

Medications

Frequent transfusions increase the risk of iron overload, which can damage the heart and liver. Iron-chelating drugs can bind with excess iron and extract it from the body. Prophylactic antibiotics are often also prescribed for children with thalassemia to make up for the early loss of splenic function.

🖑 Massage Considerations

Risks

- Thalassemia can range from subtle to severe. Severe versions of thalassemia can involve the loss of spleen function and heart failure; both of these conditions carry cautions for massage therapy.

Benefits
- Clients with milder versions of thalassemia may benefit from bodywork sessions that are designed to stay within their ability to adapt to the changes that massage brings about.

thoracic outlet syndrome

Thoracic outlet syndrome (TOS) is an entrapment of brachial plexus nerves, blood vessels (the subclavian and axillary veins or arteries), or both at the thoracic outlet (the area behind the clavicle between the insertions of the trapezius and sternocleidomastoid muscles).

The classic version of thoracic outlet involves a collapsed posture with muscular imbalances between tight or atrophied scalenes and pectoralis minor and stretched and irritated upper back muscles (rhomboids, serratus posterior superior, trapezius). This allows the neck to jut forward and the shoulders to roll anteriorly. Bone and muscle can mechanically compress the nerves and blood vessels, leading to TOS symptoms.

Part of getting a useful evaluation of TOS involves assessing the site or sites of impingement. Some confusing conditions (that can certainly occur alongside true TOS) include cervical misalignment, **disc disease**, **double crush syndrome**, irritated spinal ligaments, cervical ribs, **spondylosis** with bone spurs in the neck, rib misalignment, rotator cuff **tendinopathy**, **impingement syndrome** at the shoulder, **carpal tunnel syndrome**, and other wrist injuries.

Signs and Symptoms
- Nerve symptoms: shooting pain, numbness, loss of sensation, weakness, tingling, paresthesia
- Vascular symptoms: feeling of fullness, coldness, difference in coloration and temperature
- Symptoms are exacerbated by sleeping on the affected side or lifting the affected arm over the head

Treatment Options

The treatment for TOS depends on the cause and location of the impingement. TOS caused by muscle atrophy or tightness responds best to strengthening exercises and stretching. A small percentage of TOS patients are good candidates for surgery, which has the goal of releasing pressure on the affected nerves. This can mean the removal of a cervical rib or resectioning of the first rib.

Medications

TOS is not typically treated with medication.

Massage Considerations

Risks
- Any technique that causes nerve sensations in the arm contraindicates massage.
- Clients with TOS must be positioned in a way that doesn't exacerbate their symptoms.

Benefits
- If TOS is related to muscular imbalance, massage can be an important tool to create better balance between anterior and posterior muscular tension and to increase the client's awareness of his or her postural and movement patterns.

- If TOS is related to issues that massage cannot affect, the muscular impact of careful stretching and bodywork may offer some temporary relief but won't necessarily have long-term benefits.

thrombophlebitis, deep vein thrombosis

Thrombophlebitis and deep vein thrombosis (DVT) refer to inflammation of a vein caused by clots. These clots can form anywhere in the venous system, but they develop most often in the calves, thighs, and pelvis. Thrombophlebitis is a term used for clots in superficial leg veins (lesser and greater saphenous), and DVT develops in deeper leg veins, specifically the popliteal, femoral, and iliac veins.

DVT and thrombophlebitis can develop in any circumstance that involves venous stasis (slowed movement of venous blood), increased coagulability, or blood vessel damage. Physical trauma, **varicose veins**, local infections, physical restriction (tight knee braces or socks), immobility, **pregnancy**, some blood diseases, recent surgery, and high estrogen birth control pills can all contribute to this risk.

Of the two conditions, DVT is by far the most dangerous. Clots that form in the superficial vessels tend to be smaller (because the vessels themselves are smaller), and they tend to melt more readily; both of these features make thrombophlebitis much less threatening than DVT.

If a clot in a deep vein breaks or becomes dislodged (often because of sudden movement after a period of immobility), fragments flow through the bloodstream until they are caught in vessels that get smaller in diameter leading to the lungs. DVT is a predisposing factor for a potentially deadly pulmonary **embolism**.

Signs and Symptoms

- May be silent or subtle
- Pain, heat, redness, swelling may be present
- Possible pitting edema
- Deep, aching pain
- Flaking, discoloration, skin ulcers

Treatment Options

Thrombophlebitis and DVT are typically treated with medication. If the patient is bedridden, he or she may be given pneumatic compression in which a machine mimics the pumping action of exercise by inflating and deflating a tubular balloon around the affected leg. Support hose to prevent the accumulation of postoperative edema are also recommended.

Self-care measures for thrombophlebitis, such as hot packs, analgesics, and gentle exercise, may be recommended to resolve episodes of vein inflammation.

Some patients may have a filter implanted in the vena cava to prevent clots from reaching the lungs.

Medications

The treatment for both thrombophlebitis and DVT is anticoagulant medication.

 Massage Considerations

Risks

- DVT carries very significant risks for massage. It may be silent or have only subtle symptoms, and mechanical disruption (e.g., with a vigorous pétrissage to the calf) may trigger the release of a clot that could cause a life-threatening pulmonary embolism.

- Thrombophlebitis tends to involve smaller clots and a lower risk of pulmonary embolism, but massage therapists are well advised to avoid this risk whenever possible.
- Clients with a history of blood clots may be taking anticoagulant medications. It is important to bear in mind that these drugs increase the risk of bruising.

Benefits
- Massage has no specific benefits for clients with thrombophlebitis or DVT; these conditions require immediate attention and should be cleared up before a client receives any but the lightest possible bodywork.
- Clients who have a history of thrombophlebitis or DVT but no current risks can enjoy the same benefits from massage as the rest of the population.

thrombosis: see embolism, thrombus, thrombophlebitis

thrush: see candidiasis

thyroid cancer

Thyroid cancer is the development of malignant cells in the thyroid gland (either the cells that make thyroid hormone or the cells that manufacture calcitonin mutate and multiply). It is distinguished from thyroid nodules and cysts by the tendency for the cancerous cells to spread into other tissues, usually through the lymph system.

Several types of thyroid cancer have been identified, including papillary carcinoma, follicular carcinoma, anaplastic thyroid cancer, and medullary thyroid cancer. These range from slow-growing, easily treatable forms to aggressive types that can metastasize before palpable tumors develop.

Although it is unclear why some people develop thyroid cancer, a number of risk factors have been found in many patients. These include a history of exposure to radiation from nuclear fallout, nuclear accidents, or childhood radiation treatment for adenoids and **acne**; an insufficient amount of iodine in the diet; and an inherited genetic predisposition for medullary thyroid cancer.

Signs and Symptoms
- Palpable lump in the throat
- Dysphagia (difficulty swallowing)
- Hoarseness, chronic cough
- Dyspnea (shortness of breath)
- Enlarged lymph nodes in the neck

Treatment Options
Treatment for thyroid cancer depends on what type is present and how far it has progressed. Surgery to remove the affected parts of the thyroid is a common intervention. Late-stage thyroid cancer may be treated with external-beam radiation to the specific growth areas.

Medications
Some types of thyroid cancer are treated with doses of radioactive iodine, which can kill off tumor cells. Chemotherapy is suggested to access cancer cells that have invaded the lymph system.

All thyroid cancer treatments are then followed by a lifetime commitment to replacing the thyroid hormones, which are vital to regulate the metabolism of fuel and calcium.

 ## Massage Considerations

Risks
- The risks of massage for thyroid cancer patients are the same as with other types of cancer; they are related to side effects of cancer treatment, including infection; poor immunity; and in the case of thyroid cancer, a particularly high risk of skin damage from radiation treatments.

Benefits
- Carefully administered massage can be a useful adjunct to cancer treatment by helping improve sleep, reduce pain perception, increase immune system activity, and generally offer support and nurturing to clients undergoing an extremely challenging process.
- Clients who have had thyroid cancer and have completed their treatment with no long-term problems can enjoy the same benefits from massage as the rest of the population.

tic douloureux: see trigeminal neuralgia

tinea: see fungal infections

tinnitus

Tinnitus is the technical term for ringing in the ears. Several factors can contribute to this condition, but a history of repeated exposure to loud noises (gunfire, fireworks, loud music) is a common predisposing factor. These experiences can damage the nerve endings that are sensitive to sound vibrations. Aging and the accompanying stiffening of the tiny inner ear bones may also contribute to tinnitus.

Tinnitus can be a free-standing disorder, but it is sometimes a symptom of an underlying problem. **Hyper- or hypotension, Ménière disease, temporomandibular joint disorders, traumatic brain injury, allergic reactions, diabetes, hyper- or hypothyroidism**, and reactions to medications can all cause a sensation of ringing in the ears. Taking too much aspirin can cause this sensation, and some people develop it in response to other medications such as anti-inflammatory drugs, antidepressants, and antibiotics.

Signs and Symptoms
- Sense of a dull roar, crickets chirping, ocean waves
- Can be high or low pitched
- Can be constant or intermittent
- Can be lessened with background noise
- Can interfere with sleep, leading to other complications

Treatment Options

Treatment for tinnitus depends on the underlying causes. For many people, treatment means finding ways to live with this condition. Hearing aids or tinnitus maskers (devices that resemble hearing aids but that produce low-level white noise that competes with the ringing to cancel it out) may help. Some patients find that working with a counselor to help deal with this condition is important. Other interventions include white noise machines, biofeedback, gentle exercise to increase circulation, and guided relaxation.

Medications

Tinnitus is typically not treated with medication.

 Massage Considerations

Risks
- After underlying factors have been ruled out, massage has no specific risks for clients with tinnitus.

Benefits
- It is possible that the relaxation and decrease in blood pressure associated with massage may at least temporarily ease the symptoms of tinnitus.
- Some clients with tinnitus have found that craniosacral therapy eases their symptoms.

Practitioner Advice
- Some clients may be more comfortable receiving massage with music or other background noise to dull their sensation of noise.

---

torticollis

Torticollis, also called wryneck, is an umbrella term for any condition that causes the head to be pulled to one side.

Torticollis can be a simple matter of having "slept wrong" so that the neck is stiff and painful all day, or it could be a symptom of a more serious underlying problem. Several types of torticollis have been classified, including congenital torticollis (a genetic anomaly resulting in the development of only one sternocleidomastoid muscle); infant torticollis (a complication of head twisting late in gestation); spasmodic torticollis (a type of **dystonia**); a stiff neck caused by cervical subluxation, ligament irritation, and trigger points in neck muscles; or other more rare and serious conditions that may involve infection or cancer.

Signs and Symptoms
- Imbalance in the neck rotators so that the head is involuntarily turned to one side
- Can involve pain, cramping

Treatment Options

Treatment for torticollis depends on the underlying cause. Congenital or infantile situations call for exercise to strengthen the auxiliary muscles. Wryneck from subluxated vertebrae can be addressed with bony manipulation. Torticollis related only to muscle spasm and trigger points responds well to massage.

Medications

Most torticollis is not treated with medication. Spasmodic torticollis may be treated with sedatives to limit spasm or botulinum toxin to temporarily paralyze the affected muscles.

 Massage Considerations

Risks
- Torticollis that is not related to a musculoskeletal imbalance may contraindicate massage; this is particularly true when inflamed lymph nodes or any signs of infection are present.

- Other risks for massage in the context of torticollis must be assessed individually and addressed with both the client and the client's health care provider for best outcomes.

Benefits

- Torticollis related to muscle spasms, trigger points, or ligament irritation indicates massage, which can have a positive influence on these problems.

Tourette syndrome

Tourette syndrome is a neurologic disorder that results in tics, which are sudden, rapid, nonrhythmic, recurrent, predictable movements. Tics may be primarily motor (a twitch, shrug, or grimace) or vocal (a grunt, yell, clearing of the throat, or barking).

Tourette syndrome is usually diagnosed in early childhood. Patients may begin with one kind of tic (often a facial twitch) that may become a more complicated tic, or it may be replaced by a different type of tic altogether. Most people with Tourette syndrome experience both motor and vocal tics. Motor tics can be quite complex, involving the facial muscles or muscles in the shoulder or arms. Vocal tics are usually fairly simple, but a rare (and frequently publicized) version of Tourette syndrome is a tic called coprolalia, which is an involuntary utterance of obscenities or inappropriate words.

Many people with Tourette syndrome also have **attention-deficit hyperactivity disorder** or **obsessive–compulsive disorder**.

Signs and Symptoms

- Mild to extreme motor and vocal tics
- May come in episodes of increased severity, frequency
- Symptoms persist for at least a year with no more than a 3-month break in that time

Treatment Options

A variety of medications can help control Tourette syndrome tics, but the side effects can be severe, so if the tics are mild, many patients don't undergo treatment for this condition.

Medications

Drugs for Tourette syndrome include neuroleptics, antidepressants, antianxiety medication, anticonvulsants, and some antihypertensive drugs.

✋ Massage Considerations

Risks

- Massage has no specific risks for clients with Tourette syndrome.

Benefits

- Although massage is unlikely to improve Tourette syndrome, it can certainly improve the quality of life of clients with the disorder.
- A client's motor tics may involve muscles that end up being tight and uncomfortable; massage can help reduce muscle tone in these overused areas.

toxemia: see pregnancy-induced hypertension

toxoplasmosis

Toxoplasmosis is an infection with a protozoan parasite called *Toxoplasma gondii*. This microorganism invades target cells in the body (the most common sites are the brain, skeletal muscle, and the heart), and if the immune system doesn't eradicate it, cysts full of protozoan eggs (oocysts) may develop.

Toxoplasmosis can infect several species of mammals, but it is especially active in humans and domesticated cats. Most people are never aware of their infection, but for three population groups, it is potentially dangerous. During **pregnancy**, women can pass the parasite to the fetus (this is the only form of human-to-human transmission of toxoplasmosis); unborn babies and newborns are vulnerable to eye and brain damage from the pathogen; and people who are immune compromised (**HIV** patients, organ transplant recipients, and people undergoing chemotherapy) are at risk for very extreme toxoplasmosis infections.

Toxoplasmosis is spread through oral contact with the organism. It is concentrated in cat feces and is present in undercooked meat, especially pork, lamb, and venison. This is why it is especially important for pregnant women and immunocompromised people to avoid handling cat litter and raw meat (or any tool or surface that raw meat has touched).

Signs and Symptoms
- Usually silent
- In high-risk populations: inflamed lymph nodes, muscle aches, invasion of other tissue

Treatment Options
Most people with toxoplasmosis don't require treatment. People in high-risk groups are treated with medication.

Medications
Toxoplasmosis can be treated with medication. Drugs used for this condition include antimalaria drugs and a selection of antibiotics.

✋ Massage Considerations

Risks
- If this condition is silent, massage has no specific risks for toxoplasmosis.
- For clients with symptomatic toxoplasmosis, rigorous circulatory massage should be delayed until treatment is complete.

Benefits
- Massage has no specific benefits for people with toxoplasmosis.
- Clients who have recovered from this infection can enjoy the same benefits from massage as the rest of the population.

transient ischemic attack: see stroke

traumatic brain injury

Traumatic brain injury (TBI) is brain damage that is not brought about by congenital or degenerative conditions. It leads to altered states of consciousness; cognitive impairment; and disruption of physical, emotional, and behavioral function.

TBI is usually the result of an external force such as from a direct blow or a rapid acceleration–deceleration incident. Motor vehicle accidents, gunshot wounds, falls, sports, and physical violence are leading causes. TBI can also be the result of a hemorrhagic **stroke** or central **sleep apnea** that leads to anoxia or hypoxia in the brain.

Signs and Symptoms

- Vary according to the severity and the area of the brain affected
- Frontal lobe: language, motor dysfunction
- Close to the brain stem: massive loss of autonomic function
- Acute injury
    - Leakage of cerebrospinal fluid from the ears, nose
    - Dilated, asymmetrical pupils; visual disturbance
    - Dizziness, confusion
    - Apnea, slowed breathing
    - Slow pulse, low blood pressure
    - Loss of bowel, bladder control
    - Seizure
    - Motor, sensory paralysis
    - Loss of consciousness
- Long-term consequences
    - Mild to severe cognitive dysfunction
    - Hypertonicity, spasticity
    - Seizures
    - Changes in behavioral, emotional function
    - Brain stem injuries: coma, persistent vegetative state

Treatment Options

TBI is treated with surgery to remove pressure on the brain if necessary followed by intensive physical, recreational, occupational, and speech therapy to preserve or recover function.

Medications

Medications for TBI survivors usually address behavioral and mood issues (antidepressants, antianxiety medication) or controlling seizures (anticonvulsants).

Massage Considerations

Risks

- Paralysis and loss of sensation have cautions for massage because overtreatment can occur without client feedback.
- If a client with a TBI cannot communicate verbally, the massage therapist must become sensitive to his or her nonverbal signals about comfort or distress.

Benefits

- If sensation is present and the client is able to communicate clearly about his or her comfort, massage can be an important part of the rehabilitation picture for TBI patients to assist in the maintenance of healthy muscles and connective tissues.

tremor

Tremor is a movement disorder that can indicate a variety of central nervous system problems. The key characteristics of tremor disorders are that the movements are rhythmic oscillations of antagonistic muscle groups and the movement occurs in a fixed plane. Some of the most common types of tremor are essential tremor, **Huntington disease**, St. Vitus' dance (see **rheumatic fever**), **Parkinson disease**, alcohol withdrawal, and **peripheral neuropathy**.

Signs and Symptoms

- Rhythmic oscillations on a fixed plane of movement
- Most often affects the head and forearms

Treatment Options

Tremor is treated according to the underlying causes. Surgical interventions may be used if the tremor is debilitating and unresponsive to medication; these interventions include surgical interruptions at the thalamus or globus pallidus.

Medications

Dopamine precursors, beta-blockers, tranquilizers, antiseizure medications, botulinum toxin (if it affects the muscles of the voice or head), and small doses of alcohol may be suggested for various types of tremor.

Massage Considerations

Risks

- Tremor is often an indicator of an underlying problem that should be identified and addressed before bodywork is pursued.
- Any massage technique that exacerbates the person's symptoms must be adjusted; otherwise, massage has no specific risks for uncomplicated tremor.

Benefits

- Massage has no specific benefits for most types of tremor.
- Some clients find that craniosacral therapy provides some relief from uncomplicated tremor symptoms.

trichinosis

Trichinosis is an infestation with one of a variety of species of roundworms called trichinella. The most common agent is *Trichinosis spiralis*, which is found in the muscle tissue of domesticated livestock. Pigs are the most likely carriers, but the organisms can also be found in sheep, goats, and horses when these animals have been fed uncooked meat products in the form of meal or kibble. Other species of trichinosis are found in wild carnivores, including swine, cougars, bears, walrus, seals, and wild dogs.

Blood-borne trichinosis worms invade a variety of tissues, where they cause an inflammatory reaction that is marked by high numbers of eosinophils. Symptoms of trichinosis can be traced to both the activity of the worms and the inflammatory response against them. This can be dangerous because this inflammation increases the risk of tiny blood clots (microthrombi) that may damage the heart or brain.

Most trichinosis infections are eradicated by immune system activity or culminate in the creation of connective tissue cysts in striated muscle tissue. It is possible, however, for the worms to invade other tissues with more serious consequences, including the heart, brain, lungs, and kidneys.

Trichinosis is rare in the United States, where regulations about the processing and cooking of pork are well known and usually followed. However, large outbreaks of this disease are commonly reported in other countries. Travelers to these places who eat the local food may be at risk for this parasite.

Signs and Symptoms

- Early signs: gastrointestinal discomfort (nausea, vomiting, diarrhea, fever, chills)
- Later signs: depend on the location of worm colonies
    - Edema, especially around the eyelids
    - Muscle aches, weakness
    - Loss of coordination
    - Meningitis, encephalitis
    - Arrhythmia, heart failure
    - Renal failure
    - Pneumonia

Treatment Options

Trichinosis is treated with medication.

Medications

If trichinosis is identified before connective tissue cysts in muscle tissue have formed, it is treatable with a variety of antiparasitic medications. Inflammation is treated with steroidal anti-inflammatory drugs. After the parasites have become encysted, however, medication has little effect on them. Analgesics may be suggested for chronic muscle pain, but no other treatment options have much impact.

Massage Considerations

Risks

- Early-stage trichinosis contraindicates massage.
- Later-stage infections may present some cautions for bodywork, especially if they involve any damage to the heart, brain, or kidneys.

Benefits

- Massage has no specific benefits for clients with trichinosis.
- Clients who have successfully undergone treatment for trichinosis with no lasting problems can enjoy the same benefits from massage as the rest of the population.

trigeminal neuralgia

Trigeminal neuralgia (TN) is damage or irritation to one or more of the three branches of cranial nerve V, the trigeminal nerve. It is also called tic douloureux, which is French for "painful spasm" or "unhappy twitch."

Primary TN is considered to be idiopathic (the cause or source of the nerve irritation may never be identified). Secondary TN is caused by mechanical pressure on the nerve or some other structural problem. Contributing factors include tumors, bone spurs, a recent infection, complications of dental surgery, or other diseases. Perhaps the most common cause of TN is the growth of tiny blood vessels that may strangulate or otherwise irritate the nerve.

Episodes of trigeminal nerve pain can be triggered by speaking, chewing, swallowing, sitting in a draft, a light touch to the wrong spot, and sometimes by no stimulus at all.

TN is sometimes an indicator of another disorder. **Multiple sclerosis** and **temporomandibular joint disorders** can both cause TN. Sinus and tooth infections can create similar symptoms, but they are treated differently.

Signs and Symptoms
- Brief, repeating episodes of sharp, electrical, stabbing pain on one side of the face
- Episodes may last 10 seconds to a minute or several jabs may occur in rapid succession
- Muscle tic may accompany nerve pain

Treatment Options

TN treatment begins with medication to control pain and nerve impulses. Sometimes a portion of the nerve is destroyed to interrupt the pain signals it sends. This results in permanent numbness but also results in a cessation in sometimes debilitating symptoms. If noninvasive measures are insufficient to control TN symptoms, surgery to decompress the nerve or remove the strangulating artery that wraps around it may be recommended.

One alternative intervention for TN is acupuncture. This approach often has some success with problems of nerve conduction.

Medications

Mainstream treatment for TN typically starts with analgesics and then proceeds to antiseizure drugs.

🖐 Massage Considerations

Risks
- TN contraindicates any massage or bodywork that exacerbates symptoms; this may include pressure on the face or positioning the client in a face cradle that irritates this condition.

Benefits
- If a client with TN can be comfortable, massage may address the peripheral stresses that go along with this painful condition. Chronic tension in the head, neck, and upper back muscles that guard against pain can be relieved with good results.
- If a client can tolerate it, craniosacral therapy may help reduce the severity and duration of TN episodes.

trisomy 21: see Down syndrome

trophic ulcers: see decubitus ulcers

tuberculosis

Tuberculosis (TB) is a bacterial infection leading to the development of pus- and bacteria-filled cysts ("tubercles") in the lungs and other tissues. It is caused by *Mycobacterium tuberculosis*, an air-borne bacterium with a protective waxy coat that allows it to survive for prolonged periods outside a host.

TB moves in the body in two phases. The primary phase is TB exposure. It occurs when a person inhales bacteria into the lungs. The bacteria are protected from the immune system by their waxy coating, so the body effectively builds a connective cyst or wall around them. The lungs are the most common site, but these tubercles may also develop on the bones, kidneys, and other tissues as well. For about 90% of people exposed to TB, this is the extent of the infection.

About 10% of exposed people eventually develop TB as an active infection. The bacteria reactivate and escape their connective tissue cysts. Larger fibrous capsules are built to try to contain the infection, leading to permanent scarring in the lung. Tubercles may join together to make large cavities in the lungs or other infected tissues. Inside the cysts, the bacteria destroy healthy tissue. The cysts fill with pus, necrotic cells, and active bacteria. When any of this is expelled in coughing, the disease can spread into the community.

Signs and Symptoms

- Primary phase: usually silent; may look like the flu
- Active disease: fever, sweating, weight loss, exhaustion, cough with bloodstained phlegm

Treatment Options

TB is treated with antibiotics and lots of rest, sunshine, and good nutrition.

Medications

Antibiotic treatment is effective against common TB, but any course of medication must be consistently used for several weeks or even months. Failure to do so results in the development of a drug-resistant strain of TB called multidrug resistant TB (MDR-TB). This strain is directly communicable to uninfected people, is much more difficult and expensive to treat, and has a mortality rate about equal to untreated regular TB. XDR-TB ("extremely drug-resistant TB") is a relatively new form of the bacterium that has essentially no drug treatment options.

Massage Considerations

Risks

- Active TB infection is communicable through casual contact. This condition contraindicates any massage until the risk of communicability has been eradicated.
- Massage has no specific risks for clients with primary TB who are being treated with antibiotics.

Benefits

- Massage has no specific benefits for clients with TB.
- Clients who have had TB or who have a silent infection that is being treated with antibiotics can enjoy the same benefits from massage as the rest of the population.

ulcerative colitis

Ulcerative colitis (UC) is an autoimmune disease of the colon involving progressive inflammation, scar tissue, and ulcerations. It occurs in unpredictable flares followed by periods of remissions, a pattern similar to other autoimmune conditions.

UC begins in the rectum, where immune system cells attack the most superficial layer of the colon. The resulting inflammation kills tissue and results in the formation of shallow ulcers. Colon function is impaired, which causes chronic diarrhea. The sores may become infected, leading to a release of blood and pus in the stool.

UC is a progressive disease. Although it begins in the rectum, it may spread to affect the whole colon. The lesions are continuous, however, rather than appearing in disconnected patches.

The tissue changes seen with UC are limited to the large intestine. This distinguishes it from **Crohn disease**, a similar condition that affects the whole gastrointestinal (GI) tract. UC and Crohn disease are referred to together as inflammatory bowel disease.

The inflammatory nature of acute UC often affects other systems in the body. A person in a flare of UC may also experience **hepatitis, osteoarthritis, osteoporosis, anemia** from blood loss, and **kidney stones** from the disruption in electrolyte balance and chronic dehydration that accompany long-term diarrhea. The chronic damage and repair cycle seen with UC leads to a significantly increased risk of **colorectal cancer**. In very rare situations, the colon may swell up to the point that it is in danger of rupture. This is called toxic megacolon and is a medical emergency.

Signs and Symptoms

- During flare:
    Painful, chronic diarrhea
    Blood in the stool
    Abdominal cramping
    Loss of appetite
    Fever
    Inflammation in other tissues
- During remission:
    Minimal abdominal pain
    Sensitivity to triggers for cramping, discomfort

Treatment Options

If medication is unsuccessful in controlling UC, surgery to remove the bowel is a permanent solution for this problem.

Medications

Treatment options for UC begin with medications that lessen the severity of flares and prolong periods of remission. Corticosteroids may be prescribed for short periods. Immunosuppressive drugs and nicotine patches have also been found to improve symptoms.

Massage Considerations

Risks
- During flare, rigorous circulatory massage may exacerbate symptoms.
- During flare or remission, deep abdominal massage is a local contraindication.

Benefits
- Energetic or reflexive techniques that support a healthy immune response and the sympathetic/parasympathetic balance may be appropriate if the client is comfortable.
- Clients with UC in remission can enjoy benefits of any massage that doesn't intrusively manipulate tissues or organs deep in the abdomen.

Practitioner Advice
- For clients with a colostomy bag, the therapist must be careful about positioning to avoid disrupting their equipment. The best way to work in this situation is to invite the client to explain how he or she is most comfortable. External colostomy bags may be adhered to the skin with oil-soluble glue; this is another reason they are a local contraindication.

---

ulcers

An ulcer is the result of tissue damage that, because it is subject to constant irritation or poor circulation, doesn't heal. Cells die and are sloughed off, and a crater develops but doesn't crust over. Ulcers in the stomach or small intestine are called peptic ulcers.

Three main factors contribute to the development of peptic ulcers: the fluctuation between sympathetic and parasympathetic response, the presence of *Helicobacter pylori* bacteria, and the use of nonsteroidal anti-inflammatory drugs (NSAIDs). Although a "flight or fight" sympathetic response tends to inhibit gastric activity, function is restored in a parasympathetic state. Unfortunately, corrosive gastric juices are often replaced faster than protective mucus, so frequent swings between stress and relief can radically alter the environment inside the stomach. Small erosions may then be colonized by special spirochetal bacteria (*H. pylori*) that thrive in the acidic surroundings. NSAIDs can contribute to ulcers by inhibiting the formation of mucus that protects the wall of the GI tract.

Ulcers that penetrate deep into the wall of the stomach or small intestine can cause significant bleeding, leading to **anemia**. Perforation of the GI tract wall can cause **peritonitis**. Scarring can completely block the digestive tract. Having a peptic ulcer increases the risk of developing **stomach cancer**, and the presence of *H. pylori* is associated with an increased risk for some types of **lymphoma**.

Signs and Symptoms
- Gnawing, burning pain in the chest or abdomen
- Episodes last 30 minutes to 3 hours
- The pattern of pain in relation to eating varies by individual
- Nausea, vomiting, loss of appetite, bleeding into the GI tract

Treatment Options

Most ulcer treatment protocols begin with medication, but ulcers caused by the use of NSAIDs do not respond to antibiotic therapy. The only way to limit them is to suspend the use of the medications that damage the stomach lining.

Surgeries for ulcers can involve severing a branch of the vagus nerve, removing a section of the stomach, enlarging the pyloric valve, or any combination of the three.

Medications

Treatment for most ulcers includes antibiotics for the *H. pylori*; bismuth, which protects the delicate stomach lining; and proton pump inhibitors, which limit acid production.

Massage Considerations

Risks

- If relaxation massage temporarily masks ulcer symptoms, a client could be delayed in getting an important diagnosis. Any GI symptoms that persist for more than a couple of weeks should be pursued with a primary care provider.
- A client with peptic ulcers may find that rigorous manipulation of the abdomen is painful; peptic ulcers contraindicate this kind of work.
- If a client moves into a parasympathetic state during massage and gastric activity increases, it is possible that symptoms of a peptic ulcer could be exacerbated. These clients may be better off with shorter sessions, possibly using a massage chair rather than a table.

Benefits

- If a client tolerates massage well, it could be a stress management intervention that, along with appropriate medication and other care, can help prevent or repair peptic ulcers.

upper respiratory tract infection: see common cold

urinary tract infection

Urinary tract infections (UTI) are infections that may occur anywhere in the urinary system from the kidneys to the bladder to the urethra. Because kidney infections are a separate entity, the term *UTI* usually refers to infections of the lower urinary tract, which includes the urethra (urethritis) and bladder (cystitis).

Escherichia coli is the causative agent behind most UTIs. These strains of bacteria live normally and harmlessly in the digestive tract but cause problems in the urinary tract. Certain varieties of staphylococcus and other agents, including *Klebsiella*, chlamydia, and mycoplasma are the cause of some infections. It's important to identify the correct causative agent because they respond to the different antibiotics.

Chronic irritation can also contribute to the development of UTIs; "honeymoon cystitis" refers to inflammation and subsequent infection brought about by repeated irritation of the urethra from sexual activity.

When men develop a UTI, it is usually a sign of prostate problems (**prostatitis, benign prostatic hyperplasia, prostate cancer**) or a symptom of a sexually transmitted infection (**gonorrhea, syphilis,** or **chlamydia**).

Untreated UTIs are associated with a risk that bacteria could invade the rest of the urinary tract, culminating in **pyelonephritis**. Pathogens from the kidneys then have access to the bloodstream, and life-threatening **septicemia** can follow.

Signs and Symptoms

- Painful, burning, frequent urination
- Reduced bladder capacity
- Blood-tinged or cloudy urine
- For men: pain in the penis or scrotum

Treatment Options

UTIs are usually treated with medication. Structural problems with the way urine drains from the bladder may contribute to chronic infections; surgery may be recommended to correct these problems.

When a person has a UTI, it is important for him or her to hydrate well because frequent urination helps flush bacteria from the system. Supplementing cranberries or blueberries creates an environment in the bladder that is hostile to bacteria, but the sweeteners added to these juices can undo this benefit.

Medications

UTIs typically respond well to a short course of antibiotics. People who experience low-grade chronic UTIs that don't clear up with normal treatments are sometimes successfully treated with long-term, low-dose antibiotics.

Massage Considerations

Risks

- Acute UTIs contraindicate rigorous massage because of unresolved infection and general discomfort.

Benefits

- Massage has no specific benefits for clients in the midst of a UTI.
- After antibiotic treatment has begun, massage may support immune system activity and promote general comfort to assist in eradicating the infection.
- Clients with a history of UTI but no current symptoms can enjoy the same benefits from massage as the rest of the population.

urticaria: see hives

---

uterine cancer

Uterine cancer is the development of malignant growths in the uterus. The two types of uterine cancer are endometrial carcinoma (cancer of the glandular tissue) and uterine sarcoma (cancer of the muscle or connective tissue).

Endometrial carcinoma is by far the most common type of uterine cancer. It involves cancer cells in the endometrial lining of the uterus. These cells easily metastasize through direct contact with other tissues or through the pelvic lymph supply.

Uterine sarcoma is relatively rare and arises from muscle or connective tissue in the uterus. It can also metastasize through direct contact or through the lymph system.

A number of nonmalignant conditions can affect the uterus and cause symptoms that mimic uterine cancer. These include uterine **fibroid tumors, endometriosis,** and endometrial hyperplasia (a condition in which the endometrium thickens as a woman approaches menopause). Endometrial hyperplasia can be a precursor of uterine cancer but is not a consistent predictor.

Whenever a woman experiences disruption in her menstrual cycle or vaginal bleeding after menopause, she should consult a doctor to determine whether the cause of her symptoms are benign or malignant.

Signs and Symptoms

- Vaginal bleeding in peri- and postmenopausal women
- Pelvic pain
- Palpable abdominal mass

Treatment Options

Treatment for uterine cancer is determined by what stage it is in at diagnosis. Surgery to remove the uterus, ovaries, or both is usually the first step. This may be followed by external or internal radiation.

Medications

Chemotherapy for uterine cancer is typically only used when the cancer is found in the later stages with metastasis. Hormone therapy may be recommended as a long-term strategy to bind up estrogen receptor sites on any leftover cancer cells.

Massage Considerations

Risks

- The risks for massage and uterine cancer are more related to cancer treatment than the cancer itself. Surgery, chemotherapy, and radiation all have side effects that influence choices about massage, including reduced immunity, infection, bruising and bleeding, and many others.

Benefits

- Carefully administered massage can boost immune system function, promote good-quality sleep, improve appetite, and be generally supportive for the healing process.

uveitis: see iritis

V

vaginitis

Vaginitis is an umbrella term for any inflammation of the vagina. Several factors can contribute to this condition, but bacteria, yeasts, protozoa, and tissue changes that occur after menopause are responsible for most cases. The major types of vaginitis include bacterial vaginosis, yeast infection (**candidiasis**), trichomoniasis infection, and atrophic vaginitis.

   Vaginitis is usually caused by a particular pathogen (with the exception of atrophic vaginitis), but some habits can increase the risk of developing this condition. The use of hot tubs or baths, douching, wearing tight pants or damp underwear, and using vaginal products (sprays, spermicides, lubricants, perfumed tampons) can all irritate the vaginal lining.

   Tests show that both bacterial vaginosis and trichomoniasis infection increase the risk of HIV transmission.

Signs and Symptoms

- Vary, depending on the causative factor
- Itching, burning, pain in the vagina
- Painful intercourse
- Vaginal discharge

Treatment Options

Vaginitis is treated with medication.

Medications

All types of vaginitis are easily treated with antibiotics, topical creams, or vaginal suppositories. It is important to treat the correct disorder, however, so women with new symptoms should consult a doctor before using any over-the-counter preparations.

Massage Considerations

Risks
- Massage has no specific risks for clients with vaginitis.

Benefits
- Massage has no specific benefits for clients with vaginitis.
- Clients who have had vaginitis can enjoy the same benefits from massage as the rest of the population.

---

varicocele

A varicocele is a distended vein surrounding the scrotum, spermatic cord, or both. The veins that carry blood out of the testicles are not symmetrical. The right spermatic vein drains into the vena cava, and the left side drains into the renal vein. This asymmetry, along with more acute angles and differences in valves, puts the left testicle at risk for reflux and distension of the veins that would ordinarily carry blood back into the body.

Varicoceles are associated with low numbers of sperm, poor motility, and a high percentage of malformed sperm. Although many men develop varicoceles without having problems with fertility, a high percentage of men with infertility also have varicoceles. The leading theory is that these varicosities increase the temperature inside the scrotum, leading to problems with spermatogenesis.

Varicoceles can be progressive. When they develop at adolescence and are untreated, atrophy of the testicle with poor sperm production and reduced testosterone production may result.

Most varicoceles are slowly progressive. When one develops rapidly, especially on the right side, a kidney tumor (**renal cancer**) should be suspected.

Signs and Symptoms
- Usually painless
- Possible infertility
- Sensation of heaviness in the scrotum
- May be palpable or visible

Treatment Options

In adult men, varicoceles that cause no symptoms or problems in fertility require no treatment, but a variety of surgeries to correct varicoceles have been developed.

Medications

Varicoceles are not treated with medication.

Massage Considerations

Risks
- Massage has no specific risks for clients with varicoceles.

Benefits
- Massage has no specific benefits for clients with varicoceles.
- Clients with varicoceles can enjoy the same benefits from massage as the rest of the population.

varicose veins

Varicose veins are distended, often twisted or "ropey," superficial veins. They are caused by dysfunctional internal valves that promote the movement of blood against gravity. When blood backs up in the system, the affected vein is stretched, distorted, and generally weakened.

Damage to the valves in the veins can be brought about by wear and tear, mechanical obstruction (tight knee socks, a knee brace, or a fetus pressing on the femoral vein), systemic congestion from poor kidney or liver function, or congenital weakness.

Varicose veins can occur at other sites around the body. At the anus, they are called **hemorrhoids**. At the esophagus, they are called esophageal varices. And at the scrotum, they are called **varicoceles**.

Chronically impaired circulation may result in **thrombophlebitis** or varicose ulcers.

Signs and Symptoms
- Lumpy, bluish, wandering lines visible through the skin
- Often on the back of the calf or medial leg
- Itching, throbbing pain
- Possible distal edema
- Possible sores or ulcers on the skin from poor circulation

Treatment Options

Mild varicose veins are usually treated with support hose or elastic bandages for external support. Reclining with the feet slightly elevated also reduces the symptoms. Hydrotherapy (alternating hot and cold water on the affected area) may help strengthen the smooth muscle tissue in the veins and slow the progression of varicose veins. If these interventions are insufficient, patients may consider a variety of surgical options that remove or shut down varicose veins; new blood vessels quickly grow in to replace their function.

Medications

Varicose veins are not treated with medication, although some patients may use analgesics for pain relief.

Massage Considerations

Risks
- Varicose veins locally contraindicate deep or sharp pressure, especially when the veins are elevated from the skin and have visibly been distorted from their original pathway.
- Heavy massage distal to extreme varicose veins is also a caution.

Benefits
- If pressure is gentle and diffuse (flat hands as opposed to pointed fingertips) and as long as the skin in the area is intact, careful massage over mild varicose veins is appropriate and can ease pain and itching.
- Tiny reddened "spider veins" (telangictasias) are slightly dilated venules and are safe for massage.

vasculitis

Vasculitis is a general term for any inflammation of a blood vessel. Vasculitis can be a free-standing disorder, but it is often a symptom or indicator of an underlying condition, especially autoimmune diseases, that involve systemic inflammation. It is typically classified according to the size of blood vessels that are affected: large vessel vasculitis, medium-sized vessel vasculitis, and small vessel vasculitis.

- Large vessel vasculitis: This is any vasculitis that affects major arteries. The most common version of this condition is called giant cell arteritis or temporal arteritis, which is closely associated with **polymyalgia rheumatica**. This involves inflammation that may begin at the aorta but concentrates in the arteries of the head and face and may lead to permanent vision loss.
- Medium-sized vessel vasculitis: The most common version of this disorder is **polyarteritis nodosa**.
- Small vessel vasculitis: Several different conditions can cause inflammation and rupture of small blood vessels. Complications of **hepatitis** B and C, **HIV**, **allergic reactions** to some medications, and Churg-Strauss syndrome (a complication of **asthma**) can all involve small vessel vasculitis.

Many other conditions list vasculitis among their symptoms, including **lupus, rheumatoid arthritis**, **scleroderma**, and **Behçet disease**.

Signs and Symptoms

- Vary, depending on the location and severity
- Fatigue, weakness, fever
- Joint pain, abdominal pain
- Kidney dysfunction
- Neuropathy
- Rashes, hemorrhages in the skin
- Proinflammatory markers in the blood (high erythrocyte sedimentation rate, C-reactive protein)

Treatment Options

Vasculitis is treated with medication.

Medications

Very mild vasculitis can be treated with nonsteroidal anti-inflammatory drugs, but severe cases require more powerful medication. Steroidal anti-inflammatory drugs (especially prednisone) can be useful but have serious side effects. Cytotoxic drugs may be used to quell immune system overactivity, but they also have serious side effects and so are typically recommended for short-term dosages.

Massage Considerations

Risks

- Untreated vasculitis can be dangerous, with a risk of blood clots, ruptured vessels, and kidney damage. In these situations, vasculitis contraindicates rigorous circulatory massage.
- Other risks for massage in the context of vasculitis are connected to medications that may quell an inflammatory response or suppress immune system activity.

Benefits

- Reflexive or energetic techniques can be supportive for immune system response and to decrease pain and anxiety for clients who are being treated for vasculitis.

---

vertigo

Vertigo is the sensation of the world being in whirling movement while the person is still. It is brought about by a difference between what the eyes perceive and what the sensors in the inner ear relay about position in space.

Several factors can contribute to vertigo, but the most common one is a condition called benign paroxysmal positional vertigo (BPPV). In this condition, tiny crystals of calcium carbonate called otoconia detach from sensory nerve endings that detect back-and-forth movement and fall into other parts of the inner ear, where they stimulate sensors for balance. The result is a strong sensation that the world is spinning, along with nystagmus (rhythmic oscillation of the eyes) and other symptoms. Episodes of BPPV usually last for several seconds or minutes, and they occur after a change of position of the head. Tipping the head back is such a common trigger that this condition is sometimes called "top-shelf vertigo."

BPPV is often age related, but it can also be a result of head trauma, viral infection, or a complication of ear surgery.

Other causes of vertigo include labyrinthitis, infection of the bony labyrinth (**otitis interna**), **Ménière disease**, **multiple sclerosis**, ischemic or hemorrhagic **stroke**, toxic damage to the brain, **traumatic brain injury**, migraine **headache**, **acoustic neuroma**, or leakage of perilymphatic fluid.

Signs and Symptoms

- Dizziness
- Sensation of spinning
- Lightheadedness
- Loss of balance
- Blurred vision
- Nausea
- Nystagmus

Treatment Options

BPPV is usually treated with maneuvers of the head that allow the calcium carbonate crystals to fall back into the appropriate chamber of the bony labyrinth. This intervention is almost always successful, although repeated applications may have to be tried, and the patient needs to keep the head upright for up to 48 hours after a treatment.

In rare cases, surgery to "plug" the chamber where the otoconia belong may be conducted. Other causes of vertigo are treated according to the factors that contribute to the symptoms.

Medications

Medical intervention for vertigo include antianxiety drugs and drugs for motion sickness to reduce the feeling of nausea.

Massage Considerations

Risks
- A client with vertigo in a new pattern should be referred to a primary care provider for evaluation.
- Many clients with BPPV find that they need to avoid lying flat, especially if they have had a recent episode. Massage therapists should be prepared to work with clients in a semireclining position or in a massage chair if being horizontal causes symptoms.

Benefits
- Carefully applied head holds may help ease the symptoms of BPPV.
- Massage has no specific benefits for other forms of vertigo.
- If a client with a form of vertigo that has no cautions for massage can be made comfortable, then he or she can enjoy the same benefits from massage as the rest of the population.

Practitioner Advice
- BPPV is managed with a series of positional head holds that allow the calcium carbonate crystals to fall back into the appropriate chamber of the bony labyrinth. Massage therapists who have clients with BPPV may be able to consult with their health care providers to learn these maneuvers as well.

---

vitiligo

Vitiligo is an idiopathic disorder in which melanocytes of the skin, mucous membranes, and retina are prematurely destroyed. It is unclear whether this is an autoimmune disorder or a problem with the lifespan of certain skin cells.

When melanocytes die, they leave a pink or white patch on the skin. The hair that grows from the area also turns white or gray. Vitiligo usually appears in one of three major patterns: a focal pattern, a segmental pattern, or a generalized pattern. Focal pattern vitiligo involves one patch or just a few small areas. Segmental pattern vitiligo has patches that all appear on one side of the body. Generalized vitiligo has patches all over the body. Patches frequently develop in areas with exposure to sunlight, including the hands, arms, and face. Other areas that may be affected include the axilla, groin, and abdomen.

Most people with vitiligo find that it is a slowly progressive disease. Patches may get larger or spread to other places on the body. Some patients report that physical or emotional stress can exacerbate the disease.

Vitiligo often appears with other autoimmune disorders or in families that deal with these conditions. Disorders associated with an increased incidence of vitiligo include Graves disease (**hyperthyroidism**), **Addison disease**, pernicious **anemia**, and alopecia areata (bald patches).

Signs and Symptoms
- Depigmented areas on the skin or mucous membranes

Treatment Options

Several treatments have been developed for vitiligo patients. The most successful option for most people is a combination of oral psoralen and careful doses of ultraviolet (UV) radiation, which causes the depigmented skin to become darker. Other options include topical psoralen with UV radiation, skin grafts, and careful tattooing in isolated areas to mimic unaffected skin.

People with vitiligo are very vulnerable to sunburn, so they need to use sunscreen carefully and consistently.

Medications

Oral psoralen (a group of medications that increase skin pigmentation) is the medication used most frequently with vitiligo.

Massage Considerations

Risks

• Massage has no specific risks for clients with vitiligo.

Benefits

• Massage has no specific benefits for clients with vitiligo other than those enjoyed by the rest of the population.

Practitioner Advice

• This relatively benign disease can feel massively disfiguring. It is common for people with vitiligo have an extremely negative self-image. Massage, through nonjudgmental nurturing touch, may help counteract some of the worst aspects of this disorder.

von Willebrand disease: see hemophilia

warts

Warts are small, benign neoplasms caused by a type of the human papilloma virus that targets keratinocytes. These cells then produce extra keratin. The result is a pile-up of hard, crusty, water-proofing protein that is also known as verruca vulgaris, or common warts.

Warts can be contagious if the edges are roughened; the virus is in the blood and in the shedding skin cells. Warts are usually self-limiting, although the process of clearing them up can take a long time. In very healthy people, warts can be expected to disappear within 1 year. For others, it can take even longer.

Verruca vulgaris is the most common type of wart, but other types have also been identified. A short list includes plane warts (small, brown, smooth warts seen most often on the faces of children), flat warts (similar to verruca vulgaris, they appear on the face and can be spread by shaving), and **molluscum contagiosum**.

Signs and Symptoms

• Hard, cauliflower-shaped growths on the skin
• Often on the hands, elbows, knees, plantar surfaces of the feet
• Plantar warts can resemble calluses and often show "speckling" as a result of supplying capillaries

Treatment Options

Warts can be treated with topical applications of salicylic acid, but they may recur in a circular pattern around the original wart. Liquid nitrogen, electrosurgery, carbon dioxide lasers, injections, excision, and covering the warts with duct tape are other options.

Medications

Warts may be treated with topical medications to remove them.

🖐 Massage Considerations

Risks

- Warts locally contraindicate massage, mainly because it is inappropriate to irritate them.
- Warts that are bleeding or shedding are potentially contagious, although this risk is probably low.

Benefits

- Massage has no specific benefits for warts.
- Clients who have warts can enjoy the same benefits from massage as the rest of the population, as long as the warts themselves are avoided.

Practitioner Advice

- Plantar warts that appear on the soles of the feet can resemble calluses, but it is important not to treat them like calluses. Clients may be tempted to try to snip them off or rub them with pumice stone, but these interventions can cause the warts to bleed and spread. Massage therapists, while not providing a diagnosis, can at least point out that plantar warts have some features that distinguish them from calluses: they don't necessarily appear in places with the most wear and tear, they aren't symmetrical from one foot to the other, and they often have a "speckled" appearance that shows the capillary supply to the new growth.

West Nile disease: see encephalitis

whiplash

Whiplash, or cervical acceleration–deceleration (CAD) is a broad term used to refer to a mixture of injuries, including **sprains, strains,** and joint trauma to structures in and around the neck. Bone **fractures, disc disease,** and concussion (a type of **traumatic brain injury**) are commonly seen along with these soft tissue injuries and may be addressed simultaneously. Whiplash can also contribute to arthritis in the spine (**spondylosis**) or jaw (**temporomandibular joint disorders**).

Whiplash injuries are often (but not always) associated with car accidents in which the head "whips" backward and forward in rapid succession.

Signs and Symptoms

- Vary according to the injured structures and severity
- May be delayed by days, weeks, or months
- Headache
- Stiffness in the neck and elsewhere
- Pain in the neck, arms
- Symptoms of associated injuries (e.g., fractures, temporomandibular joint disorders, traumatic brain injury)

Treatment Options

Neck collars are used for acute whiplash to take the stress off wrenched ligaments and to try to reduce muscle spasm. But collars are strictly for short-term use because this kind of immobilization can create more long-term problems than benefits.

Further treatment for whiplash depends on the type and severity of specific injuries that have occurred. This can include medication, chiropractic or osteopathic care, physical therapy, psychological counseling, massage therapy, or other interventions.

Medications

Many people recovering from whiplash injuries use analgesics, anti-inflammatory drugs, and muscle relaxants to help manage their symptoms.

Massage Considerations

Risks

- Some of the injuries that can occur in a whiplash accident contraindicate massage until more information can be gathered. These include herniated discs, concussion or other nerve tissue injury, bone fractures, and damage to soft tissues in the anterior neck.
- Intrusive massage can promote blood flow, which is inappropriate in inflamed tissues. Working too soon or too deeply, especially with clients who are taking analgesics or muscle relaxants, can do more harm than good.

Benefits

- When a whiplash injury is acute, very gentle massage can help decrease pain and anxiety, and lymphatic techniques may help limit inflammation.
- Later in the healing process, massage can be a powerful aid in the resolution of muscle spasms, trigger points, and scar tissue in accessible ligaments.

Practitioner Advice

- Small, incremental improvements in function and range of motion are safer goals than dramatic progress when a client is in the process of recovering from a whiplash injury.

whooping cough: see pertussis

wryneck: see torticollis

Z

zygomycosis

Zygomycosis is an infection with any of three species of fungi that is particularly dangerous to people with severely compromised immune system function. These infections hold no threat for people with intact immune systems but can be fatal to people without adequate protection.

The fungi associated with zygomycosis typically gain access to the body through the nose or mouth. They readily invade the blood vessels, leading to the formation of blood clots and the death of surrounding tissue. The most common presentation is an infection of the sinuses, which then can affect the cranial nerves, the brain, or both. Pulmonary infections can infiltrate the thoracic cavity and affect the heart. Fungi can also invade the gastrointestinal tract, the urinary tract, and the skin.

People most at risk for zygomycosis are those with disorders that interfere with immune system function. Poorly managed **diabetes** mellitus, especially with acidosis, is a major risk factor for this disease. Other predisposing conditions include long-term steroid use, organ transplant, **leukemia**, **lymphoma**, **AIDS**, and **burns**.

Zygomycosis can cause cerebral thrombosis (**stroke**) and blindness.

Signs and Symptoms
- Vary according to which tissues are affected
- Sinus infection: fever, bulging eyes, red skin over the sinuses, black scabbing around the nose
- Lung infection: coughing, shortness of breath, hemoptysis (coughing up blood), fever
- Skin infection: single hard, painful area; black center where tissue dies
- Additional signs and symptoms: abdominal pain, vomiting, kidney pain

Treatment Options
Zygomycosis has a high mortality rate, so it is treated aggressively. The affected areas are surgically removed, and systemic medication is administered.

Medications
Intravenous antifungal medication is used for zygomycosis as quickly as possible.

Massage Considerations

Risks
- Any client who is immunocompromised and who shows signs of fever and skin discoloration should consult a doctor before undergoing massage.

Benefits
- Massage has no specific benefits for clients with zygomycosis.
- Zygomycosis is not contagious for people with healthy immune systems, so clients with this condition can receive gentle massage for palliative care without risk to the massage therapist.

Glossary

A

ablate (ah-BLATE): To remove or destroy function.

abrasion (ah-BRA-zhun): A scrape involving injury to the epithelial layer of the skin or mucous membranes.

absence seizure (AB-sens SE-zhur): A type of seizure characterized by lack of activity with occasional clonic movements.

acetaminophen (ah-set-ah-MIN-o-fen): A drug with antifever and analgesic effects similar to aspirin but with limited anti-inflammatory action.

acetylcholine (ah-set-il-KO-lene): The neurotransmitter at cholinergic synapses. It causes cardiac inhibition, vasodilation, gastrointestinal peristalsis, and other parasympathetic effects.

acral lentiginous melanoma (AK-ral len-TIH-jih-nus mel-ah-NO-mah): Pigmented lesions usually seen on the nailbed, fingers, palms, soles, or between the toes.

acromegaly (ak-ro-MEG-ah-lee): A disorder that is linked to excessive secretion of growth hormone marked by progressive enlargement of peripheral parts of the body.

acromioclavicular joint sprain (ah-KRO-me-o-klah-VIK-yu-lar joynt sprane): An injury to the ligaments that support the acromioclavicular joint.

actinic keratosis (ak-TIN-ik ker-ah-TO-sis): A premalignant warty lesion occurring on the sun-exposed skin of the face or hands in aged light-skinned persons.

acute exertional compartment syndrome (ah-KUTE eg-ZER-shun-al kom-PART-ment SIN-drome): A serious injury involving excessive swelling of the leg muscles that may dangerously compress the blood vessels and peripheral nerves.

acute idiopathic polyneuritis (ah-KUTE ih-de-o-PATH-ik pol-e-nu-RI-tis): Guillain-Barré syndrome.

acute inflammatory demyelinating polyneuropathy (AIDP) (ah-KUTE in-FLAM-ah-tor-e de-MI-el-ih-na-ting pol-e-nu-ROP-ath-e): A form of Guillain-Barré syndrome.

acyclovir (a-SI-klo-vir): An antiviral agent often used in the treatment of herpes simplex.

adenocarcinoma (ah-den-o-kar-sih-NO-mah): A malignant neoplasm of epithelial cells in glandular or glandlike pattern.

adenoma (ad-en-O-mah): A benign neoplasm usually occurring in epithelial tissue.

adhesive capsulitis (ad-HE-siv kap-su-LI-tis): A condition involving inflammatory thickening of a joint capsule, usually at the shoulder, leading to loss of range of motion. Also known as frozen shoulder.

aflatoxin (AF-lah-tok-sin) B_1: A toxin produced by some strains of *Aspergillus flavus* that causes cancer in some animals.

agglutination (ah-glu-tin-A-shun): The process by which suspended red blood cells or other particles adhere to each other and form clumps.

agoraphobia (ah-gor-ah-FO-be-ah): A mental disorder characterized by an irrational fear of leaving the familiar setting of home or venturing into the open; often associated with panic attacks.

allergic rhinitis (ah-LER-jik ri-NI-tis): Hay fever.

alpha-1-antitrypsin (AL-fah 1 an-te-TRIP-sin): A protein that protects the inner lining of alveoli.

alpha-blockers (AL-fah BLOK-erz): A class of medications used to help control hypertension.

alveolus, alveoli (al-VE-o-lus, al-VE-o-li): A small cavity or socket; specifically, the terminal epithelial structures in the lungs where gaseous exchange takes place.

amantadine (ah-MAN-tah-dene): An antiviral agent sometimes used to treat influenza.

ambulatory (AM-bu-lah-tor-e): Able to walk.

amenorrhea (ah-men-or-E-ah): Absence or abnormal cessation of menses.

amyloidosis (am-ih-loyd-O-sis): A disease characterized by extracellular accumulation of amyloid proteins in various organs and tissues.

angiogenesis (an-je-o-JEN-eh-sis): Development of new blood vessels.

angioneurotic edema (an-je-o-nu-ROT-ik eh-DE-mah): Hives on the face and neck and swelling to the point that breathing becomes difficult.

angioplasty (AN-je-o-plas-te): Recanalization of a blood vessel, usually by means of balloon dilation or the placement of a stent.

anoxia (an-OX-e-ah): Absence of oxygen.

antibody (AN-ti-bod-e): An immunoglobulin molecule produced by B cells and designed to react with specific antigens.

anticholinergic (an-ti-kol-ih-NER-jik): Antagonistic to the action of parasympathetic or other cholinergic nerve fibers (e.g., atropine).

anticoagulant (an-ti-co-AG-yu-lent): An agent that prevents or inhibits clotting of the blood.

antidiuretic hormone (an-ti-di-ur-EH-tik HOR-mone): A hormone that suppresses the output of urine. Also called vasopressin.

antigen (AN-tih-jen): Any substance that elicits an immune response on contact with sensitive cells.

antihelminthic (an-te-hel-MIN-thik): An agent used to treat or eradicate infestation with intestinal vermiform parasite (i.e., worms).

anulus fibrosis (AN-u-lus fi-BRO-sis): Fibrous ring of tissue in an intervertebral disc.

aphasia (ah-FA-zha): Impaired or absent comprehension or production of, or communication by, speech, writing, or signs; due to an acquired lesion of the dominant cerebral hemisphere.

aphtha, aphthae (AF-thah, AF-the): Small ulcer on a mucous membrane, usually in the mouth.

aplastic (a-PLAS-tik): Conditions characterized by defective regeneration (e.g., varieties of cancer).

apnea (AP-ne-ah): Absence of breathing.

apoptosis (ap-op-TOE-sis): Programmed cell death.

arachnoid (ah-RAK-noyd): A delicate membrane of spider web–like filaments that lies between the dura mater and the pia mater.

arrhythmia (ah-RITH-me-ah): Irregularity of the heartbeat.

ascites (ah-SI-teze): An accumulation of serous fluid in the peritoneal cavity.

ataxic (ah-TAX-ik): Unable to coordinate muscle activity for smooth movement.

athetoid (ATH-eh-toyd): Slow, writhing, involuntary movement of the fingers and hands and sometimes of the toes and feet.

atopic (a-TOP-ic): Relating to an allergic reaction.

atrial fibrillation (A-tre-al fib-rih-LAY-shun): Fibrillation in which the normal rhythmical contractions of the cardiac atria are replaced by rapid, irregular twitchings of the muscular wall.

atrium, atria (A-tre-um, A-tre-ah): A chamber or cavity connected to other cavities; specifically the superior chambers of the heart.

atrophic (a-TRO-fik): Denoting tissue or organ wasting.

atrophy (AT-ro-fe): A wasting of tissues from a number of causes, including diminished cellular proliferation, ischemia, malnutrition, and death.

autodigestion (aw-to-di-JES-chun): Enzymatic digestion of cells (especially dead or degenerate) by enzymes present within them.

autoimmune (AW-to-ih-MUNE): Arising from and directed against the individual's tissues.

autonomic hyperreflexia (aw-to-NOM-ik hi-per-re-FLEX-e-ah): A syndrome occurring in some persons with spinal cord lesions and resulting from functional impairment of the autonomic nervous system. Symptoms include hypertension, bradycardia, severe headaches, pallor below and flushing above the cord lesion, and convulsions.

avascular (a-VAS-ku-lar): Without blood or lymphatic vessels.

avulsion (ah-VUL-zhun): A tearing away or forcible separation.

B

babesiosis (bah-be-ze-O-sis): An infection with a species of protozoan parasites that is transferred to humans by tick bites.

bariatric (ba-re-AT-rik): Medicine concerned with the management of obesity.

barrel chest (BA-rel chest): An occasional symptom of emphysema, in which the intercostal muscles hold the rib cage out as wide as possible.

Barrett esophagus (BA-ret e-SOF-ah-gus): Chronic ulceration of the lower esophagus that is often associated with gastroesophageal reflux disorder; sometimes a precursor to adenocarcinoma of the esophagus.

basal layer (BA-sal LA-er): Also called the stratum basale; the deepest layer of the epidermis.

Bence Jones proteins (bence-jones PRO-teens): Protein fragments found in association with multiple myeloma.

benign (be-NINE): Denoting the mild character of an illness or nonmalignant character of a neoplasm.

benign paroxysmal positional vertigo (be-NINE pah-rok-SIZ-mal po-SIH-shun-al VER-tih-go): A recurrent form of vertigo caused by otoliths outside of the vestibule.

beta-amyloid (BAY-tah AM-ih-loyd): A type of protein associated with formation of plaque in the brain.

beta-blocker (BAY-tah BLOK-er): A type of drug that limits sympathetic reactions, specifically as they relate to the cardiovascular system.

beta cell (BAY-tah sel): Cell in the pancreas that secretes insulin.

bile (BI-ul): Yellowish-brown or green fluid produced in the liver, stored in the gallbladder, and released into the duodenum to aid in the digestion of fats.

bilharzia (bil-HAR-zee-ah): Infection with any variety of *Schistosoma*.

biliary colic (BIL-e-a-ree KOL-ik): Intense spasmodic pain in the right upper quadrant of the abdomen from impaction of a gallstone in the cystic duct.

bilirubin (BIL-ih-ru-bin): A dark bile pigment formed from the hemoglobin of dead erythrocytes.

biologic response modifiers (bi-o-LOJ-ik-ul re-SPONS MOD-ih-fi-erz): Substances that alter the interaction between the body's immune defenses and cancer cells to boost, direct, or restore the body's ability to fight the disease.

bipolar disease (bi-PO-lar dih-ZEZE): Manic-depressive psychosis.

bismuth (BIZ-muth): A metallic element used in several medicines, specifically in those designed to affect stomach acidity.

blepharitis (blef-ah-RI-tis): Inflammation of the eyelids.

blepharospasm (BLEF-ah-ro-spazm): Involuntary spasmodic contraction of the orbicularis oculi muscles.

blood–brain barrier (blud-brane BA-re-er): A selective filter in a continuous layer of endothelial cells connected by tight junctions; prevents or inhibits the passage of ions or large compounds from the blood to the brain tissue.

Borrelia burgdorferi (bo-RE-le-ah burg-DOR-fer-i): A species of bacteria that causes Lyme disease; transferred to humans through tick bites.

botulinum (BOT-yu-lin-um): A potent neurotoxin from *Clostridium botulinum*.

bovine spongiform encephalopathy (BO-vine SPUN-jih-form en-sef-ah-LOP-ath-e): A disease of cattle first reported in 1986 in Great Britain; characterized clinically by apprehensive behavior, hyperesthesia, and ataxia and histologically by spongiform changes in the gray matter of the brainstem; caused by a prion, such as spongiform encephalopathies of other animals (e.g., scrapie in sheep and Creutzfeldt-Jakob disease in humans).

Bowman capsule (BO-man KAP-sule): The beginning of a nephron that surrounds the glomerulus.

bradykinesia (brad-e-kin-E-se-a): A decrease in the spontaneity of movement.

bruit (BRU-e): An abnormal swishing, blowing, or murmuring sound.

bruxism (BRUK-sizm): Jaw clenching that results in rubbing and grinding of the teeth, especially during sleep.

bulla, bullae (BUL-ah, BUL-ee): A bubblelike structure, specifically the air-filled blisters on the lung formed by fused alveoli in emphysema.

Burkitt lymphoma (BUR-kit lym-FO-mah): A form of malignant lymphoma frequently involving the jaw and abdominal lymph nodes. The geographic distribution of Burkitt lymphoma suggests that it is found in areas with endemic malaria. It is primarily a B-cell neoplasm and is believed to be caused by Epstein-Barr virus, a member of the family *Herpesviridae*.

bursectomy (bur-SEK-to-me): Surgical removal of a bursa.

C

calcitonin (kal-sih-TO-nin): A hormone that increases the deposition of calcium and phosphate in bone.

calcium channel blockers (KAL-se-um CHAN-el BLOK-erz): A class of medications that prevents the passage of calcium through membranes; used to treat hypertension, angina pectoris, and arrhythmia.

calcium oxalate (KAL-se-um OK-sah-late): A sediment in urine and renal calculi.

calcium phosphate (KAL-se-um FOS-fate): Calcium salts of phosphoric acid.

callus (KAL-us): A thickening of the keratin layer of the epidermis as a result of repeated friction or intermittent pressure.

Campylobacter jejuni (KAM-pih-lo-bak-ter jeh-JU-ni): A species that causes acute gastroenteritis of sudden onset with constitutional symptoms (malaise, myalgia, arthralgia, and headache) and cramping abdominal pain.

Campylobacter pylori (KAM-pih-lo-bak-ter pi-LOR-i): *Helicobacter pylori.*

Candida albicans (KAN-di-dah AL-bih-kanz): A genus of yeastlike fungi.

carcinoma (kar-sih-NO-mah): Any of a variety of malignant neoplasms deriving from epithelial tissue.

cardiomyopathy (kar-de-o-mi-OP-ath-e): Disease of the myocardium; a primary disease of heart muscle in the absence of a known underlying etiology.

cataplexy (KAT-ah-plex-e): A transient attack of extreme generalized muscular weakness that is often precipitated by an emotional state such as laughing, surprise, fear, or anger.

catheter atherectomy (KATH-eh-ter ath-er-EK-to-me): Removal of atherosclerotic plaque through a catheter; usually applied to carotid arteries.

cauda equina (KAW-dah e-KWI-nah): Bundle of spinal nerve roots that runs through the lumbar cistern; it comprises the roots of all the spinal nerves below L1. From Latin for *horse tail.*

cervical rib (SER-vih-kal rib): An abnormally wide transverse process of a cervical vertebra or a supernumerary rib that articulates with a cervical vertebra but does not articulate with the sternum. C7 is the vertebra most often affected.

chancre (KAN-ker): The primary lesion of syphilis, which begins at the site of infection after an interval of 10 to 30 days as a papule or area of infiltration that is a dull red color, hard, and insensitive; the center usually becomes eroded or breaks down into an ulcer that heals slowly after 4 to 6 weeks.

chemonucleolysis (ke-mo-nu-kle-OL-ih-sis): Injection of chymopapain into the nucleus pulposus of a herniated disc.

chemotherapy (ke-mo-THER-ah-pe): The treatment of disease by chemical means (i.e., drugs).

childhood disintegrative disorder (child-hood dis-IN-teh-gra-tiv dis-OR-der): A type of autism spectrum disorder involving a dramatic loss of motor skills, vocabulary, and communication skills.

Chlamydia trachomatis (klah-MIH-de-ah trak-o-MAH-tis): Spherical organism that causes a variety of infections, including conjunctivitis and pelvic inflammatory disease.

cholecyst (KO-leh-sist): The gallbladder.

cholinesterase inhibitors (ko-lin-ES-ter-ase in-HIB-ih-torz): Class of drugs that improves myoneural function; used to treat patients with myasthenia gravis and Alzheimer disease.

chronic exertional compartment syndrome (KRON-ik eg-ZER-shun-al kom-PART-ment SIN-drome): An accumulation of fluid pressure in one or more of the tough fascial compartments of the lower leg.

circadian rhythm (sir-KA-de-an RITH-em): Biologic variations or rhythms that last approximately 24 hours. From Latin *circa* (*about*) and *dies* (*day*).

clonic spasm (KLON-ik spazm): Alternating involuntary contraction and relaxation of a muscle.

coagulability (ko-ag-yu-lah-BIL-ih-te): Ability to clot.

collagen (KOL-ah-jen): A major protein forming the white fibers of connective tissue.

collagenase (ko-LAJ-eh-nase): A proteolytic dissolving enzyme that acts on one or more of the collagens.

colonoscopy (kol-o-NOS-ko-pe): A visual examination of the internal surface of the colon by means of a long fiberoptic endoscope.

colostomy (ko-LOS-to-me): An artificial opening from the skin to the colon.

comedo (ko-ME-do): A dilated hair follicle filled with bacteria; the principal lesion of acne vulgaris. Plural, comedos, comedones.

comminuted (KOM-ih-nu-ted): Broken into several pieces, especially denoting a fractured bone.

comorbidity (ko-mor-BID-ih-te): Condition of having multiple pathologies simultaneously.

congenital (kon-JEN-ih-tal): Mental or physical traits that exist at birth.

cor pulmonale (kor pul-mo-NAL): Right-sided ventricular hypertrophy that often arises from disease of the lungs.

corpus callosum (KOR-pus kal-LOS-um): The plate of nerve fibers interconnecting the cortical hemispheres.

corpus luteum (KOR-pus LU-te-um): The site of egg release on follicles of the ovaries immediately after ovulation.

corticosteroid injection (kor-tih-ko-STER-oyd in-JEK-shun): An injection of a specific steroid into an injured area for its anti-inflammatory or connective tissue–dissolving properties.

cortisol (KOR-tih-sol): A glucocorticoid secreted by the adrenal cortex. It acts on carbohydrate metabolism and influences the growth and nutrition of connective tissue.

cortisone (KOR-tih-sone): A form of cortisol that may be injected into specific areas to act as an anti-inflammatory agent or to help dissolve connective tissue.

COX-2 inhibitors (cox 2 in-HIB-i-tors): A class of nonsteroidal anti-inflammatory drugs that work by blocking COX (cyclo-oxygenase) 2 enzyme, which is involved in the inflammation pathway.

***Coxsackie* virus** (kok-SAK-e VI-rus): A group of viruses first isolated in Coxsackie, New York. They may be responsible for several human diseases, including meningitis and juvenile diabetes.

C-reactive protein (c re-AC-tive PRO-teen): A beta-globulin found in the serum of various persons with certain inflammatory, degenerative, and neoplastic diseases.

crepitus (KREP-ih-tus): A crackling sound resembling the noise heard on rubbing hair between the fingers.

CREST syndrome (crest SYN-drome): A group of signs commonly associated with scleroderma, calcinosis, Raynaud phenomenon, esophageal motility disorders, sclerodactyly, and telangiectasia.

crisis (KRI-sis): A sudden change, usually for the better, in the course of an acute disease.

cruciate ligament sprain (KROO-she-ate LIG-ah-ment sprane): Major ligaments that crisscross the knee in the anteroposterior direction, providing stability in that plane.

crust (krust): A hard outer covering; a scab.

cyanosis (si-ah-NO-sis): A bluish or purplish coloration of the skin and mucous membranes caused by deficient oxygenation of the blood.

cyclo-oxygenase-2 (si-klo-OX-ih-jen-ase 2): See COX-2 inhibitors.

cystoscope (SIS-to-skope): A lighted tubular endoscope used for examining the interior of the bladder.

cytokine (SI-to-kine): Hormone-like proteins secreted by many cells and involved in cell-to-cell communication.

cytomegalovirus (si-to-MEG-ah-lo-vi-rus): A group of viruses in the *Herpesviridae* family infecting humans and animals.

cytotoxic drug (si-to-TOX-ik drug): A drug that is detrimental or destructive to certain cells.

D

de Quervain tenosynovitis (deh kare-VA ten-o-sin-o-VI-tis): Inflammation of the tendons of the first dorsal compartment of the wrist, which includes the extensor pollicis brevis and the abductor pollicis longus.

debridement (da-brede-MONH): Excision of dead tissue and foreign matter from a wound.

degenerative joint disease (de-JEN-er-ah-tiv JOYNT dih-ZEZE): Osteoarthritis.

dementia (de-MEN-sha): The loss, usually progressive, of cognitive and intellectual functions without impairment of perception or consciousness.

dendrite (DEN-drite): The process of a nerve cell that carries impulses toward the cell body.

dermatome (DER-mah-tome): The area of skin supplied by cutaneous branches from a single spinal nerve.

dermatophyte (der-MAT-o-fite): A fungus that causes superficial infections of the skin, hair, and nails.

dermatophytosis (der-mat-o-fi-TO-sis): An infection of the hair, skin, or nails caused by any one of the dermatophytes. The lesions are characterized by erythema, small papular vesicles, fissures, and scaling.

dermoid cyst (DER-moyd SIST): A tumor consisting of displaced ectodermal structures along lines of embryonic fusion. The wall is formed of epithelium-lined connective tissue, including skin appendages and containing keratin, sebum, and hair.

dextroamphetamine (dex-tro-am-FET-ah-mene): A medication for central nervous system stimulation.

diaphoresis (di-ah-for-E-sis): Perspiration.

dilatation (di-la-TAY-shun): The enlargement of a hollow structure or opening.

dilatation and curettage (di-la-TAY-shun and ku-reh-TAHJH): Dilatation of the cervix and scraping of the endometrium.

diplegia (di-PLE-je-ah): Paralysis of corresponding parts on both sides of the body.

disease-modifying antirheumatic drugs (DMARDs) (DI-sease mod-i-fying an-ti-ROO-matic drugs): Agents that apparently alter the course and progression of rheumatoid arthritis; other substances (not DMARDs) suppress inflammation and decrease pain but do not prevent cartilage or bone erosion or progressive disability.

diskectomy (dis-KEK-to-me): Excision of part or all of an intervertebral disc.

diuretic (di-u-REH-tik): A chemical agent that increases urine output.

diverticulum, diverticula (div-er-TIK-u-lum, div-er-TIK-u-lah): A pouch or sac opening from a tubular or saccular organ (e.g., the colon or urinary bladder).

dopamine (DO-pah-mene): A neurotransmitter in the basal ganglia.

drusen (DRU-zen): Small, bright structures seen in the retina and optic disc.

dura mater (DU-rah MA-ter): A tough, fibrous membrane forming the outer covering of the central nervous system.

dyshidrosis (dis-hi-DRO-sis): A skin eruption with blisters and itching that usually appears on the volar surface of the hands or feet.

dysmotility (dis-mo-TIL-ih-te): Inefficient or uncoordinated peristalsis in the gastrointestinal tract.

dysphagia (dis-FA-je-a): Difficulty in swallowing.

dysphonia (dis-FO-ne-ah): Any disorder of phonation affecting voice quality or ability to produce the voice.

dysplasia, dysplastic (dis-PLA-zha, dis-PLAS-tik): Abnormal tissue development.

dyspnea (disp-NE-ah): Shortness of breath.

dysthymia (dis-THI-me-ah): Chronic mood disorder involving long-term, low-grade depression.

dystonia (dis-TO-ne-ah): A state of abnormal (too much or too little) muscle tone.

dystrophic (dis-TRO-fik): Relating to progressive changes that may result from defective nutrition of a tissue or organ.

dystrophin (dis-TRO-fin): A protein found in the sarcolemma of normal muscle tissue; it is missing in individuals with some forms of muscular dystrophy.

E

E. coli, Escherichia coli (E-KO-li, esh-er-IK-e-ah KO-li): A species of bacteria linked with infections of the gastrointestinal or urinary tracts.

ecchymosis (ek-ih-MO-sis): A purplish patch caused by blood leaking into the skin; a bruise.

eclampsia (e-KLAMP-se-ah): One or more convulsions not attributable to other cerebral conditions. May be related to pregnancy-induced hypertension.

elastin (e-LAS-tin): A yellow, elastic fibrous protein that contributes to the connective tissue of elastic structures.

electrocauterization (e-lek-tro-kaw-ter-i-ZA-shun): Cauterization by passage of high-frequency current through tissue or by metal that has been electrically heated.

embolization (em-bo-li-ZA-shun): Therapeutic introduction of various substances into the circulation to occlude vessels, either to arrest or prevent hemorrhaging or to devitalize a structure or organ by occluding its blood supply.

emollient (e-MOL-i-ent): An agent that softens or soothes the skin.

empyema (em-pi-E-mah): Pus in a body cavity; usually refers to the thorax.

endarterectomy (en-dar-ter-EK-to-me): Excision of the diseased layers of an artery along with atherosclerotic plaques.

endocarditis (en-do-kar-DI-tis): Inflammation of the innermost tunic of the heart.

endogenous (en-DOJ-en-us): Originating or produced within the organism or one of its parts.

endolymph (EN-do-limf): The fluid in the membranous labyrinth of the inner ear.

endometritis (en-do-meh-TRI-tis): Inflammation of the endometrium.

endometrium (en-do-ME-tre-um): The inner layers of the uterine wall.

endomysium (en-do-MI-ze-um): The connective tissue sheath surrounding muscle fibers.

epimysium (ep-ih-MIS-e-um): The connective tissue membrane surrounding a skeletal muscle.

epinephrine (ep-ih-NEF-rin): The chief hormone of the adrenal medulla; a potent stimulant of the sympathetic response.

epistaxis (ep-ih-STAK-sis): Profuse bleeding from the nose.

epithelium (ep-ih-THE-le-um): A purely cellular avascular layer covering all free surfaces, including the skin, mucous, and serous membranes.

Epstein-Barr virus (EP-stine BAR VI-rus): A herpesvirus that causes infectious mononucleosis and is implicated in Burkitt lymphoma.

Ernest syndrome (ER-nest SIN-drome): A condition involving a weakened and irritated stylomandibular ligament; frequently mistaken for temporomandibular joint disorder.

erythema (er-i-THE-mah): Redness of the skin caused by capillary dilatation.

erythrocyte (e-RITH-ro-site): A mature red blood cell.

exenteration (ek-sen-ter-A-shun): Removal of internal organs and tissues, usually to ablate cancer.

exogenous (eg-ZOJ-en-us): Originating or produced outside the organism.

exophthalmus (ex-of-THAL-mus): Protrusion of one or both eyeballs.

F

fasciculation (fash-ik-u-LA-shun): Involuntary contractions or twitchings of muscle units.

fetal alcohol syndrome (fe-tal AL-ko-hol SIN-drome): A specific pattern of fetal malformation and health problems among offspring of mothers who abuse alcohol.

fibrillation (fib-ril-A-shun): Exceedingly rapid contractions or twitching of muscular fibrils.

fibrillin (FIB-ril-in): A protein of connective tissue.

fibrin (FI-brin): An elastic filamentous protein that aids in coagulation of the blood.

fibrinogen (fi-BRIN-o-jen): A globulin of the blood plasma that is converted into fibrin by the action of thrombin in the presence of ionized calcium to produce coagulation of the blood.

fibroadenoma (fi-bro-ad-en-O-mah): A benign neoplasm of glandular epithelium in which fibroblasts and other connective tissue proliferate.

fibroblast (FI-bro-blast): A cell capable of forming collagen fibers.

fimbria, fimbriae (FIM-bre-ah, FIM-bre-a): Any fringelike structure. Ovarian fimbriae extend over the ovaries.

fistula, fistulae (FIS-tu-lah, FIS-tu-lay): An abnormal passage from one epithelial surface to another.

flaccid paralysis (FLAS-sid pah-RAL-ih-sis, FLAS-id pah-RAL-ih-sis): Paralysis with a loss of muscle tone, although sensation is present.

focal dystonia (FO-kal dis-TO-ne-ah): A movement disorder that affects only one region of the body.

folate (FO-late): A form of folic acid.

folic acid (FO-lik AS-id): Member of the vitamin B complex necessary for the normal formation of red blood cells.

furuncle (FYU-runk-el): A local bacterial infection in a hair shaft; a boil.

G

gamma globulin (GAM-ah GLOB-u-lin): A preparation of proteins of human plasma containing the antibodies of normal adults.

gamma-aminobutyric acid (GABA) (GAM-ah ah-me-no-bu-TIR-ik AS-id): A principal inhibitory neurotransmitter.

gastritis (gas-TRI-tis): Inflammation, especially mucosal, of the stomach.

Giardia (je-AR-de-ah): A genus of parasitic flagellates that colonizes the gastrointestinal tract of many mammals.

globus pallidus (GLO-bus PAL-id-us): The inner and lighter gray portion of the lentiform nucleus.

glomerulus (glo-MARE-yu-lus): A tuft of capillary loops surrounded by the Bowman capsule at the beginning of each nephric tubule in the kidney.

glucagon (GLU-kah-gon): A hormone secreted by the pancreas that elevates the blood sugar concentration.

glucocorticoid (glu-ko-KOR-ti-koyd): Any steroid-like compound capable of influencing metabolism; also exerts an anti-inflammatory effect. Cortisol is the most potent of the naturally occurring glucocorticoids.

gluten (GLU-ten): The insoluble protein constituent of wheat and other grains.

glycogen (GLI-ko-jen): A substance found primarily in the liver and muscles that is easily converted into glucose.

goiter (GOY-ter): Chronic enlargement of the thyroid gland not caused by a neoplasm; may be related to both hyperthyroidism and hypothyroidism.

grand mal seizure (grand MAL SE-zhur): Sudden onset of tonic contraction of the muscles, giving way to clonic convulsive movements. Also called generalized tonic-clonic seizure.

granuloma (gran-u-LO-mah): A nodular inflammatory lesion; includes epithelial cells along with phagocytes, macrophages, and lymphocytes.

H

HACE: High-altitude cerebral edema.

hallux valgus (HAL-lux VAL-gus): A deviation of the great toe toward the lateral side of the foot; a bunion.

HAPE: High-altitude pulmonary edema.

Hashimoto thyroiditis (hah-shih-MO-toes thi-royd-I-tis): Diffuse infiltration of the thyroid gland with lymphocytes, resulting in diffuse goiter, progressive destruction of the parenchyma, and hypothyroidism.

Helicobacter pylori (hel-ik-o-BAK-ter pi-LOR-i): Species of bacteria associated with peptic ulcers.

HELLP: A mnemonic for hemolysis, elevated liver enzymes, and low platelet count; associated with pregnancy-induced hypertension.

hematuria (he-mah-TYU-re-ah): Any condition in which the urine contains blood or red blood cells.

hemiplegia (hem-ih-PLE-je-ah): Paralysis of one side of the body.

hemochromatosis (he-mo-kro-mah-TO-sis): A genetic disorder characterized by the absorption of too much iron in the blood; sometimes associated with liver cancer.

hemodialysis (he-mo-di-AL-ih-sis): Dialysis of soluble substances and water from the blood by diffusion through a semipermeable membrane.

hemolysis (he-MOL-ih-sis): Destruction of blood cells.

hemolytic (he-mo-LIH-tik): Destructive to blood cells.

hemophilic arthritis (he-mo-FIL-ik arth-RI-tis): Joint damage and inflammation associated with bleeding into joint cavities seen with hemophilia.

hemoptysis (he-MOP-tis-is): Expectoration of blood derived from the lungs or bronchi as a result of pulmonary or bronchial hemorrhage.

hemorrhage (HEM-or-aj): An escape of blood through ruptured vessels.

heterotopic ossification (het-er-o-TOP-ik os-if-ih-KA-shun): The formation of calcium deposits in soft tissues, particularly seen in spinal cord injury patients.

hidradenitis suppurativa (hi-drad-en-I-tis SUP-per-a-tee-va): Chronic suppurative folliculitis of apocrine sweat gland–bearing skin, producing abscesses with scarring.

high-density lipoprotein (HDL) (hi-DEN-sih-te LI-po-pro-tene): A compound in plasma containing both lipids and proteins; HDLs are associated with a reduced risk of cardiovascular disease.

hirsutism (HIR-zu-tizm): Presence of excessive bodily and facial terminal hair in a male pattern, especially in women; may develop in children or adults as the result of androgen (male hormone) excess caused by tumors, drugs, or medications.

histamine (HIS-tah-mene): A secretion of some cells that is a powerful stimulant of gastric secretion, a constrictor of bronchial smooth muscle, and a vasodilator.

homeostasis (ho-me-o-STA-sis): A state of equilibrium in the body with respect to various functions and the chemical compositions of fluids and tissues.

human papillomavirus (HPV) (HU-man pap-il-O-mah vi-rus): Class of DNA viruses that cause genital and cutaneous warts.

hydrocephalus (hi-dro-SEF-ah-lus): A condition marked by an excessive accumulation of cerebrospinal fluid resulting in dilatation of the cerebral ventricles and increased intracranial pressure; may also result in enlargement of the cranium and atrophy of the brain.

hyperacusis (hi-per-ah-KU-sis): Abnormal acuteness of hearing caused by irritability of the sensory nerves.

hyperalgesia (hi-per-al-JE-ze-ah): Extreme sensitivity to painful stimuli.

hyperglycemia (hi-per-gli-SE-me-ah): An abnormally high concentration of glucose in the circulating blood.

hyperkinesia (hi-per-kin-E-ze-ah): Excessive muscular activity.

hyperosmolality (hi-per-oz-mo-LAL-ih-te): Increased concentration of a solution expressed as osmoles of solute per kilogram of serum water.

hyperplasia (hi-per-PLA-zha): An increase in the number of cells in a tissue or organ, outside of tumor formation.

hyperreflexia (hi-per-ree-FLEX-e-ah): A condition in which the deep tendon reflexes are exaggerated.

hypersensitivity (hi-per-sen-sih-TIV-ih-te): An exaggerated response to the stimulus of a foreign agent.

hyperthermia (hi-per-THER-me-ah): High body temperature; fever.

hypertonic (hi-per-TON-ik): Having an increased degree of tension.

hypertrophic scar (hi-per-TRO-fik SKAR): An elevated scar resembling a keloid but that does not spread into surrounding tissues.

hypertrophy (hy-PER-tro-fe): General increase in bulk of a part or organ caused by an increase in size but not in number of the individual tissue elements.

hypokinesia (hi-po-kih-NE-zha): Diminished or slowed movement.

hypothermia (hi-po-THER-me-ah): In humans, a body temperature significantly below 98.6°F (37°C).

hypotonic (hi-po-TON-ik): Having a reduced degree of tension.

hypoxia (hi-POX-e-ah): Below-normal levels of oxygen in the body.

I

idiopathic (id-e-o-PATH-ik): Denoting a disease of unknown cause.

incision (in-SIH-zhun): A cut or surgical wound.

infantile paralysis (IN-fan-tile pah-RAL-ih-sis): Polio.

infarction (in-FARK-shun): Sudden insufficiency of arterial or venous blood supply caused by emboli, thrombi, vascular torsion, or necrosis.

inflammatory bowel disease (in-FLAM-mah-tor-e BOW-el dih-ZEZE): Umbrella term for Crohn disease and ulcerative colitis.

insulin (IN-su-lin): A hormone secreted by beta cells in the pancreas that promotes the utilization of glucose in tissue cells.

interferon (in-ter-FE-ron): A class of proteins with antiviral properties.

interleukin-1 (IN-ter-lu-kin): A cytokine that enhances the proliferation of T helper cells and the growth and differentiation of B cells.

ischemia (is-KE-me-ah): Local anemia caused by a mechanical obstruction of the blood supply.

IUD: Intrauterine device. A plastic or metal device that is inserted into the uterus for contraception.

Ixodes (ik-SO-dez): A genus of hard ticks, many of which are parasitic to humans and the vector for the spread of some diseases.

K

Kaposi sarcoma (kah-PO-seze sar-KO-mah): A malignant neoplasm occurring in the skin and sometimes in the lymph nodes or viscera; clinically manifested by cutaneous lesions consisting of reddish purple to dark-blue macules, plaques, or nodules; seen most commonly in men older than age 60 years of age and in AIDS patients.

keratin (KER-ah-tin): A substance present in cuticular structures (e.g., hair, nails, and horns).

keratinocyte (ker-AT-in-o-site): A cell of the epidermis that produces keratin.

ketoacidosis (ke-to-as-id-O-sis): Acidosis caused by enhanced production of ketonic acids.

ketogenic (ke-to-JEN-ik): Giving rise to ketones in the metabolism.

ketone (KE-tone): A potentially toxic product of metabolism. The most widely recognized ketone is acetone.

kinin (KI-nin): Any of a variety of chemicals with physiologic effects on cell activity, including visceral muscle contraction along with vascular muscle relaxation, which leads to vasodilation.

Klebsiella (kleb-se-EL-ah): A genus of bacteria that may or may not be pathogenic, depending on the individual type.

L

labyrinthitis (lab-ih-rin-THI-tis): Inflammation of the labyrinth of the inner ear; may be associated with vertigo or hearing loss.

laceration (las-er-A-shun): A torn or jagged wound.

Lactobacillus (lak-to-bah-SIL-us): A genus of bacteria that is part of the normal flora of the mouth, intestinal tract, and vagina.

lamivudine (lah-MIH-vu-dene): A reverse transcriptase inhibitor used to treat patients with HIV and hepatitis B.

lanugo (lah-NU-go): Fine, soft, lightly pigmented hair that is associated with fetal development and advanced anorexia nervosa.

laparoscopy (lap-ah-ROS-ko-pe): Examination of the abdominal contents with a scope passed through the abdominal wall.

laparotomy (lap-ah-ROH-to-me): Incision into the abdominal wall.

leaky gut syndrome (LE-ke GUT SIN-drome): Relating to dysfunctional permeability and absorption in the small intestines.

leiomyoma (li-o-mi-O-mah): A benign neoplasm derived from smooth muscle tissue.

lesion (LE-zhun): A wound or injury; a pathogenic change in tissues.

leukocyte (LU-ko-site): A type of blood cell formed in several types of tissues that is involved in immune reactions; a white blood cell.

levulose (LEV-yu-lose): Fructose; fruit sugar.

lipoprotein (lip-o-PRO-tene): Complexes or compounds containing lipid and protein. Plasma lipoproteins are characterized as very low density (VLDL), intermediate density (IDL), low density (LDL), high density (HDL), and very high density (VHDL). Levels of lipoproteins are used to assess the risk of cardiovascular disease.

lithium (LITH-e-um): An element of the alkali metal group used to treat depression and other mood disorders.

lordosis (lor-DO-sis): A deformity of the spine characterized by excessive extension.

low-density lipoprotein (LDL) (lo-DEN-sih-te lip-o-PRO-tene): A compound in plasma containing both lipids and proteins; associated with an increased risk of cardiovascular disease.

lymphadenitis (lim-FAD-en-I-tis): Inflammation of a lymph node or nodes.

lymphadenoma (lim-FAD-en-O-mah): Enlarged lymph node; may be associated with cancer.

lymphangion (lim-FAN-je-on): A lymphatic vessel.

lymphocyte (LIM-fo-site): A white blood cell formed in lymphatic tissues.

lymphokines (LIM-fo-kinez): A group of hormonelike substances that mediate immune responses; released by lymphocytes.

M

macrophage (MAK-ro-fahj): A type of phagocytic white blood cell.

malaise (mah-LAZE): A feeling of general discomfort or uneasiness.

malar rash (MA-lar rash): A rash of the cheeks or cheekbones that is often associated with lupus or erysipelas.

malignant (mah-LIG-nant): Having the property of locally invasive and destructive growth and metastasis.

malignant hypertension (mah-LIG-nant hi-per-TEN-shun): Severe hypertension that runs a rapid course, causing necrosis of arteriolar walls in the kidney and retina, hemorrhages, and death most frequently because of uremia or rupture of a cerebral vessel.

mast cell (mast sell): A white blood cell found in connective tissue that contains heparin and histamine.

matrix (MA-trix): The intercellular substance of a tissue.

medial tibial stress syndrome (ME-de-al TIB-e-al STRES SIN-drome): Pain at the posteromedial border of the tibia that occurs in conjunction with exercise.

melanin (MEL-ah-nin): Dark brown to black pigment formed in the skin and some other tissues.

melanocyte (mel-AN-o-site): A pigment-producing cell in the basal layer of the epidermis.

melatonin (MEL-ah-to-nin): A substance secreted by the pineal gland that suppresses some glandular function; associated with circadian rhythm.

meniscus (men-IS-kus): A crescent-shaped fibrocartilaginous structure of the knee, the acromioclavicular and sternoclavicular joints, and the temporomandibular joints.

menses (MEN-seze): Periodic hemorrhage from the uterine mucosa; usually preceded by ovulation but not by fertilization.

metastasis (met-AS-tah-sis): The spread of a disease process from one part of the body to another, as with the spread of cancer.

methylphenidate (meth-il-FEN-ih-date): A central nervous system stimulant often used to treat patients with attention-deficit hyperactivity disorder.

monocyte (MON-o-site): A relatively large leukocyte; normally makes up 3% to 7% of the leukocytes in the circulating blood.

mononeuropathy (mon-o-nur-OP-ath-e): Disorder involving a single nerve.

motility (mo-TIL-ih-te): The power of spontaneous movement.

mucolytic (myu-ko-LIT-ik): Capable of dissolving, digesting, or liquefying mucus.

Mycobacterium (mi-ko-bak-TE-re-um): Genus of bacteria that causes tuberculosis in humans.

Mycoplasma (mi-ko-PLAZ-mah): A specialized type of bacteria that does not possess a true cell wall but is bound by a three-layered membrane.

mycosis (mi-KO-sis): Any disease caused by a fungus.

myelin (MI-eh-lin): A membrane composed of fat and protein molecules that surrounds nerve fibers.

myoclonic (mi-o-KLON-ik): Related to one or a series of shocklike contractions of a group of muscles of variable regularity, synchrony, and symmetry generally caused by a central nervous system lesion.

myopia (mi-O-pe-ah): Optical condition in which only rays from a finite distance from the eye focus on the retina; nearsightedness.

myotonia (mi-o-TO-ne-ah): Delayed relaxation of a muscle after a strong contraction.

myxedema coma (mik-seh-DE-mah KO-mah): A state of profound unconsciousness related to extreme hypothyroidism.

N

necrosis (nek-RO-sis): Pathologic death of one or more cells or of a portion of tissue or organ.

Neisseria gonorrhoeae (ni-SE-re-a gon-o-RE-a): A species that causes gonorrhea and other infections in humans; the type species of the genus *Neisseria*.

neoplasm (NE-o-plazm): An abnormal tissue that grows by cellular proliferation more rapidly than normal and continues to grow after the stimuli that initiated the new growth cease.

nephrolithiasis (nef-ro-lih-THI-ah-sis): Presence of renal calculi.

nephron (NEF-ron): A long, convoluted tubular structure; the functional unit of the kidney.

neuraminidase (nur-am-IN-ih-daze): One of a group of proteins found in the external surface of influenza viruses.

neurofibrillary tangle (nur-o-FIB-rih-la-re TANG-el): Intraneural accumulations of filaments with twisted, contorted patterns associated with Alzheimer disease.

neurogenic bladder (NUR-o-jen-ik BLAD-er): Bladder dysfunction that originates with nervous system damage.

neuroma (nur-O-mah): General term for any neoplasm derived from cells of the nervous system, especially Morton neuroma.

neuron (NUR-on): The functional unit of the nervous system; consists of the nerve cell body, the dendrites, and the axon.

neutrophil (NU-tro-fil): A type of mature white blood cell formed in the bone marrow.

nit: The ovum of a head or body louse.

nocturia (nok-TUR-e-ah): Urinating at night.

nodular (NOD-u-lar): having nodes or knotlike swellings.

nonseminoma (non-sem-ih-NO-mah): A type of testicular cancer.

nonsteroidal anti-inflammatory drug (NSAID) (non-ster-OYD-al AN-te-in-FLAM-ah-tor-e drug): Any collection of anti-inflammatory drugs that do not include steroidal compounds. Examples include aspirin, acetaminophen, ibuprofen, and naproxen.

norepinephrine (nor-ep-ih-NEF-rin): A hormone produced in the adrenal medulla; secreted in response to hypotension and physical stress.

nosocomial (no-so-KO-me-al): A disease acquired while being treated in a hospital, specifically applied to some varieties of pneumonia.

noxious (NOK-shus): Injurious, harmful.

nucleus pulposus (NU-kle-us pul-PO-sus): The soft fibrocartilage central portion of an intervertebral disk.

numb-likeness (num-LIKE-niss): A condition characterized by reduced sensation but not total numbness.

O

occult (o-KULT): hidden, concealed, or not manifest.

onycholysis (on-ih-KOL ih-sis): Loosening of the nails, beginning at the free border and usually incomplete.

onychomycosis (on-ih-ko-mi-KO-sis): Fungal infection of the nails.

oocyte (o-o-site): A female sex cell.

oophorectomy (o-o-for-EK-to-me): Surgical removal of the ovaries.

orchiectomy (or-ke-EK-to-me): Removal of one or both testes.

orchitis (or-KI-tis): Inflammation of the testes.

oscillation (os-il-A-shun): A to-and-fro movement.

osteoblast (OS-te-o-blast): A bone-forming cell.

osteoclast (OS-te-o-klast): A cell functioning in the absorption and removal of osseus tissue.

osteonecrosis (os-te-o-nek-RO-sis): The death of bone en mass, as distinguished from caries ("molecular death") or relatively small foci of necrosis in bone.

osteopenia (os-te-o-PE-ne-ah): Pathologic thinning of bones; may be a precursor to osteoporosis.

osteophyte (OS-tee-o-fite): A bony outgrowth or protuberance.

osteotomy (os-tee-OT-o-me): The cutting of bone, usually using a saw or chisel.

ostomy (OS-to-me): Artificial opening (stoma) into the trachea, urinary tract, or gastrointestinal tract.

otolith (O-tuh-lith): Tiny "ear stone" of hardened material that is found in the vestibule of the inner ear.

P

pain–spasm–ischemia cycle: Self-perpetuating cycle of pain, which causes spasm, which increases pain, ad infinitum.

palliative (PAL-le-ah-tiv): Alleviation of symptoms without curing the underlying disease.

palpable (PAL-pah-bel): Perceptible to touch.

palpitation (pal-pih-TA-shun): Forcible or irregular pulsation of the heart perceptible to the patient, usually with an increase in frequency or force with or without an irregularity in rhythm.

Pap test: Microscopic examination of cells scraped usually from the uterine cervix and stained with Papanicolaou stain to look for signs of cancer.

paraplegia (pare-ah-PLE-je-ah): Paralysis of both lower extremities and generally the lower trunk.

paresis (pah-RE-sis): Partial or incomplete paralysis.

paresthesia (pare-es-THE-zha): An abnormal sensation, such as burning, prickling, tickling, or tingling.

pedunculate (peh-DUNK-u-late): Having a pedicle; suspended by a stalk.

perforation (per-for-A-shun): Abnormal opening in a hollow organ.

pericarditis (per-ih-kar-DI-tis): Inflammation of the pericardium.

perimenopause (per-ih-MEN-o-pawz): The 3- to 5-year period before the final cessation of the menstrual cycle, during which estrogen levels begin to decrease.

periodic limb movement disorder (PLMD): A disorder characterized by periodic episodes of repetitive and highly stereotyped limb movements that occur during sleep.

periosteum (per-ee-OS-te-um): The thick fibrous membrane covering every surface of a bone except the articular cartilage.

periostitis (per-ee-os-TI-tis): Inflammation of the periosteum.

phlegm (flem): Abnormal amounts of mucus, especially as expectorated from the mouth.

photosensitivity (fo-to-sen-sih-TIV-ih-te): Abnormal sensitivity to light, especially of the eyes.

phyllodes tumor (FIL-odez TU-mor): A low-grade, rarely metastasizing form of breast neoplasm.

pia mater (PI-ah MA-ter): A delicate fibrous membrane firmly adherent to the brain and spinal cord.

pilonidal cyst (pi-lo-NI-dal sist): An abscess in the sacral region containing hair, which may act as a foreign body leading to chronic inflammation.

pinna (PIN-na): A feather, wing, or fin; used to describe the ear.

pitting edema (PIT-ing eh-DE-mah): Edema that retains for a time the indentation produced by pressure.

placenta abruptio (plah-SEN-tah ab-RUP-te-o): Premature separation of the placenta.

plaque (plak): A small differentiated area on a surface; atheromatous plaques form well-defined yellow areas or swellings on the intimal surface of an artery.

plasmapheresis (plaz-mah-fer-E-sis): Removal of whole blood from the body, separation of its cellular elements, and reinfusion of them suspended in saline or another plasma substitute.

platelet (PLATE-let): An irregularly shaped fragment of a megakaryocyte that aids in blood clotting.

plexus (PLEK-sus): A network or interjoining of nerves, blood vessels, or lymphatic vessels.

polyneuropathy (pol-e nu-ROP-ath-e): A disease process involving a number of peripheral nerves.

popliteal cyst (pop-LIT-e-al sist, pop-lit-E-al sist): A Baker cyst.

popliteal fossa (pop-LIT-e-al fos-ah, pop-lit-E-al fos-ah): The diamond-shaped space posterior to the knee bounded superficially by the diverging biceps femoris and semimembranosus muscles above and inferiorly by the two heads of the gastrocnemius muscle.

postherpetic neuralgia (post-her-PET-ik nu-RAL-je-ah): Pain that lasts after the lesions related to herpes zoster have healed.

prednisone (PRED-nih-zone): An analog of cortisol; used as a steroidal anti-inflammatory drug.

preeclampsia (pre-e-KLAMP-se-ah): Development of hypertension with proteinuria or edema, or both caused by pregnancy.

pretibial myxedema (pre-TIB-e-al mik-seh-DE-mah): A rash that occurs in the tibial region, specifically associated with hyperthyroidism.

prion (PRI-on): Small infectious proteinaceous particle on nonnucleic acid; the causative agent for bovine spongiform encephalopathy, Creutzfeldt-Jakob disease, kuru, and others.

prodromic (pro-DRO-mik): Relating to the early or premonitory symptom of a disease, especially herpes simplex.

progestin (pro-JEST-in): A hormone of the corpus luteum.

proliferants (pro-LIF-er-ants): Injected substances that are designed to stimulate the growth of new collagen fibers, which with appropriate stretching and exercise, lie down in alignment with the original fibers.

prophylaxis (pro-fil-AK-sis): Prevention of a disease or of a process that can lead to a disease.

proprioceptor (pro-pre-o-SEP-tor): Sensory end organs that relay information about position and muscle tension.

prostadynia (pros-tah-DIN-e-ah): Chronic pelvic pain syndrome; associated with prostate pain.

prostaglandins (PROS-tah-glan-din): Substances in many tissues with effects such as vasodilation, vasoconstriction, and stimulation of smooth muscle tissue.

pruritus (pru-RI-tis): Itchiness.

pseudohypertrophy (SU-do-hy-PER-tro-fe): An increase in the size of an organ or a part not caused by an increase in size or number of the specific functional elements but by another fatty or fibrous tissue.

psoralen (SOR-ah-len): A phototoxic drug used in the treatment of psoriasis.

pustule (PUS-tyule): A small, circumscribed elevation of the skin containing purulent material.

PUVA (POO-va): Oral administration of psoralen and subsequent exposure to long-wavelength ultraviolet A light; used to treat psoriasis.

Q

quadriplegia (kwoh-drih-PLE-je-ah): Paralysis of all four limbs.

R

radiation (ra-de-A-shun): The sending forth of light, short radio waves, ultraviolet or x-rays, or any other waves for treatment, diagnosis, or other purpose.

radicular pain (rah-DIK-u-lar pane): Pain felt along the pathway of a spinal nerve.

radiculopathy (rah-dik-u-LOP-ath-e): Any disorder of the spinal nerve roots.

radioimmunotherapy (ra-de-o-ih-my-no-THER-ah-pe): The use of radiation with medication to target specific tumor cells.

reduction (re-DUK-shun): The restoration, by surgical or manipulative procedures, of a part to its normal anatomic relation.

renal calculus (RE-nal KAL-kyu-lus): A stone or pebble formed in the kidney collection system.

renal colic (RE-nal KOH-lik): Severe pain caused by the impaction or passage of a calculus in the ureter or renal pelvis.

retinoin (RET-ih-no-in): A class of keratolytic drugs derived from retinoic acid and used for treatment of severe acne and psoriasis.

rhinitis (ri-NI-tis): Inflammation of the nasal mucous membrane.

rhinophyma (ri-no-FI-mah): Hypertrophy of the nose with follicular dilatation, resulting from hyperplasia of sebaceous glands with fibrosis and increased vascularity.

Rickettsia rickettsii (rih-KET-se-ah rih-KET-se-i): The agent of Rocky Mountain spotted fever and its geographic variants; transmitted by infected *Ixodid* ticks, especially *Dermacentor andersoni* and *Dermacentor variabilis*.

Ringworm (ring-werm): A fungal infection of the keratin component of hair, skin, or nails; tinea.

rodent ulcer (RO-dent UL-ser): A slowly enlarging ulcerated basal cell carcinoma usually on the face.

rotavirus (RO-tah-vi-rus): A group of RNA viruses, some of which cause human gastroenteritis. These viruses are major causes of infant diarrhea throughout the world.

rotoscoliosis (ro-to-sko-li-O-sis): Combined lateral and rotational deviation of the vertebral column.

S

Salmonella (sal-mo-NEL-ah): A group of bacteria associated with gastrointestinal tract infections and food poisoning.

salpingitis (sal-pin-JI-tis): Inflammation of the fallopian (uterine) tube.

sarcoma (sar-KO-mah): A neoplasm of connective tissue.

sarcomere (SAR-ko-mere): The segment of a myofibril between Z lines; the functioning contractile unit of striated muscle.

Sarcoptes scabiei (sar-KOP-teze SKA-be-i): The itch mite; varieties are distributed worldwide and affect humans and many animals. The mite burrows into the skin and lays eggs within the burrow; intense itching and rash develop near the burrow in about 1 month.

Schwann cells (shwahn selz): Cells forming a continuous envelope around each fiber of peripheral nerves.

sclerodactyly (skler-o-DAK-tih-le): Stiffness and tightness of the skin of the fingers, with atrophy of the soft tissue and osteoporosis of the distal phalanges of the hands and feet; a limited form of progressive systemic sclerosis.

sebaceous gland (seh-BAY-shus gland): Gland in the dermis that usually opens into hair follicles and secretes an oily semifluid; sebum.

seborrheia (seb-o-RE-ik): Overactivity of the sebaceous glands resulting in an excessive amount of sebum.

sebum (SE-bum): The secretion produced by sebaceous glands.

selective serotonin reuptake inhibitors (SSRIs) (seh-LEK-tiv SER-o-to-nin re-UP-take in-HIB-ih-torz): A class of drugs used in the treatment of depression that selectively prevent the reuptake of serotonin in the brain.

self-limited disease: A disease that resolves spontaneously with or without treatment.

seminiferous tubules (sem-ih-NIF-er-us TU-byulez): The glandular part of testicles that contains the sperm-producing cells.

seminoma (sem-ih-NO-mah): A type of germ cell tumor.

serotonin (ser-o-TO-nin): A chemical found in many tissues. In the brain, it is a neurotransmitter associated with mood disorders; in the body, it can be a vasoconstrictor, can stimulate smooth muscle contraction, and can inhibit gastric secretion.

Shigella (shih-GEL-ah): A genus of bacteria associated with gastrointestinal infection.

sigmoidoscopy (sig-moid-OS-ko-pe): Endoscopic inspection of the sigmoid flexure of the colon.

spastic paralysis (SPAS-tik pah-RAL-ih-sis): Central nervous system damage resulting in permanent muscle contraction; combines the aspects of hypertonia, hypokinesia, and hyperreflexia.

spasticity (spas-TIS-ih-te): A state of increased muscle tone with exaggerated muscle tendon reflexes.

specific immunity (speh-SIF-ik ih-MYU-nih-te): The immune state in which an altered reactivity is directed solely against the antigens that stimulated it.

specific muscle weakness: Degeneration and weakening of the muscles supplied by specifically damaged motor neurons, as opposed to general muscle weakness, which may be unrelated to nerve damage.

sphincter (sfink-tur): A muscle that encircles a duct, tube, or orifice.

spirochete (SPI-ro-kete): A type of bacteria shaped like undulating spiral rods.

splenomegaly (splen-o-MEG-ah-le): Enlargement of the spleen.

sputum (SPYU-tum): Expectorated matter, especially mucus or mucopurulent matter, expectorated in diseases of the air passages.

squamous (SKWA-mus): Relating to or covered with scales.

St. Anthony's fire (saynt AN-thon-ee's fyre): Any of several inflammatory infections of the skin, especially erysipelas.

staging (STA-jing): The classification of distinct phases or periods in the course of a disease.

Staphylococcus (staf-ih-lo-KOK-us): A type of bacteria formed of spherical cells that divide to make irregular clusters.

status epilepticus (STAT-us ep-ih-LEP-tih-kus): Repeated seizure or a seizure prolonged for at least 30 minutes; may be convulsive tonic-clonic, nonconvulsive absence, complex partial, partial epilepsia partialis continuans, or subclinical electrographic status epilepticus.

stenosis (sten-O-sis): A stricture or narrowing of any canal.

stent: A device to hold tissue in place or provide support.

steroids (STER-oydz): A large group of chemical compounds including some hormones and drugs of a particular molecular composition. Some steroids include gonadal and adrenal hormones.

stoma (STO-mah): An artificial opening between two cavities or between a hollow area and the surface of the body.

strabismus (strah-BIS-mus): A lack of parallelism in the visual axes of the eyes.

stratum basale (STRAT-um bah-SAL): The deepest layer of the epidermis; composed of dividing stem cells and anchoring cells.

Streptococcus (strep-to-KOK-us): A type of bacteria formed of spherical cells that occur in pairs or in long or short chains.

Streptococcus pneumoniae (strep-to-KOK-us nu-MO-ne-a): A species diplococci frequently occurring in pairs or chains. This species is a normal inhabitant of the respiratory tract and the cause of lobar pneumonia, otitis media, meningitis, sinusitis, and other infections.

stroma (STRO-mah): The framework, usually made of connective tissue, of an organ, gland, or other tissue.

stromal cell tumor (STRO-mal sel TU-mur): A tumor that arises from connective tissue stroma rather than epithelium.

struvite (STRU-vite): A compound of magnesium ammonium phosphate found in some renal calculi.

subacute (sub-ah-KYUTE): Between acute and chronic, denoting medium duration or relatively mild severity.

subcutaneous (sub-kyu-TA-ne-us): Beneath the skin.

subluxation (sub-luk-SA-shun): An incomplete dislocation. Although a relationship is altered, contact between joint surfaces remains.

superficial fascia (su-per-FISH-al FASH-a): A loose fibrous envelope of connective tissue under the skin containing fat, blood vessels, and nerves.

sympathectomy (sim-pa-THEK-to-me): Excision of a section of a sympathetic nerve or one or more of the sympathetic ganglia.

syncope (SIN-ko-pe): Loss of consciousness and postural tone through diminished cerebral blood flow (fainting).

syncytial (sin-SIH-shal): Relating to a mass formed by the secondary union of originally separated cells.

systole (SIS-tole): Contraction of the heart, specifically of the ventricles.

T

tachycardia (tak-e-KAR-de-a): Rapid heartbeat, usually applied to rates greater than 100 bpm.

tau (tow): A protein that helps maintain the structure of the cytoskeleton.

telangiectasia (tel-an-je-ek-TA-ze-ah): Dilatation of previously existing small vessels, most commonly in the skin. Also called spider veins.

tender point (TEN-der poynt): One of many predictable bilateral pairs of points that produce a painful response with a minimum of pressure 4 kg; used to help diagnose fibromyalgia.

tendinosis (ten-din-O-sis): The condition of chronic tendon injury without inflammation.

teratoma (ter-ah-TO-mah): A neoplasm that contains tissues not normally found in the tissue in which it arises; usually found as benign ovarian cysts in women and malignant testicular growths in men.

testosterone (tes-TOS-teh-rone): A naturally occurring androgen found in the testes and other tissues.

thenar (THE-nar): The fleshy mass on the lateral side of the palm; the ball of the thumb.

thrombocyte (THROM-bo-site): Platelet.

thrush: Infection of the oral tissues with *Candida albicans*; often an opportunistic infection in persons with AIDS or other conditions that depresses the immune system.

thyroxin (thi-ROK-sin): Tetraiodothyronine (T_4), a secretion of the thyroid gland.

tinea (TIN-e-ah): A fungal infection of the keratin component of hairs, skin, or nails.

tinea barbae (TIN-e-ah BAR-ba): Tinea of the beard, occurring as a follicular infection or as a granulomatous lesion; the primary lesions are papules and pustules.

tinea capitus (TIN-e-ah KAP-ih-tus): A common fungus infection of the scalp caused by various species of *Microsporum* and *Trichophyton* on or within the hair shafts.

tinea corporis (TIN-e-ah KOR-por-is): A well-defined, scaling, macular eruption of dermatophytosis that frequently forms annular lesions and may appear on any part of the body.

tinea cruris (TIN-e-ah KRU-ris): A form of tinea imbricata occurring in the genitocrural region, including the inner side of the thighs, the perineal region, and the groin.

tinea manus (TIN-e-ah MAN-us): Ringworm of the hand, usually referring to infections of the palmar surface.

tinea pedis (TIN-e-ah PED-is): Dermatophytosis of the feet, especially of the skin between the toes, caused by one of the dermatophytes, usually a species of *Trichophyton* or

Epidermophyton. The disease consists of small vesicles, fissures, scaling, maceration, and eroded areas between the toes and on the plantar surface of the foot.

tinea unguium (TIN-e-ah UNG-we-um): Ringworm of the nails caused by a dermatophyte.

tinea versicolor (TIN-e-ah VER-sih-koh-lor): An eruption of tan or brown branny patches on the skin of the trunk, often appearing white in contrast to hyperpigmented skin after exposure to the summer sun; caused by growth of *Malassezia furfur* in the stratum corneum with minimal inflammatory reaction.

tonic spasm (TON-ik SPAZ-em): Continuous involuntary spasm of the skeletal muscle.

tonic-clonic seizure (TON-ik KLON-ik SE-zher): The sudden onset of tonic contraction of muscles, giving way to clonic convulsive movements. Also called grand mal seizure.

topical immunomodulators (TINs) (TOP-ih-kal im-u-no-MOD-u-la-torz): A class of anti-inflammatory ointments used as an alternative to steroidal applications in the treatment of atopic dermatitis.

torsion (TOR-shun): A twisting of a structure along its long axis.

transcutaneous (tranz-kyu-TA-ne-us): The passage of substances through unbroken skin.

transcutaneous electrical nerve stimulation (TENS): A device used to control pain with electrical stimulation applied through the skin to the nerves.

Treponema pallidum (trep-o-NE-mah PAL-ih-dum): A species of spirochetal bacteria that causes syphilis in humans.

Trichophyton (trih-KOF-ih-ton): A genus of pathogenic fungi that cause dermatophytosis in humans and animals.

tricyclic antidepressants (tri-SIK-lik an-te-de-PRES-ants): A chemical group of drugs that share a three-ringed nucleus (e.g., amitriptyline, imipramine).

trigger point (TRIG-er poynt): A small area in which myofibrils maintain involuntary contractions. Pressure on a trigger point elicits moderate to severe pain in specific referring patterns.

triiodothyronine (tri-I-o-do-THI-ro-nene): T_3, a secretion of the thyroid gland.

trophic (TRO-fik): Relating to or dependent on nutrition; resulting from interruption of the nerve supply.

tubercle (TU-ber-kel): A nodule or bump; may refer to bony prominences, elevations on the skin or other tissues, or the lesions caused by infection with *Mycobacterium tuberculosis*.

tumor (TU-mor): Any swelling, usually denoting a neoplasm.

tunica intima (TU-nih-kah IN-tih-mah): The innermost coat of a blood or lymphatic vessel.

tunica media (TU-nih-kah ME-de-ah): The middle, usually muscular coat of a blood vessel or lymphatic vessel.

U

unilateral (u-nih-LAT-er-al): Confined to one side only.

uremia (yu-RE-me-a): An excess of urea and other nitrogenous waste in the blood.

ureteroscopic stone removal (u-re-ter-o-SKOP-ik STONE re-mu-val): Removal of a calculus in the mid- to lower ureters with a ureteroscope.

V

valgus (VAL-gus): Laterally deviated.

vapocoolant (VA-po-koo-lant): A topical anesthetic aerosol spray used for pain relief and stretching of muscles affected by trigger points.

varix, varices (VAR-ix, VAR-ih-sez): A dilated vein.

varus (VAR-us): Medially deviated.

venule (VEN-yule, VE-nyule): A venous branch continuous with a capillary.

verruca (veh-RU-ka): A wart composed of a thickened keratin layer of the epidermis.

vesicle (VES-ih-kul): A small, circumscribed, fluid-filled elevation of the skin; a blister.

villus, villi (VIL-us, VIL-i): A projection from the surface, especially of a mucous membrane.

virulent (VIR-u-lent): Extremely toxic, denoting a markedly pathogenic microorganism.

W

wheal (wele): A reddened, itchy, changeable edematous area of the skin that is caused by exposure to an allergenic substance in a susceptible individual.

X

xeroderma (ze-ro-DER-mah): Excessively dry skin; a mild form of ichthyosis.

xeroderma pigmentosum (ze-ro-DER-mah pig-men-TO-sum): A genetic disorder that impedes the ability to heal from overexposure to ultraviolet radiation.

Index